Textbook for
OPHTHALMIC ASSISTANTS

PREFACE

There is no dearth of books for undergraduates and postgraduates in ophthalmology, ranging from slime paperbacks costing only a few hundred to a plethora of hard-bound volumes costing thousands of rupees. In contrast to this number of books for paramedics, who have chosen to be ophthalmic assistants, there is a chronic shortage of books for them. They generally refer to smaller books meant for undergraduate medical students. Most of the time, such books are beyond their comprehension. The situation is worsened by their lack of knowledge of the basics of human anatomy and physiology, compounded by their poor grasp of chemistry and physics. Unfortunately, the qualifications for students to join such courses are not uniform among all universities. It is a sad scenario when teachers find candidates with arts and commerce among their students.

The present work has been designed to overcome these lacunae. The book draws an outline of ocular anatomy, physiology, and ophthalmic optics in simple English that such students can understand. The book has separate chapters on disorders of different parts of the eyes in simple language. Only the outline of treatment has been given sufficient importance as has been given to preventive methods. No attempt has been made to describe surgical steps that are out of the domain of a paramedic ophthalmic assistant. The book is well illustrated with drawings, photographs, flowcharts, and tables.

Hope this book will overcome the inherent shortcomings of the books available presently.

PK Mukherjee

ACKNOWLEDGMENTS

At the very beginning, I wish to thank Shri Jitendar P Vij (Group Chairman), M/s Jaypee Brothers Medical Publishers (P) Ltd, New Delhi, for his suggestion, which motivated me to write this book for paramedical ophthalmic assistants, a 3-year course, and permitted to use diagrams and figures published by Jaypee Brothers in other books. I am immensely thankful to Mr Ankit Vij (Managing Director), Mr MS Mani (Group President), Dr Madhu Choudhary (Director–Educational Publishing), Ms Pooja Bhandari [Director–Production (Books and Journals)], Ms Sunita Katla (Executive Assistant to Group Chairman and Publishing Manager), Ms Samina Khan (Executive Assistant to Director–Educational Publishing), Dr Sangeeta Yadav (Development Editor), Mr Ajay Kumar Sharma [DGM–Production (Books and Journals)], Mr Rajesh Sharma (Production Coordinator), Ms Seema Dogra (Cover Visualizer), Ms Neha Verma (Graphic Designer–Cover), Ms Uma Adhikari (Typesetter), Ms Geeta Barik (Proofreader), Mr Radhey Shyam (Graphic Designer); and other members of Jaypee Brothers for their assistance in getting this book printed.

I express my heartfelt gratitude to Dr SL Adile, Former Director, Medical Education, Government of Chhattisgarh; Dr AK Chandrakar, Vice Chancellor, Ayush University of Medical Science, Raipur; Dr Somen Misra, Professor and Head of the Department; Dr ML Garg, Dean, Government Medical College Kanker; Dr Nidhi Pandey, Director, Regional Institute of Ophthalmology Medical College, Raipur; and Dr Santosh Patel, Professor in Department of Ophthalmology, Pt. Jawahar Lal Nehru Medical College, for their unending help in writing the book.

I am indebted to Dr Santosh Honavar for permission to use photographs of retinoblastoma published in IJO and other publications. I extend my gratitude to Editor IJO for allowing me to access material from the journal from time to time.

I am very thankful to Sri Anil Kumar Prasad, my computer assistant, who had immense patience in typing, retyping, correcting the manuscript, drawing the pictures, and making the charts and table. Without his efforts, this book would not have been possible.

I am thankful to all the persons who have permitted me to use their clinical pictures in the book.

Lastly, I am thankful to my wife, Protima Mukherjee, who has been the driving force behind writing this book and other books published earlier. Without her forbearance, it would not have been possible to complete the project.

I appreciate the tolerance of my daughters and sons-in-law, for whom I could not spare much time during this project.

CONTENTS

1. **Anatomy of the Eye** 1
   - General Consideration   1
   - Gross Anatomy of the Eye   1
   - Nerve Supply of the Eye   22

2. **Development of the Eye** 23
   - Development of the Lens   24

3. **Physiology of the Eye** 26
   - Metabolism   26
   - Physiology of Vision   26
   - Clinical Optics   39

4. **Symptomatology** 53
   - Nonvisual Ocular Symptoms   58

5. **Examination of the Eye** 63
   - History   63
   - Examination of the Eye   64
   - Clinical Examination of the Eye   79
   - Examination Under Diffuse Light   79
   - Examination Under Focal Illumination   81
   - External Examination of the Specific Structure of the Eye   82
   - Examination of the Lacrimal System   84
   - Examination of the Eye with Watering   84
   - Examination of the Orbit   85
   - Examination of a Case of Proptosis   86
   - Examination of the Conjunctiva   86
   - Examination of the Globe and Sclera   89
   - Examination of Cornea   90
   - Examination of the Anterior Chamber   93
   - Examination of the Uvea   93
   - Examination of the Pupillary Margin   94
   - Examination of the Lens   96
   - Examination of the Squint (Strabismus)   99
   - Examination of a Case of Glaucoma   103

6. **Disorders of the Lids** 105
    - Ptosis   105
    - Epicanthus   108
    - Blepharophimosis   108
    - Ankyloblepharon   108
    - Coloboma of Lids   108
    - Distichiasis   108
    - Acquired Disorders of the Lids   109
    - Acquired Structural Anomalies of the Lids   115
    - New Growths on the Lids   116
    - Malignant Growth of the Lids   117

7. **Disorder of the Lacrimal System** 120
    - Drainage of Tears   120
    - Dryness of the Eyes   121
    - Diseases of the Lacrimal Drainage System   121
    - Diseases of the Lacrimal Gland   126

8. **Disorders of the Orbits** 128
    - Proptosis and Exophthalmos   128
    - Infectious Diseases of the Orbit   131

9. **Disorders of Conjunctiva** 137
    - Common Clinical Features of Conjunctival Disorders   138
    - Conjunctivitis   146
    - Some Specific Types of Conjunctivitis   147
    - Chlamydial Conjunctivitis   150
    - Allergic Conjunctivitis   153

10. **Disorders of the Cornea** 156
    - Disorders of the Cornea   156
    - Contact Lenses   169

11. **Disorders of Sclera** 174
    - Congenital Anomalies of Sclera   174
    - Inflammation of Sclera   175
    - Ectasia (Bulging) of Cornea and Sclera   176

12. **Disorders of the Lens** 179
    - Loss of Transparency   179
    - Congenital Anomalies of the Lens   192

13. **Disorders of the Iris, Ciliary Body and Choroid** 194
    - Aniridia   194

14. Disorders of Retina 210
- Media 213
- Common Macular Disorders 222
- Vascular Retinopathies 224
- Vascular Obstructive Disorder of Retina 227
- Tumors of Retina 233

15. Disorders of the Optic Nerve 236
- Visual Path 236

16. Glaucoma 245
- Applied Anatomy of Glaucoma 245
- Applied Physiology of Glaucoma 247
- Glaucoma 248
- Chronic Simple Glaucoma (Wide-Angle Glaucoma) 251
- Glaucoma Suspect 256

17. Squint 261
- Diplopia 264
- Amblyopia 264
- Squint 265

Index 273

PLATE 1

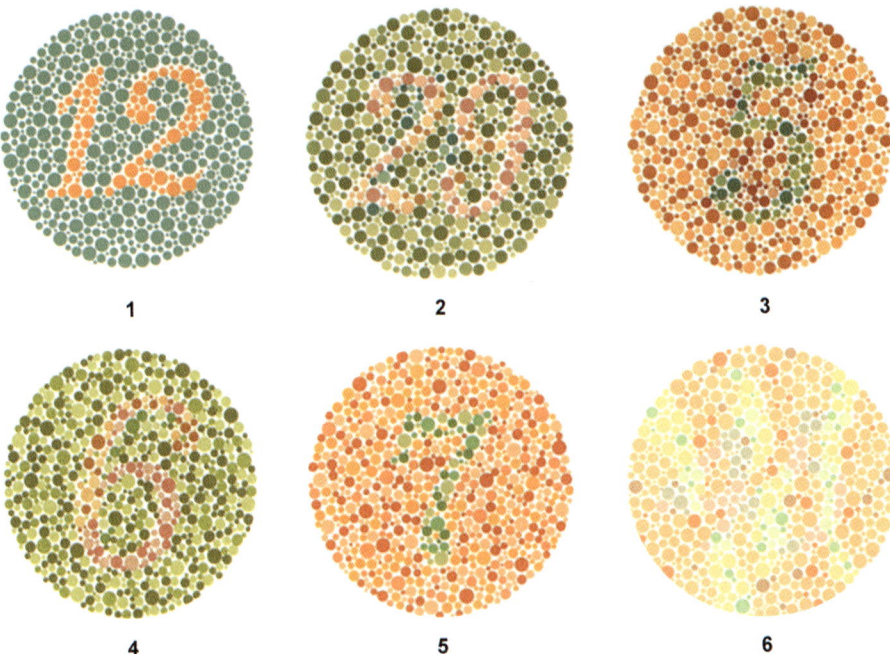

Fig. 5.11: Ishihara plates.

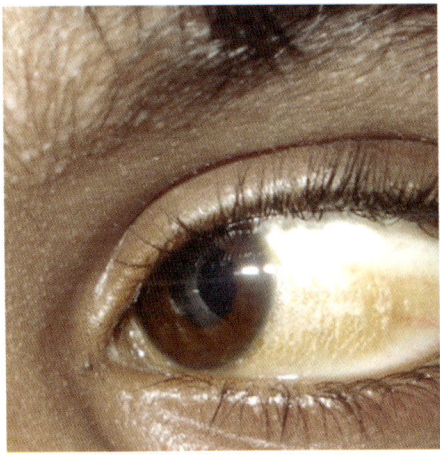

Fig. 5.25: Xerosis of conjunctiva.

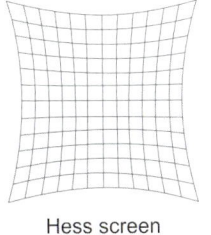
Hess screen

Blank diplopia chart

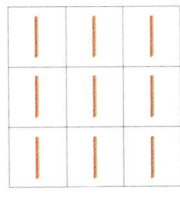
Diplopia charting in normal eye

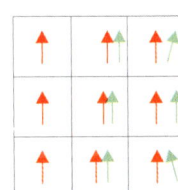
Diplopia chart lateral rectus palsy

Fig. 5.34: Diplopia chart.

PLATE 2

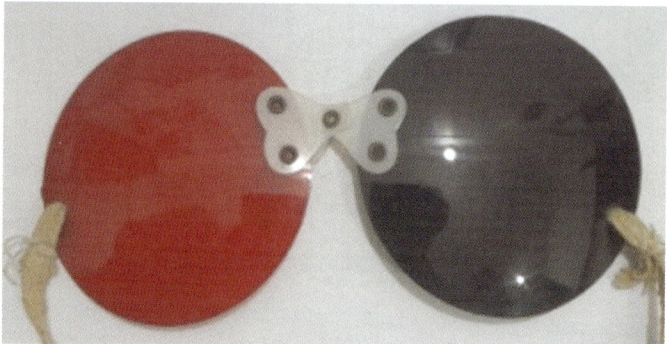

Fig. 5.35: Diplopia glasses.

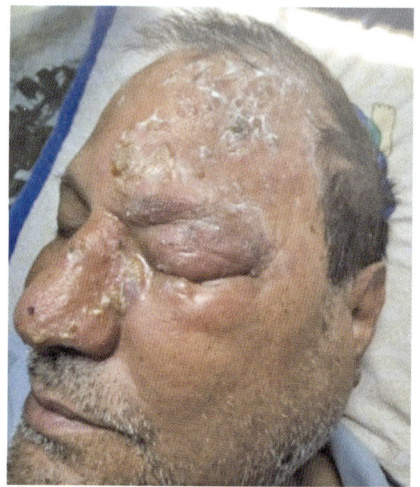

Fig. 6.9: Herpes zoster ophthalmicus.

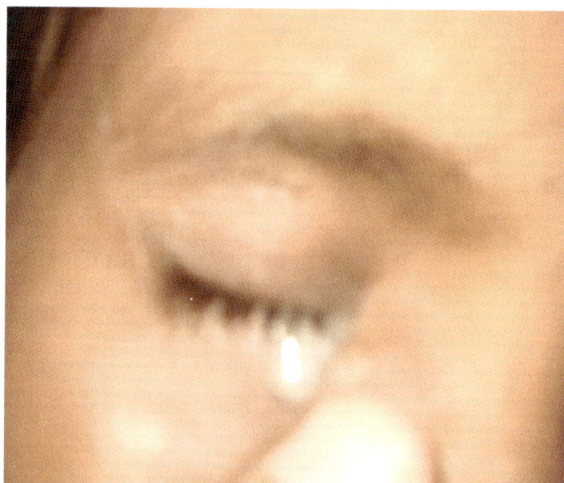

Fig. 7.2: Untreated case of congenital dacryocystitis.

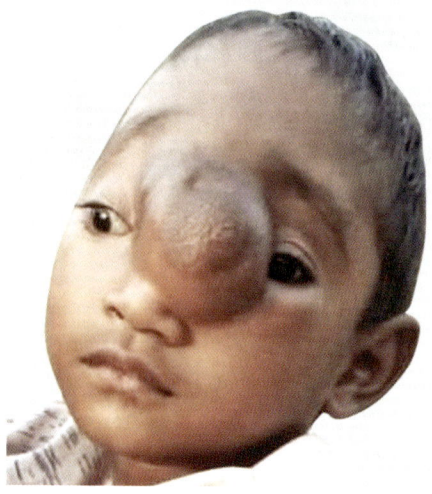

Fig. 8.2: Meningocele.

PLATE 3

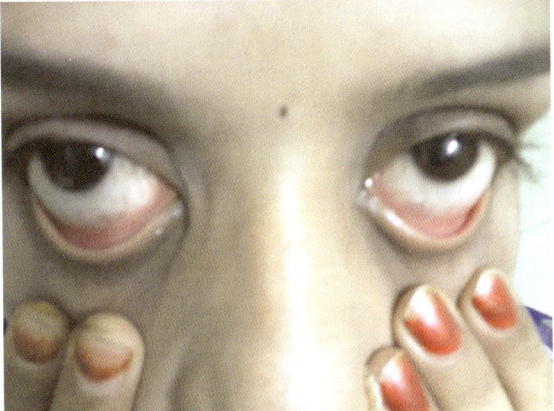

Fig. 9.3: Early conjunctival congestion.

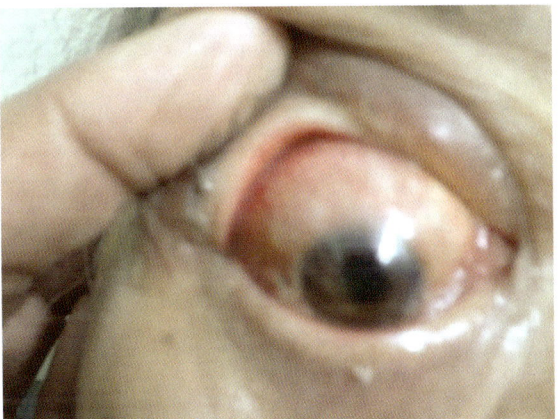

Fig. 9.5: Fully developed conjunctival congestion with subconjunctival hemorrhage.

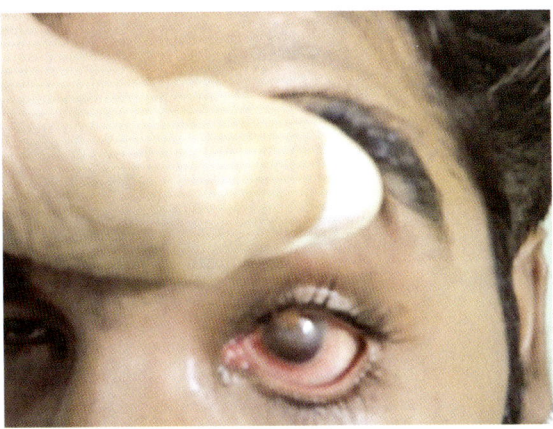

Fig. 9.6: Circumciliary congestion.

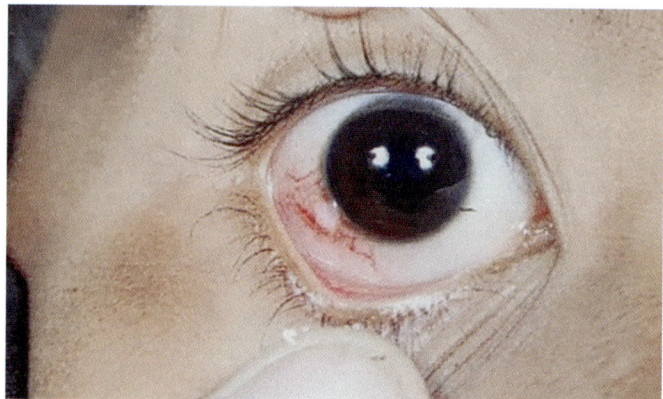

Fig. 9.12: Limbal phlycten.

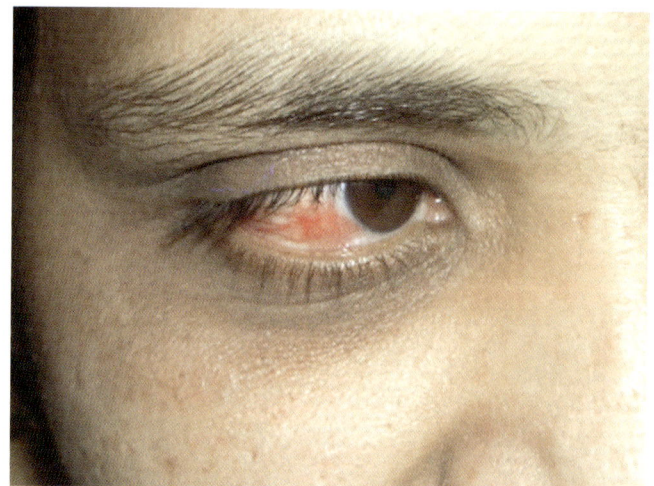

Fig. 9.13: Episcleritis.

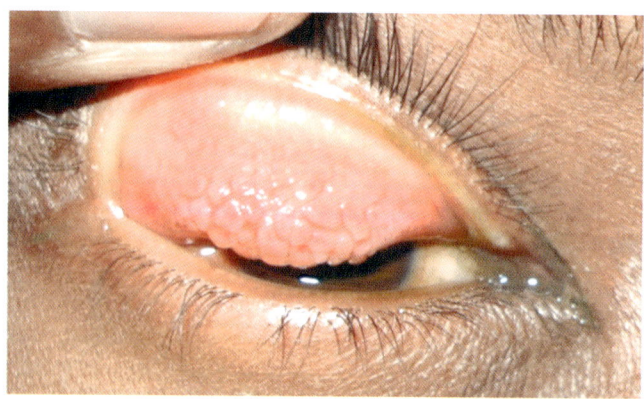

Fig. 9.19: Papillae in tarsal spring catarrh.

PLATE 5

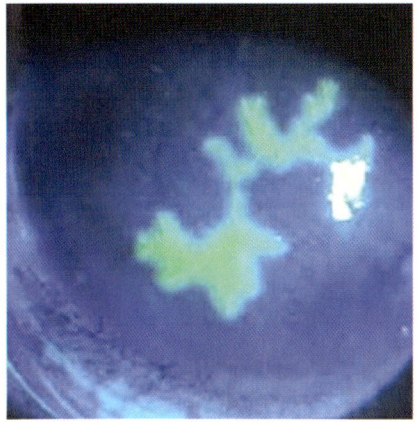

Fig. 10.5: Dendritic ulcer staining seen under cobalt blue light.

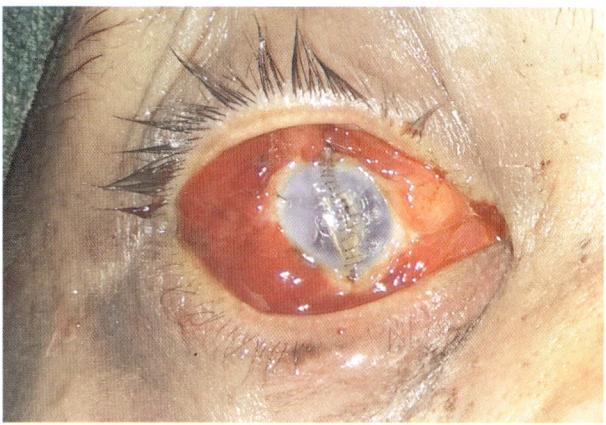

Fig. 10.10: Repaired full thickness corneoscleral wound.

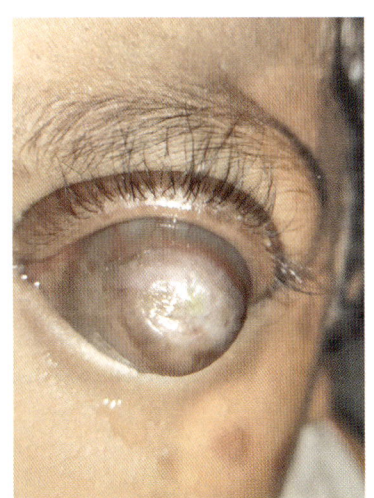

Fig. 11.5: Total corneal staphyloma with degeneration.

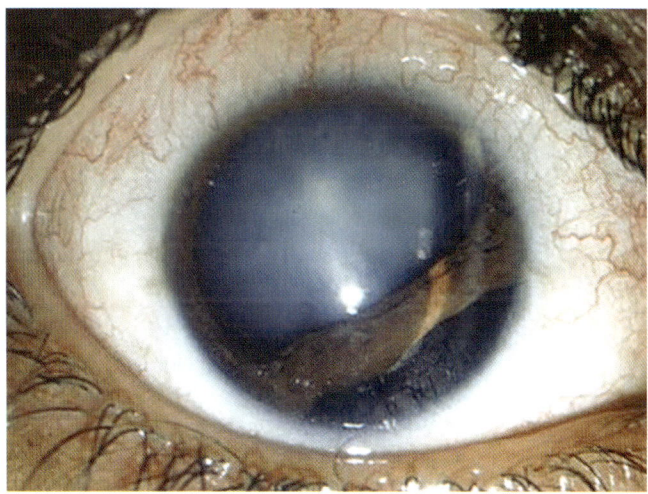

Fig. 12.11: Traumatic cataract with iridodialysis.

PLATE 6

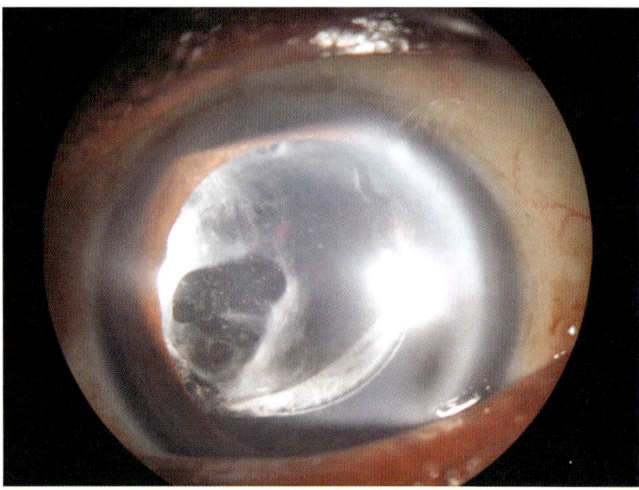

Fig. 12.15: Dense after-cataract in pseudophakia. (*Courtesy:* Dr Santosh Patel)

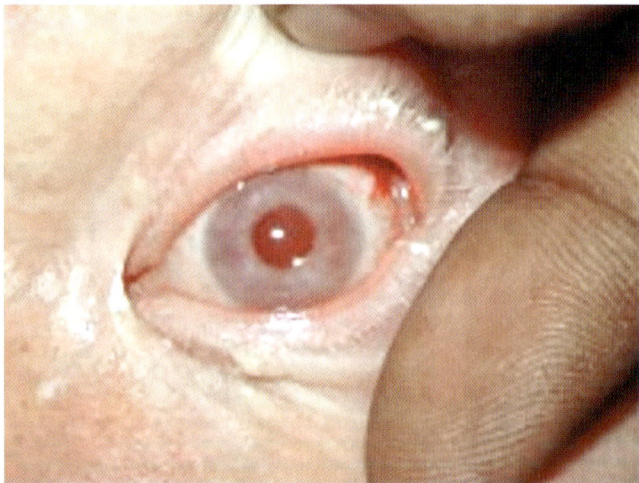

Fig. 13.8: Clinical picture of albinism showing of pigment in the iris and pink pupil. (*Courtesy:* Dr Santosh Patel)

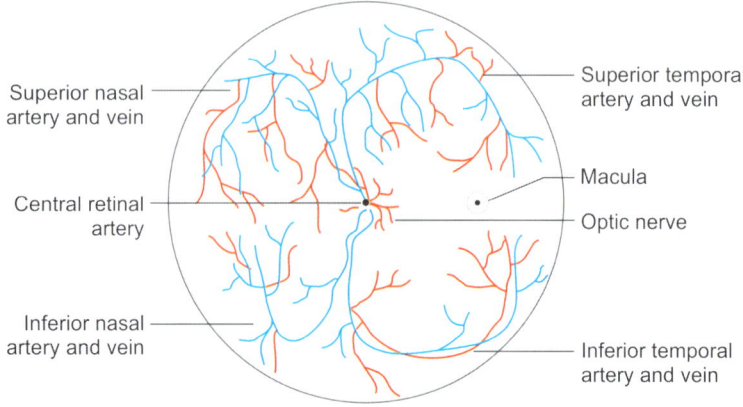

Fig. 14.5: Appearance of normal retinal vessels as seen by indirect ophthalmoscope.

PLATE 7

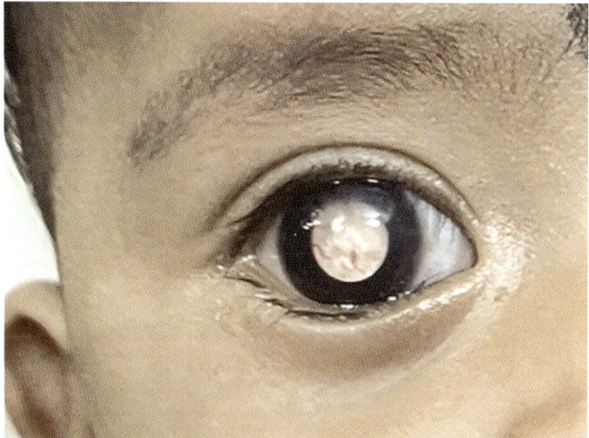

Fig. 14.10: Retinoblastoma: White reflex in the pupillary area in a blind eye.

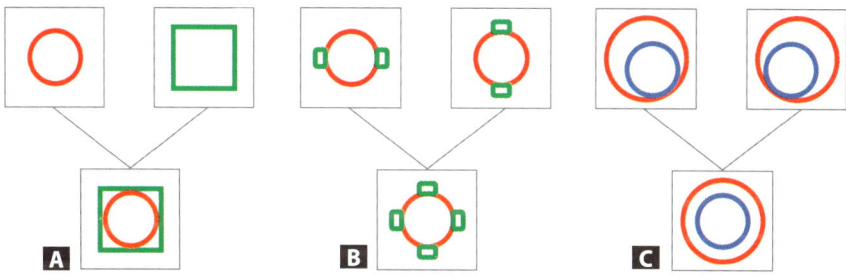

Figs. 17.3A to C: Three grades of binocular vision: (A) Simultaneous macular perception; (B) Binocular fusion; (C) Stereopsis.

CHAPTER 1

Anatomy of the Eye

GENERAL CONSIDERATION

All animals have been endowed with five senses, i.e., vision, hearing, smell, taste, and touch. All are not equally developed in all species. In humans, the vision is most developed; they have the ability to see distant and near objects with equal efficiency, good color sense, a large field of vision, depth perception, and contrast sensitivity, which makes them superior to other animals. Human beings have poor night vision when compared to animals but have excellent color sense, which animals lack. Logically, a person should be able to see an object at infinity, provided it is large and bright enough. For clinical purposes, 6 meters has been taken as the far point.

All animals and humans have a pair of almost identical eyes that are capable of acting independently of each other, coordinated with each other by the nervous system, which helps them move in a coordinated manner to give a single vision and helps to change vision from infinity to a near point of interest. Good coordination between two eyes has the following advantages:
- Increase the field of vision: The field of vision in two eyes is larger than a single field.
- Ability to change focus as per requirement
- Increased depth of focus
- Increased vision: A person who can read two lines on the vision drum with one eye and three lines with the other eye will be able to read five to six lines with both eyes open.
- A man with poor vision may not be aware of his shortcoming if the other eye has good vision.

To have such an effective faculty, the eyes must have an elaborate focusing system, coordination between two eyes, a large range of vision, and good color vision with anatomy within normal limits.

The focusing system consists of:
- Cornea, aqueous, lens, and vitreous
- Accommodation and convergence
- Binocular movement
- Neural coordination is brought about by various reflexes consisting of light, accommodation, and convergence reflexes.
- Neural control is brought about by neural centers, their tracts, supraneural paths, and coordinated binocular movement.

GROSS ANATOMY OF THE EYE

Topographically, the structures involved in vision and its other functions have been broadly divided into the following:
1. Orbit and its contents
2. The globe
3. Intraocular structures of the globe
4. Adnexa of the eye

Orbit

Orbits are not formed organs; they are two spaces on each side of the midline of the skull that protect the eyeball. The orbits are placed between the forehead above and the cheek bones (maxilla) below. The orbits are surrounded by the bones of the skull and face on all sides, except on the outer side **(Fig. 1.1)**.

The orbits are two pyramidal spaces with an apex towards the brain. The base of the pyramid is an imaginary plane that extends from all sides of the rim of the orbit.

The bones shown in **Figure 1.2** are the frontal zygomatic, maxillary, ethmoid, and sphenoid **(Fig. 1.2)**.

The walls of the orbit are not of the same size, shape, and thickness; the inner walls of the orbit are parallel to each other, the lateral wall and the roof are inclined towards the medial wall. The lower wall is called the floor of the orbit. The point where the four walls meet is called the apex of

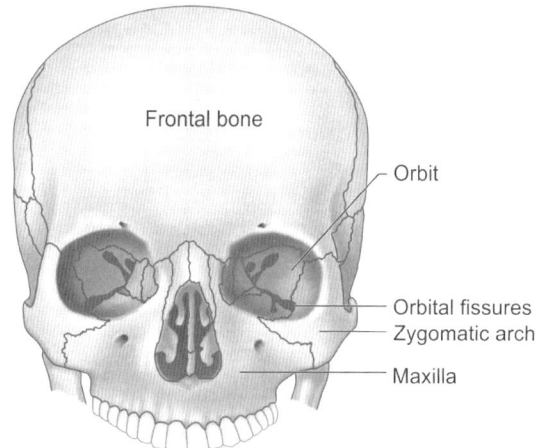

Fig. 1.1: Position of orbit in the skull.

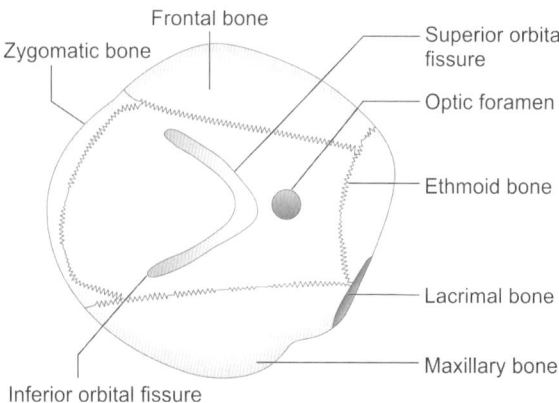

Fig. 1.2: Bones forming the orbit with the optic foramen and orbital fissures.

the orbit. There are three deficiencies in the orbit. They are the apex, superior, and inferior orbital fissures. The apex and the superior orbital fissure communicate with the brain and transmit nerves and vessels from the brain to the orbit.

Through the apex pass the optic nerve and ophthalmic artery; through the superior orbital fissure pass the third, fourth, and sixth nerves and branches of the fifth nerve. The superior and inferior ophthalmic veins pass through this fissure from the orbit towards the brain. The inferior orbital fissure communicates with the maxilla below, transmitting the second branch of the fifth nerve.

The orbits are lined by a thin layer of fibrous tissue called the periorbita, which is continuous with the periosteum of the skull and face. The orbit is divided into various surgical spaces by the various fascias **(Fig. 1.3)**.

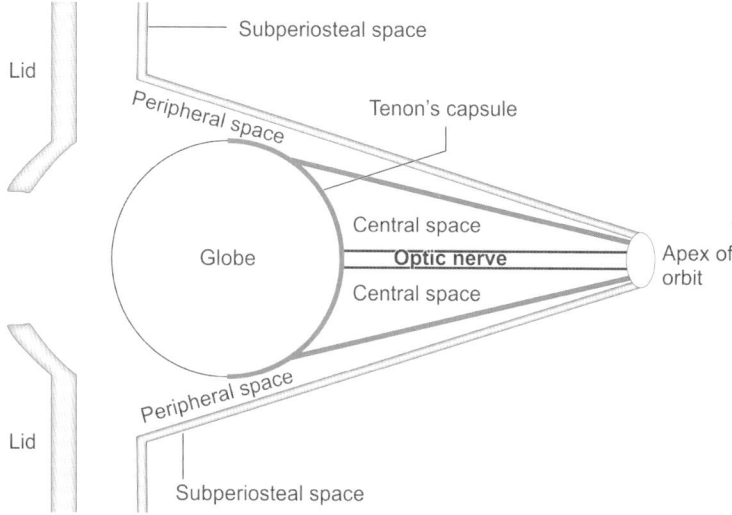

Fig. 1.3: Surgical spaces of the orbit.

The contents of the orbit are:
1. Globe.
2. Extraocular muscles.
3. Cranial nerves*: Upper and lower branches of the third nerve, the fourth nerve, branches of the fifth nerve, and the sixth nerve.
4. Branches of the ophthalmic artery
5. Ophthalmic veins.
6. Branches of the sympathetic chain with ciliary ganglion
7. Orbital fascia
8. Orbital fat
9. There are no lymphatics in the orbit.

Cranial nerves*

There are 12 cranial nerves. All of them are not related to the eye. The following chart gives the list of all cranial nerves with their functions **(Table 1.1)**.

Table 1.1: List of all cranial nerves with their functions.

Cranial nerve number	Name	Function
CN I	Olfactory nerve	Sense of smell
CN II	Optic nerve	Vision
CN III	Oculomotor nerve	Ability to move the globe – superior and inferior recti, medial rectus, inferior oblique, levator palpebrae superioris
CN IV	Trochlear nerve	Ability to move eyes up and down or back and forth, rotate the eye
CN V	Trigeminal nerve	Sensations in face and cheeks, taste and jaw movements
CN VI	Abducens nerve	Ability to move eyes outward
CN VII	Facial nerve	Facial expressions and sense of taste. Close the eye
CN VIII	Auditory/vestibular nerve	Sense of hearing and balance
CN IX	Glossopharyngeal nerve	Ability to taste and swallow
CN X	Vagus nerve	Digestion and heart rate
CN XI	Accessory nerve (or spinal accessory nerve)	Shoulder and neck muscle movement
CN XII	Hypoglossal nerve	Ability to move the tongue

Note: *Out of the 12 cranial nerves, only the second, third, fourth, fifth, sixth, and seventh have ophthalmic purposes.*

The base of the orbit is encircled by the boney rim of the orbit. The facial part of the orbit:
❖ Tenon's capsule
❖ Fascias of extraocular muscles
❖ Check ligaments
❖ Orbital septum

The orbital septum divides the orbit into two unequal parts, i.e., a preseptal (in front of the septa) and a retroseptal part. The latter is many times larger than the former **(Fig. 1.3)**.

Orbital Fat

The orbital fat fills the gap between the other contents of the orbit. The main purpose of it is to act as a cushion for the globe and stabilize it along with the extraocular muscles. It is divided into two parts, i.e., intraconal and extraconal. The extraconal is again divided into two parts, i.e., pre- and postseptal. It is white without any blood or nerve supply.

Ciliary Ganglion

The ciliary ganglion is an important ganglion of the autonomic nervous system. It is a relatively small ganglion situated between the optic nerve and the lateral rectus behind the globe. Paralysis of this ganglion causes dilatation of the pupil and the abolition of pain from the uvea. This feature is used in the retrobulbar injection of an anesthetic agent to paralyze the pupil and abolish pain during intraocular surgery.

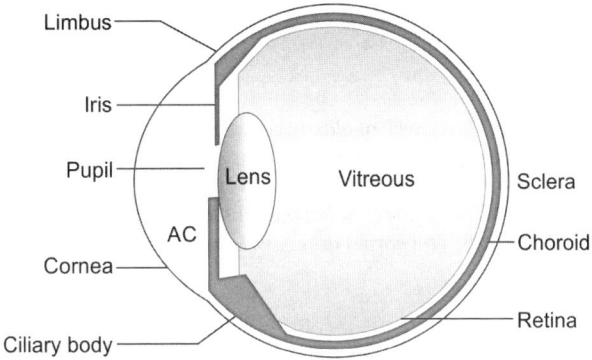

Fig. 1.4: Various parts of the globe.

Globe

The globe is the largest part of the orbit; it is commonly referred to as the eyeball. It is an imperfect sphere; it is not equally curved all over. Its anterior-posterior length is greater than other dimensions. It is formed by the bloodless structures of the sclera and the cornea (**Fig. 1.4**).

The curvature of the cornea is greater than that of the sclera. At birth, the globe is smaller, with a diameter of 16.00 mm in comparison to 24.00 mm in an adult eye. The outer wall of the globe is divided into two parts: a large part called the sclera and a small part called the cornea.

Sclera

The sclera forms the posterior 5/6 of the globe. It extends from the optic nerve up to the cornea.
The functions of the sclera are:
- The sclera is white.
- Keeps the inside of the globe dark.
- Protects the intraocular structures.
- Act as attachments for extraocular muscles.
- Act as passageways for nerves, arteries, and veins to and from the inner structures.
- It is not involved with vision.
- It is less pain-sensitive than the cornea.
- The thickness of the sclera is not uniform throughout. It is thickest around the optic nerve and is almost equally thick at the junction of the cornea with the sclera. It is thinnest at the insertion of the recti muscles.
- The junction of the cornea and sclera is called the limbus.
- There are hardly any blood vessels in the sclera, but long and short posterior ciliary vessels pass through the sclera without supplying it.
- The long and short ciliary nerves pierce the sclera to reach the uvea.
- The sclera is covered by a loose vascular structure on the outer surfaces called the conjunctiva, which is separated from the globe by Tenon's capsule*.
- The sclera is lined by the uvea on the inner surface of the globe.
- There are two holes in the sclera, i.e., a larger hole called the anterior scleral foramen and the smaller posterior scleral foramen, through which pass the optic nerve and central retinal vessels.
- The sclera is impervious to fluids except some aqueous. The passage of aqueous fluid through the sclera is called uveoscleral outflow.

❖ The uvea gets detached from the sclera if fluid or a tumor develops in between; this condition is called choroidal detachment.

Tenon's capsule*

The Tenon capsule (fascia bulbi) is a layer of elastic connective tissue that extends from the optic nerve behind to a position 3.00 mm from the limbus in front. It acts as a socket in which the globe moves freely. The capsule fusses with the sheaths of the recti. The muscles pass through the fascia to get attached to the globe. The space between the capsule and the globe is called the subtenon's space, which is utilized to give subtenon injections of antibiotics and steroids. The nerves and vessels perforate the capsule to reach the globe.

Cornea

The cornea forms the anterior 1/5 of the globe. The main function of the cornea is optical. The other function is protective, similar to the sclera, with the difference that the cornea is transparent.

The optical functions are:
1. It acts as a strong convex lens of +40 D when the rays pass through it.
2. Its refractive index is 1.37.
3. It acts as a convex mirror, which forms a small, erect, and virtual image of the object in front. This property is used to measure the curvature, power of the cornea and elicit Purkinje images*. The curvature is measured by an optical instrument called a keratometer that measures curvature both in millimeters and diopter **(Fig. 1.5)**.

Purkinje Images*

*The Purkinje images are four in number; these are reflected images from the anterior and posterior surfaces of the cornea and lens. To elicit it, light from a torch is thrown on the anterior surface of the cornea. This forms a bright, erect, and virtual image of the object that moves with the movement of the light; this is called the first Purkinje image. The second image has the same qualities but is less bright than the first. The third image is formed by the anterior surface of the lens. It too is virtual, erect, and small, moving with the movement of the light. Because the anterior surface of the lens also acts as a convex mirror. The fourth image is formed by the posterior surface of the lens. As the posterior lens surface behaves as a concave mirror, this image is real-inverted and moves against the movement of light. The absence of the third and fourth images denotes the absence of the lens (aphakia) from the pupillary area **(Fig. 1.6)**.*

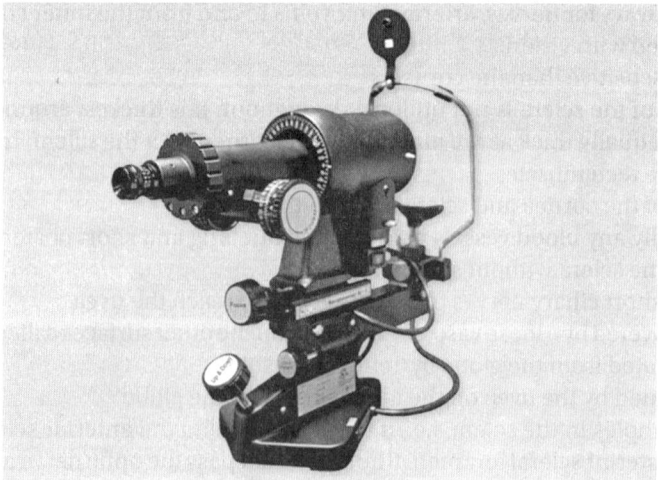

Fig. 1.5: Keratometer.
(*Courtesy:* Appasamy Associates)

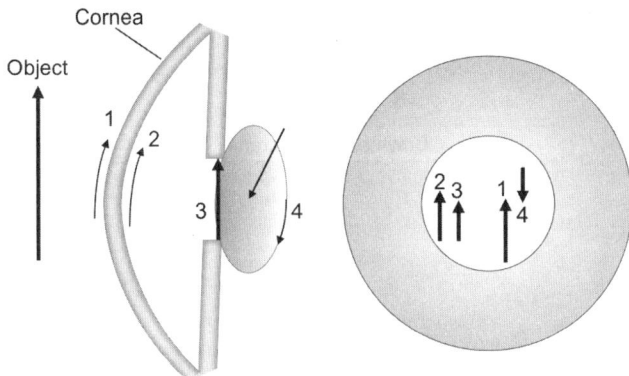

Fig. 1.6: Purkinje images.

The cornea looks circular on a cursory look, but it is really not so; its vertical diameter is 11 mm and its horizontal diameter is 12 mm. This makes the vertical meridian more curved (myopic) than the horizontal. The diameter is measured by a corneal caliper, which gives a result in millimeters. A cornea less than 9 mm in diameter is called a microcornea, and one larger than 12 mm is called a megalocornea (**Fig. 1.7A**).

The curvature is not equal on both surfaces; the posterior surface is more curved, making the central part thinner (i.e., 0.523 mm), while the peripheral part is as thick as the surrounding sclera (i.e., 0.660 mm). The thickness of the cornea is measured by an instrument called a pachymeter. That can be ultrasonic or optical. The central thinness makes the cornea prone to perforation.

The corneal surface is bright and smooth; loss of both are signs of disease. The smoothness is elicited by an instrument called a keratoscope called the Placido disc (**Fig. 1.7B**).

The cornea is devoid of blood vessels except near the limbus; the presence of blood vessels in the cornea is a sign of pathology. The cornea is very sensitive to pain, and the nerves responsible for pain originate from the nasociliary branch of the trigeminal. The pain sensation is abolished by instilling a local anesthetic agent.

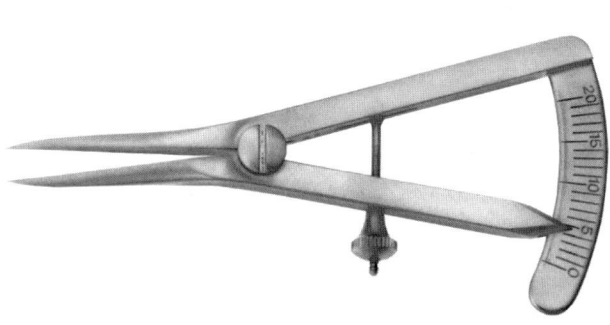

Fig. 1.7A: Common corneal calipers.

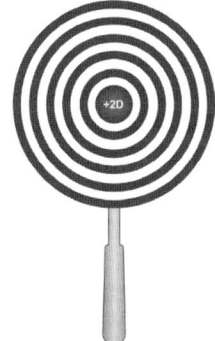

Fig. 1.7B: Placido's disc.

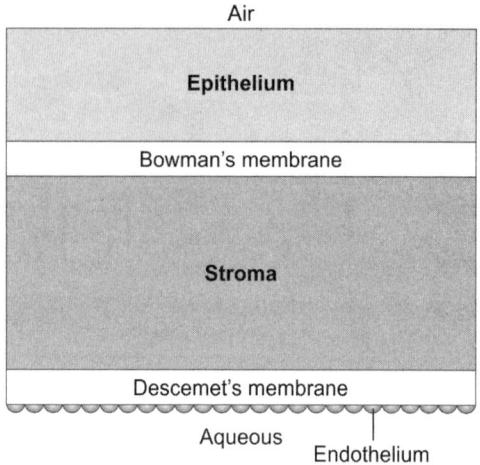

Fig. 1.8: Section of the cornea showing the relative thickness of its parts.

The cornea has five layers. They are: Epithelium, Bowman's membrane, stroma, Descemet's membrane, and endothelium. The epithelium is continuous with the conjunctiva, The stroma is continuous with the sclera, and the endothelium is an extension of the iris epithelium. It is attached to the Descemet's membrane; the Descemet's membrane has the ability to regenerate and extends in the trabecular meshwork; in contrast, the Bowmen's membrane is 1.00 mm short from the corneal periphery without the ability to regenerate. It is situated between epithelium and stroma **(Fig. 1.8)**.

Tear Film

The epithelial surfaces of the cornea and conjunctiva are always moist. The absence of moisture is a sign of a disease called ocular surface disorder (dry eye). The moisture is supplied by the tear film, which is mostly supplied by secretion from the lacrimal gland. The other sources of tear film are accessory lacrimal glands, conjunctival glands, and meibomian glands. The tear film has three layers: lipid (oil), aqueous (water), and mucin layer **(Fig. 1.9)**.

Out of the three layers, the aqueous layer is the thickest and lies between the lipid and mucus layer. The former faces the air, while the latter comes into contact with the corneal epithelium.

The functions of the tear film are:
- Keeping the cornea and conjunctiva moist.
- Remove unwanted material from the eye.
- It is an optical part of the cornea.
- It provides oxygen to the cornea.
- It provides nutrition to the cornea.

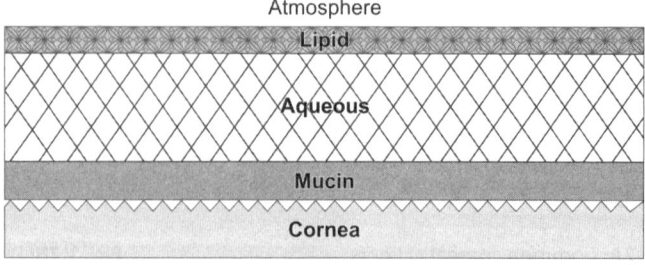

Fig. 1.9: Three layers of tear film.

- ❖ It possesses mild antimicrobial properties.
- ❖ Derangement of any layer results in changes in the cornea.

Most of the tear is formed in the main lacrimal glands on the superior lateral part of the upper fornix, where it flows down and medially across the ocular surface towards the lacrimal puncta in the lower lid. About 90% of the tear is drained by the lower puncta. From the puncta, it passes successively through the canaliculus sack, nasolacrimal duct, and nose. The amount of tear is tested by a simple test called the Schirmer's test *(see dry eye syndrome)*.

Limbus

The limbus is an important surgical landmark, it is a junction of the cornea, sclera, and conjunctiva. It is an ill-defined area about 1.00 mm around the cornea. The corneal epithelium, which has 4 layers on the cornea, is converted to 8–10 layers to mix with the conjunctiva. The Bowmen's membrane does not reach the limbus. The limbus is highly vascular.

Extraocular Muscle

There are eight extraocular striated muscles in relation to the orbit. They are:
- ❖ **Those move the eye**: Superior and inferior recti, superior and inferior oblique, medial and lateral recti.
- ❖ **Those with protective purposes**: Levator palpebrae superioris and orbicularis oculi. The first opens the lids, and the second closes the lids; they have a coordinated movement.

The four recti, levator, and superior oblique arise from the apex. The last has its effective origin on the upper medial side of the rim. The inferior oblique originates from the inferio medial aspect of the rim; the four recti are inserted in front of the equator at various distances from the limbus, as shown in **Figure 1.10**.

The superior oblique runs under the superior rectus. The inferior oblique lies under the inferior rectus, above the floor. **Table 1.2** shows the insertion, nerve supply, and action of the extraocular muscle.

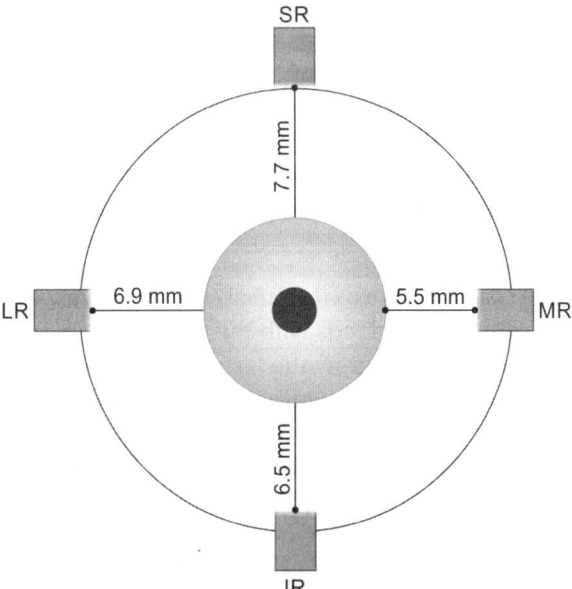

Fig. 1.10: Attachment recti to the sclera.

Table 1.2: Insertion, nerve supply, and action of the extraocular muscle.

Sl. No.	Name of the muscle	Origin	Insertion	Nerve supply	Action
1.	Superior rectus	Annulus of Zinn	8 mm behind the limbus	Third	• Elevation • Adduction • Intorsion
2.	Medial rectus	Annulus of Zinn	5.5 mm behind the limbus	Third	• Adduction
3.	Inferior rectus	Annulus of Zinn	6.5 mm behind the limbus	Third	• Depression • Abduction • Extortion
4.	Lateral rectus	Annulus of Zinn	7 mm behind the limbus	Sixth	• Abduction
5.	Superior oblique	Outside the annulus of Zinn	13.5–18.5 mm behind the limbus	Fourth	• Intorsion • Depression • Abduction
6.	Inferior oblique	Medial side of the rim of the orbit	Behind the equator 16.5 mm from the limbus	Third	• Extorsion • Elevation • Abduction
7.	Levator palpebral superior	Apex of orbit above the origin of superior rectus	Skin of the lid upper part of the tarsal plate upper fornix	Third	Elevation of the upper lid
8.	Orbicularis oculi	Rim of the orbit	No definite insertion	Seventh	Closing the lids

Conjunctiva

The conjunctiva is a specialized mucus membrane of the external eye. It extends from the lid margin to the limbus. It is transparent; white sclera is visible through it. The conjunctiva is highly vascular; only a few vessels are visible in a normal conjunctiva; an inflamed conjunctiva has many vessels that give it its red color. The conjunctiva is moist on the exposed surface and is richly supplied by sensory nerves. The sensation of the conjunctiva is less than that of the cornea. The conjunctiva is anatomically divided into the following parts without any definite demarcation in between. They are the **palpebral conjunctiva, bulbar conjunctiva, and fornices.**

Palpebral conjunctiva: It is also known as the tarsal conjunctiva, extends from the lid margin to the fornix. The tarsal conjunctiva blends with the skin at the lid margin and is called the marginal conjunctiva, through which grow the lashes. The meibomian gland opens in the marginal conjunctiva. The palpebral conjunctiva is again divided into two parts, i.e., the tarsal conjunctiva and the orbital conjunctiva. The former is firmly attached to the tarsal plate and cannot be separated from it; the tarsal glands are visible through the normal conjunctiva. The tarsal conjunctiva is the place where papillae, follicles, and fibrosis develop. The orbital conjunctiva extends from the tarsal plate to the fornix. It contains Wolfring's glands, which supply mucus to the tear film. It is very loose, the upper fornix is larger than the lower **(Figs. 1.11 and 1.12).**

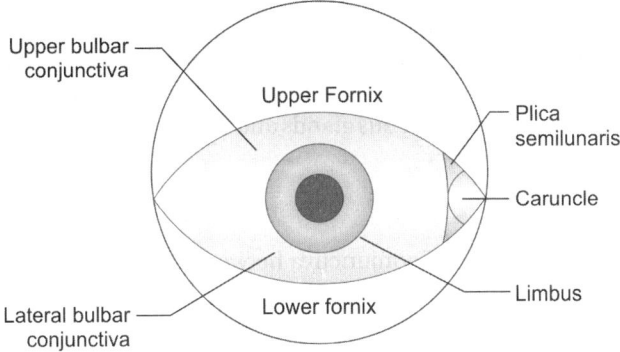

Fig. 1.11: Various parts of the conjunctiva as seen from the front.

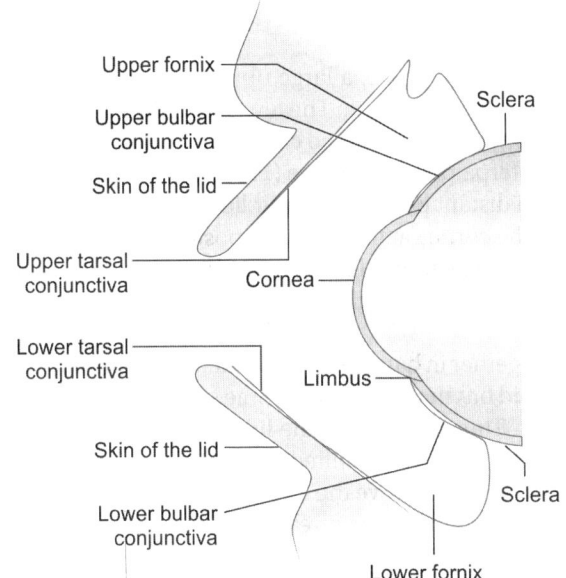

Fig. 1.12: Various parts of the conjunctiva as seen from the side.

Bulbar conjunctiva: It is the largest and most visible part. It extends from the limbus to the upper fornix above and lower fornix below, medially to the middle canthus, and laterally to the lateral canthus. It can be moved over the sclera all around except around the limbus; it is loose enough to be lifted from the sclera. Due to its looseness, it is a common site for the accumulation of fluid under it. The space between the conjunctiva and sclera is called the subconjunctival space, where antibiotics and steroids can be injected. It contains goblet cells that supply mucus to the tear film.

Fornices: The junction of the palpebral and tarsal conjunctiva is known as the fornix; there are two fornices, i.e., the upper and the lower. The upper fornix is larger than the lower and is difficult to see fully. The lower fornix is shallow both in length and depth. It can be examined by pulling the lower lid down. The lacrimal ducts and Krause's glands open in the upper fornices. The lacrimal ducts supply aqueous to the tear film; they open at the superolateral part of the fornix. The lower fornix only has Krause's glands. Both fornices can be used to deposit medicines by subconjunctival injection.

Caruncle

Caruncle is a visible part of the bulbar conjunctiva at the medial canthus; it is a about 2–3 mm rounded elevated structure covered by modified skin and conjunctival epithelium. A few lashes sprout from it, and it may contain sebaceous glands and sweat glands. It does not have any known functions.

Plica Semilunaris

It is a vertical crescent-shaped fold of conjunctiva between the caruncle and the limbus. It, too, does not have any definite purpose. It is equivalent to the nictitating membrane of many lower animals.

Ocular Adnexa

The ocular adnexa comprises two systems, i.e., the lid and the lacrimal system.

Lids

The lids are two in number in each eye: a large upper lid and a small lower lid, the upper lid extends from the eyebrow to the lid margin. The lower lid extends from the cheek to the lower lid margin. The junctions of the two lids are called canthi, i.e., medial and lateral. The space between the two lids is called the interpalpebral aperture **(Figs. 1.13A and B)**.

When the eyes look at a distant point, the upper lid covers 2.00 mm of the upper cornea, and the lower lid just touches the cornea at the 6 O'clock position. If the upper lid covers >2.00 mm of the cornea, it is called ptosis. The upper lid covers a larger area of the globe than the lower. The main function of the lids is to protect the globe; the other function is to spread the tear film evenly on the ocular surface.

The two lids function together in harmony. The structures of the two lids are similar with a few exceptions, i.e., the upper lid has the levator palpebrae superioris and the Muller's muscle, which are absent in the lower lid. The structures of the lids are the skin, tarsal plate, and conjunctiva. The skin of the lids is very thin and can be lifted up. There is no fat under the skin of the lid. The upper lid forms a horizontal groove above the level of the tarsal plate. The loss of this crease is an indication of ptosis. The lid margin is a mixture of skin and conjunctiva, with a rounded anterior border and a sharp posterior border. From the outer border arise the eyelashes; they are more numerous and longer in length on the upper lid. On the inner border, open the meibomian ducts. On the medial end of each lid, 2.00 mm from the medial canthus, open the lacrimal puncta. The lid has two striated muscles. The orbicularis oculi and the levator.

The **orbicularis** lies in the front part of the orbit in a circular fashion, in between the tarsal plate and the skin **(Fig. 1.14)**.

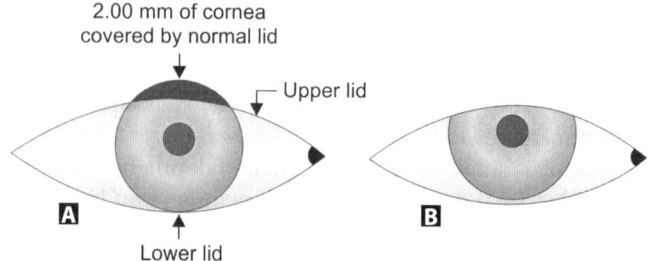

Figs. 1.13A and B: Position of the normal lid in relation to the limbus and pupil.
(A) Normal position of upper lid; (B) Ptosis.

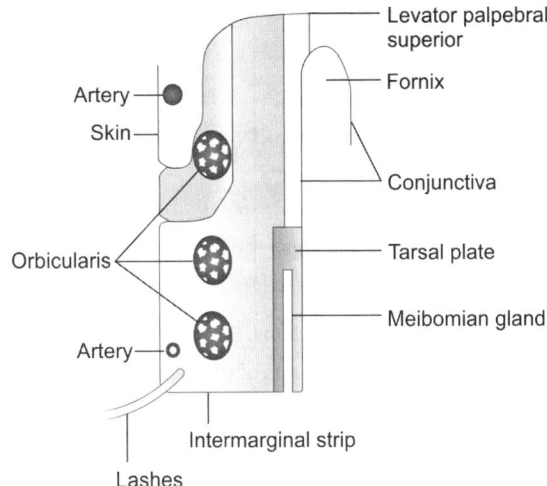

Fig. 1.14: Vertical section of the upper lid.

Its function is to close the lids. It is supplied by the seventh cranial nerve. Paralysis of the muscle prevents closure of the lid. The action of the orbicularis is opposed by the levator. Otherwise, the two muscles have a delicate balance between them. When the orbicularis contracts, the levator relaxes, and when the levator contracts, the orbicularis relaxes.

The **levator palpebrae superioris** is present only in the upper lid; it is supplied by the upper division of the third nerve. Its main function is to lift the upper lid. The levator takes its origin from the apex of the orbit, passing under the roof of the orbit in a fan shape. The nasal end is attached to the medial canthal ligament and the temporal to the lateral canthal ligament. As the levator and the superior rectus have the same nerve supply, the two act simultaneously when the lids close. As the lid comes down, the superior rectus pulls the globe up; this is called the Bell's phenomenon, which is a protective reflex.

Muller's Muscle

The Muller's muscle is a non-striated (plane) muscle supplied by a sympathetic chain without any bony origin; it is not attached to the globe and does not take part in the movement of the globe. It is a thin sheet of muscle from the inferior surface of the LPS that is inserted at the upper border of the tarsal plate. It helps the LPS keep the upper lid open.

Lacrimal System

The Lacrimal system consists of the following parts **(Fig. 1.15)**:
❖ Producing tears
❖ Spreading and draining the tears

The first part consists of the main lacrimal gland and accessory lacrimal glands. The main lacrimal gland produces almost 90% of tears; it is situated in the superior temporal part of the orbit. 10 to 20 lacrimal ducts carry the tears to the upper fornix. The gland is supplied by trigeminal, facial, and sympathetic nerves.

The accessory glands are Krause's and Wolfring's glands in the conjunctiva.

The second part consists of the lid, which plays the most important role in spreading the tear across the ocular surface to bring the tears to the drainage system. Which consists of two puncta, one in each lid, two canaliculi, a single lacrimal sac, and a nasolacrimal duct.

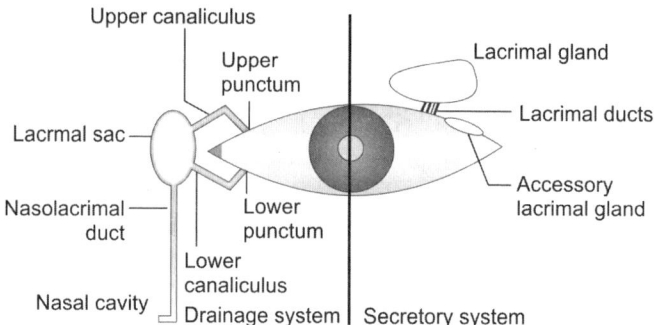

Fig. 1.15: Diagram showing various parts of the lacrimal system; the vertical line demarcates between the secretory and draining parts.

The puncta are situated 6.00 mm from the canthus; they are visible depressions in the lids. The lower punctum drains 80% of tears. They open in the canaliculi, which open in the lacrimal sac.

Lacrimal Sac

The lacrimal sac lies in the lacrimal fossa between the eye and the nasal bone. Normally, it is neither visible nor palpable unless distended. The rounded upper end is called the fundus of the sac, and the lower end of it opens the canaliculi. The sac is surrounded by bones on all sides except the front, which lies under the medial palpebral ligament. The nasolacrimal duct is a tube that joins the lacrimal sac to the nose. It is a common site of congenital anomalies of the lacrimal system, leading to congenital nasolacrimal obstruction in infants.

Intraocular Structures

The intraocular structures are more protected, compact, and specialized than the adnexa. They consist of:
- Aqueous humor
- Uvea
- Lens
- Vitreous
- Retina

Out of the two vascular structures mentioned above are the uvea and retina.

Aqueous Humor

Aqueous humor is a crystal clear vital fluid with many purposes. It fills both the anterior and posterior chambers. The lens divides the globe into two unequal parts: a small aqueous chamber and a large vitreous chamber. They do not communicate with each other as long as the lens is in place. The posterior chamber is occupied by the vitreous, which is lined by the retina. The aqueous chamber is again divided into two unequal parts by the iris. The large part in front of the iris is called the anterior chamber. The space behind the iris and in front of the lens is called the posterior chamber.

The anterior chamber is bounded by the cornea and posteriorly by the iris pupil and lens. The two surfaces of the anterior chambers meet at the periphery and are called the anterior chamber. The angle is formed by a lace-like structure called a trabecular meshwork. The apex of which opens in the canal of Schlemm's to join the episclera vein, the depth of the anterior chamber is not uniform; it is deepest in front of the pupil and narrowest at the angle. The posterior chamber is bounded by the iris, pars plicata of the ciliary body, and lens with its suspensory ligament. The ciliary processes project into the posterior chamber. The aqueous is constantly produced and continuously drained, maintaining equilibrium between the two. The volume of the aqueous is 125 µL, and the aqueous is formed at a rate of 2–3 µL per minute. It flows out at a rate of 2.5 µL per minute. 90% of aqueous drains through the trabecular meshwork, and the rest through uveoscleral flow. Both flows can be influenced by drugs that are used to treat glaucoma, but there is no method to increase the formation of the aqueous (Fig. 1.16).

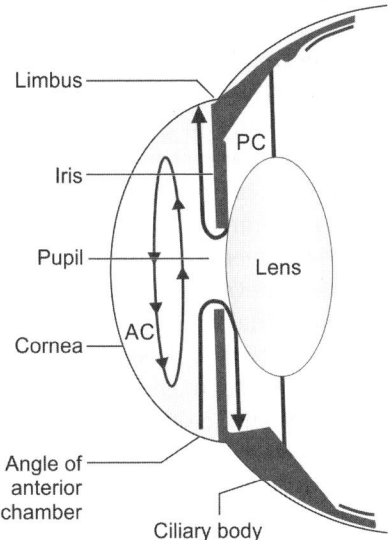

Fig. 1.16: Circulation of aqueous.

Uvea

The uvea is the most vascular of the intraocular structures. It is sandwiched between the retina on the inner side and the sclera on the other side, behind the equator. It is divided into three parts, i.e., the iris, ciliary body, and choroid.

Choroid

The choroid is the largest part of the uvea, extending from the end of the ciliary body up to the margin of the optic nerve. It is sandwiched between the outer layer of the retina and the inner surface of the sclera. The part of the choroid adjacent to the retina is Bruch's membrane. Followed by a layer of choriocapillaris; under the choriocapillaris lie the larger vessels. The choroid is heavily pigmented, which gives it its black color. The function of the sclera is to supply nutrition to the retina. The other purpose of the choroid is to keep the inside of the eye dark. Four vertex veins arise from the four quadrants of the choroid. It has no visual function. It does not contain any muscle, and due to its vasculature, it is prone to bleeding.

Ciliary Body

The ciliary body is the thickest part of the uvea, lying between the choroid and the iris. In fact, the iris arises from the ciliary body. The ciliary body is triangular in shape, with an apex towards the choroid. Its bases face the lens and vitreous; it lines the anterior part of the sclera; and it has two parts, i.e., ciliary muscle and ciliary processes. The latter produces aqueous, the former is involved in accommodation. The ciliary processes are about 70 in number and project from the anterior part of the ciliary body. The suspensory ligaments are attached to the ciliary processes.

The ciliary muscle lies in the anterior and outer parts of the ciliary body. The anterior part of the ciliary muscle is inserted into the scleral spur. The anterior surface of the ciliary body is lined by ciliary epithelium and pigment epithelium.

Iris

The iris is the smallest and thinnest part of the uvea; it hangs like a curtain in front of the lens, dividing it. The aqueous chambers in the anterior and posterior chambers communicate through an aperture in the center, called the pupil. The periphery of the iris, which is very thin, is attached to the anterior surface of the ciliary body. The normal pupil is about 3.00 mm wide in children, and in old age it becomes smaller. It also constricts in the presence of light and accommodation. The constriction of the pupil is called miosis, and dilatation is called mydriasis. Generally, the size of the pupils on both sides is equal; the difference in size between the two eyes is called anisocoria. The change in color between two eyes is called heterochromia. The dark color of the iris is due to the presence of melanin. In albinism, where there is an absence of pigment in the uvea, the color of the iris is pale. The normal color of the pupil is black; color of the pupil in aphakia is jet black. The pupillary border is lined by a layer of pigments. The surface of the pupil is rough. The anterior surface of the iris is lined by a single layer of endothelium that is continuous with the corneal endothelium. Under the endothelium lies the thickest part of the iris, which is called the stroma. It contains two plain muscles, i.e., constrictor and dilator. The dilator is situated on the periphery, and the constrictor is around the pupillary margin. The constrictor is supplied by the third nerve, while the other is supplied by the cervical sympathetic. Alongside these muscles, the iris also contains blood vessels, stroma, and fibrous tissue. The iris vessels, in contrast to the ciliary body and choroid, do not bleed on trauma, even on cutting.

Besides miotic, bright light, and inflammation of the iris, which are common causes of miosis, the following conditions also cause constriction of the pupil are:

- Light reflex
- Near reflex
- Accommodation
- Convergence

To understand the near, accommodation, and convergence reflexes, it is essential to understand the visual pathway.

The visual path is in fact a neural tract on which depend the other reflexes. The visual path extends from the retina to the visual cortex. The stimulus from the retina traverses through the optic nerve chiasma, the optic tract, and the lateral geniculate body. The retinal fibers arising from the temporal half pass straight to the chiasma, optic tract, and geniculate body. The nasal fibers cross over to the other side at the level of the chiasma. Thus, the fibers from the optic tract onward contain temporal fibers from the same side and nasal fibers from the other side. This arrangement is continuous from the lateral geniculate body to the optic cortex **(Fig. 1.17)**.

Light Reflex

The afferent fibers from the retina, along with visual fibers, go up to the lateral geniculate body; thereafter, the pupillary fibers leave the optic tract and go to the pretectal nuclei **(Fig. 1.18)**.

Fibers from each eye go to the nuclei on both sides. Light thrown into one pupil causes constriction of both pupils, which is called a direct pupillary reaction. From each pretectal nucleus. The impulses to the Edinger-Westphal nucleus on both sides of the efferent path are via the third nerve to the ciliary ganglion, from where they traverse via short ciliary nerves to the sphincter muscle of the iris.

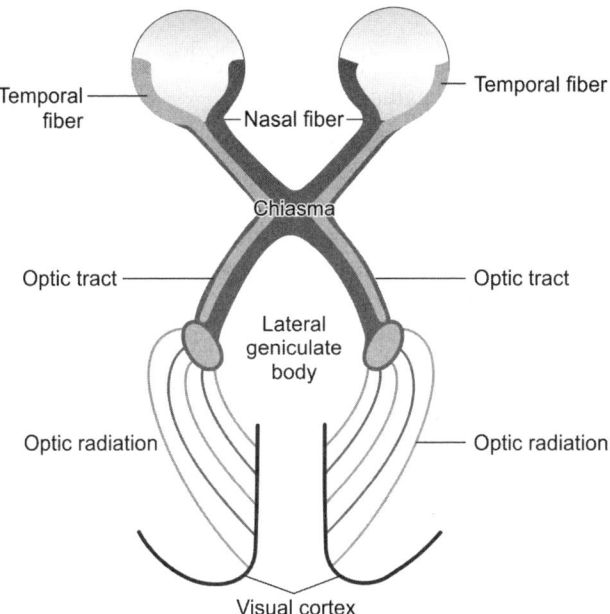

Fig. 1.17: The optic pathway.

Note: That the fibers from the medial (or nasal) half of each retina cross over to the optic tract of the opposite side.

Afferent path is that path that arises from the eye and ends in the brain. The path that arises from the brain to the eye is called the efferent path.
The afferent visual path is: retina → optic nerve → chiasma → optic tract → lateral geniculate body → visual cortex.
The efferent path of third nerve is: nucleus → lower division of third → ciliary ganglion → short ciliary nerves → pupil.

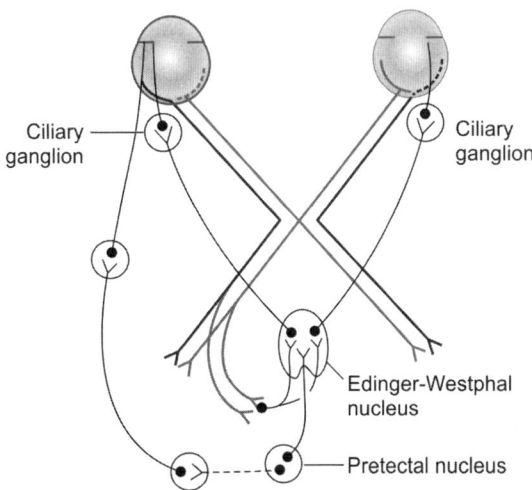

Fig. 1.18: Path of light reflex.

Near Reflex

The near reflex consists of two paths, i.e., the accommodation reflex and the convergence reflex; they act simultaneously in different paths.

Accommodation: Accommodation is the ability to bring divergent rays into focus on the retina. The accommodation reflex is initiated by difficulty in near vision. The afferent path passes through the visual fibers up to the visual cortex, from where it joins an area in the visual cortex. From where the efferent path starts by joining the Edinger-Westphal nucleus. The efferent path after this is similar to the light reflex. This is a parasympathetic reflex. It can be abolished by cycloplegics and retrobulbar anesthesia **(Fig. 1.19)**.

Convergence: Convergence is the ability to move both eyes simultaneously towards the nose. It can be done at will or happen reflexly, when accommodation is activated, the exact path of convergence is not well understood. Probably the afferent path starts from the medial rectus and goes to the third nerve, from where it goes to the mesencephalic nucleus of the fifth nerve, from there to the convergence center, and back to the third nerve nucleus to reach the ciliary ganglion. Three phenomena, i.e., constriction of the pupil, accommodation, and convergence, act together. When a small object is looked at near point.

Blood Supply to the Uvea

The uvea is one of the most vascular parts of the eye. The iris is less vascular than the choroid and the ciliary body. The uvea gets its blood supply from the posterior and anterior ciliary arteries; both are branches of the ophthalmic artery, which is the main source of blood supply to the eye and its adnexa. Out of the 12 branches of the ophthalmic artery, only two branches, i.e., the posterior ciliary and muscular branches, supply the uvea. The twigs of muscular branches that supply the uvea are called anterior ciliary arteries. There are two groups of arteries, i.e., short and long posterior ciliary arteries. The short posterior arteries are about 10–20 in number; they enter the sclera in a circular fashion around the nerve and become choriocapillaris. The long posterior ciliary arteries are two in number, i.e., nasal and temporal. They enter the sclera in front of short ciliary arteries, one on each side, to reach the ciliary body.

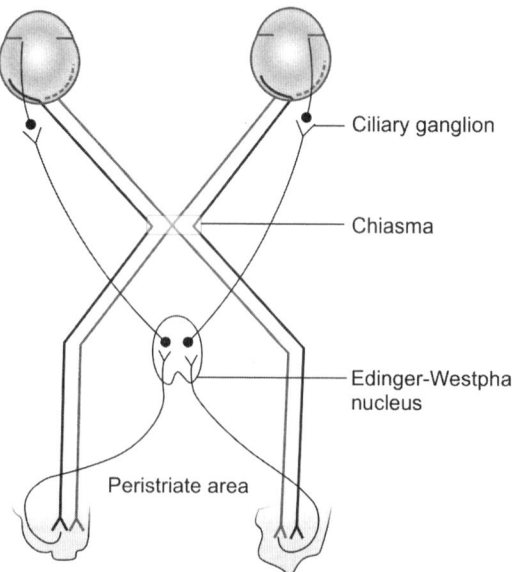

Fig. 1.19: Path of accommodation.

Lens

The total refractive power of a normal adult eye is +60D, divided into two components, i.e., the cornea and lens. The cornea imparts 2/3 of its rest to the lens. The cornea is not capable of changing dioptric power, which is the sole property of the lens. The lens can change the dioptric power to focus rays coming from infinity to a near point by a faculty called accommodation.

The lens is a specialized part of the eye; it is suspended by the suspensory ligaments between the posterior surface of the iris and the anterior surface of the vitreous. In children, there is a strong binding between the posterior surface of the lens and the anterior vitreous face. That passes off gradually as the patient ages; by 50 years, it is totally abolished. The lens viewed from the front looks circular, and from the side, it looks elliptical. The diameter of the lens is about 10.00 mm. The thickness of the lens at the center is about 3.00 mm. The lens is covered by a capsule. The capsule all around, i.e., the anterior and posterior capsules, the two merge with each other in a rounded periphery called the equator of the lens. The thickness of the capsule is not equal on both surfaces. The posterior capsule is thinner than the anterior capsule; the thinnest part is the center of the posterior capsule. The central most part of the anterior lens is called the anterior pole, and its posterior counterpart is the posterior pole. The curvature of the two surfaces is not equal. The posterior surface is more curved than the anterior surface **(Fig. 1.20)**.

The capsule is lined by lens epithelium, which is thickest at the equator and gradually thins towards the pole; it is absent at the posterior pole. The cells of epithelia grow and multiply due to repeated division. The old cells are pushed towards the center to form the nucleus. The epithelial cells lose their nuclei as they elongate. The division and elongation of the lens continue throughout life. The elongated cells formed the cortex, and the central compressed area is the nucleus, which has different zones corresponding to the age of the lens. They are embryonal, infantile, and adult. The lens of the child is soft, which gradually hardens to become semisolid. The lens of the child is almost spherical at birth, which gradually flattens to become elliptical with age. The lens is suspended by the suspensory ligaments all around the ciliary body. The lens gets its nutrition from the aqueous humor after birth. Before birth, it gets its nutrition from Tunica Vasculosa Lentis. The lens is vascular after birth and remains so unless it develops opacity. Technically, any opacity in the lens is a cataract. As the lens is vascular, it is immune to infection, inflammation, degeneration, and dystrophy. The lens does not develop malignancy; it is devoid

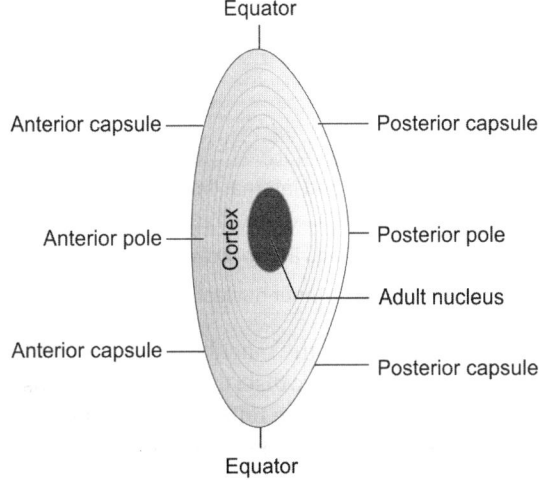

Fig. 1.20: Parts of lens.

of nerve supply. The ability of the lens to change its power is called accommodation. The refractive index of a transparent lens is 1.43.

Vitreous Chamber

Vitreous is an inner gel extending from the back of the lens to the disc. It is firmly attached to the ora serrata by a band of vitreous 4.00 mm wide called the base of the vitreous. Vitreous has a weak attachment at the macula. The attachment at the back of the lens under 40 is strong that passes off by 55 years of age. The vitreous, unlike the lens, does not have a capsule. The vitreous is a semisolid gel with 90% water, hyaluronic acid, and polysaccharides dissolved in it. The purpose of the vitreous is to prevent the lens from sagging and keep the retina pressed against the uvea. The other function of the vitreous is optical. The fully developed vitreous is devoid of blood vessels and nerves. During development, the hyaloid artery traverses between the optic disc and the posterior surface of the lens.

Retina

The retina is the most developed neural part of the eye concerned with vision, color vision, photopic vision, scotopic vision, and field of vision.

It is a transparent, delicate, thin layer of neural ectoderm lining the interior of the posterior two-thirds of the globe, with its anterior border 8.00 mm from the limbus and called the ora serrata; the posterior end surrounds the optic nerve. The retina is firmly attached to these areas. The retina lies between the vitreous on the inner side and the choroid on the outer side. It is made up of two layers of secondary optic cups; the inner part has visual properties. The outer layer of the optic cup gives rise to its pigment layers. The pigment epithelium is a single layer of cells that contains melanin. The purpose of the pigment epithelium is to absorb scattered light, which is converted to heat and dissipated by choroidal vessels. The retina internal to the pigment layer is transparent except for the blood vessels. The retinal pigment layer is attached to the Bruch's membrane of the choroid **(Fig. 1.21)**.

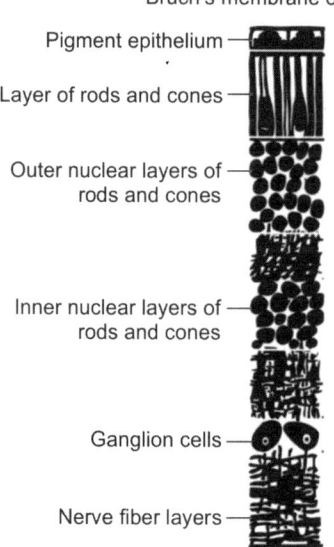

Fig. 1.21: Ten layers of retina.

The sensory retina has:

1. Three	2. Two	3. One
i. Visual cells (rods and cones)	i. External and internal limiting membrane	i. Ganglion cells
ii. Bipolar cells	ii. External and internal plexiform	ii. Nerve fiber layer
iii. Ganglion cells	iii. Outer and inner nuclear layers	

The retina is ten-layered all over, barring the macula and ora serrata. All the layers except the nerve fiber layer stop at the margin of the optic disc; the nerve fibers pass backwards through the lamina to form the optic nerve. The optic nerve represents the blind spot, which has no vision. The retina is thinnest at the ora serrata and thicker at the posterior pole. The cones, which are meant for central vision, day vision, and color sense, are maximal at the macula. The rods are at their maximum at the periphery. The peripheral retina is meant for night vision; it has very poor color vision. The macula is an ill-defined circular area at the posterior pole lateral to the disc on the horizontal raphe, 4.00 mm away.

It is 5.5 mm in diameter, and the central 0.35 mm is foveola, i.e., surrounded by a zone 1.5 mm in diameter called fovea. The foveola is a small depression; all the layers of the retina except the internal limiting membrane are absent at the fovea.

The retina has a double blood supply, i.e., from the choriocapillaris that supply the outer four layers: the inner six layers are supplied by the central retinal artery and its branches **(Fig. 1.22)**. The retinal arteries do not anastomose with each other.

The central retinal artery is a direct branch of the ophthalmic artery. The central retinal artery arises from the ophthalmic artery at the apex of the orbit under the optic nerve. It enters the optic nerve from its inferior surface, 10.00 mm behind the globe, to reach the central core of the optic nerve **(Fig. 1.23)**.

At the lamina, it divides into a superior and an inferior branch. Each of these branches again divides into medial and temporal branches in an arc over the macula. Each of these branches keeps on dividing into smaller branches until they reach the ora serrata.

The retinal arteries do not give branches to the macula, which depends solely on the underlined choriocapillaris. The retinal veins flow in the reverse direction, following the course of the arteries. At places, they cross each other. The junction is called the arteriovenous junction.

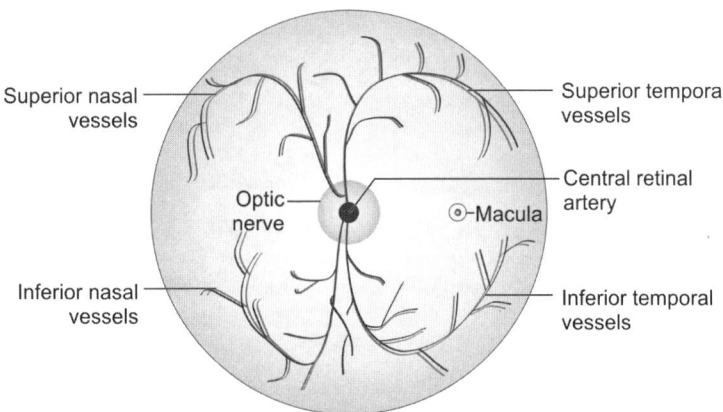

Fig. 1.22: Branches of the central retinal artery and veins.

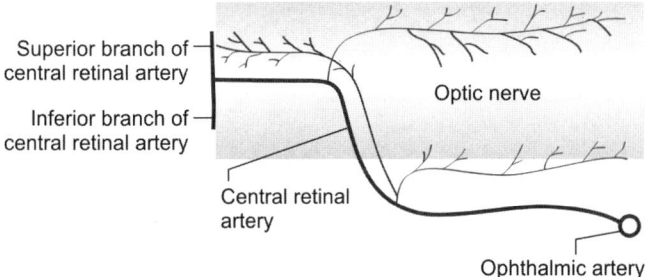

Fig. 1.23: Relation of the central retinal artery to the optic nerve.

NERVE SUPPLY OF THE EYE

The uvea is the only intraocular structure that has a pain sensation. Out of the three parts of the uvea that show movement, the retina, vitreous, and lens do not have pain sensation. The retina and choroid do not move as they do not have any muscles.

The nerve supply to the intraocular structures can be divided into the following parts:
- Sensory supply to the uvea by the nasociliary artery
- Motor supply to the iris and ciliary body by parasympathetic and sympathetic

The nerves that supply the uvea are called ciliary nerves, i.e., short posterior ciliary and long ciliary. The short posterior ciliary nerves are about 15 in number. They enter the globe around the optic nerve. The long ciliary nerves are two in number; they arise from the nasociliary. They are sensory, mostly parasympathetic, and, to a lesser extent, sympathetic. Mobility and pain sensations can be abolished by retrobulbar injections of anesthetic agents.

CHAPTER 2

Development of the Eye

The eyes are a forward extension of the brain. The development of the eyes is closely associated with the development of the brain. Both develop from the top of the neural tube.

Figure 2.1 consists of three germinal layers, i.e., ectoderm, mesoderm, and endoderm; the last is not associated with eyes. The ectoderm has two parts, i.e., the surface ectoderm and the neuroectoderm. From the surface ectoderm will develop the lens, epithelium of the conjunctiva, cornea, meibomian glands, lacrimal gland, and accessory lacrimal gland. From the neuroectoderm will develop the sensory retina, retinal pigment epithelium, ciliary body, pigment epithelium of the iris, sphincter and dilator of the iris, and neural part of the optic nerve. The mesoderm that develops in between the surface and neural ectoderm will give rise to the corneal stroma and its endothelium, Descemet's membrane, the stroma of the choroid and iris, ciliary muscles, sclera, vitreous, and bones of the orbit.

The following structures develop from both layers:
- **Lids:** Surface ectoderm and mesoderm
- **Zonules:** Surface ectoderm and mesoderm
- **Vitreous:**
  - *Primary:* Mesoderm
  - *Secondary:* Neuroectoderm

The eyes start developing at 2.6 mm (between the second and third weeks of conception). The eyes grow out of the developing forebrain. In the beginning, the developing forebrain has two layers, i.e., the outer-surface ectoderm and the inner-neuroectoderm.

Fate of the Neuroectoderm

The neuroectoderm develops two hollow projections, one on each side; the projections are called primary optic vesicles, and the narrow tube that joins the primary optic vesicles to the forebrain is called the optic stalk, which will ultimately be transformed into the optic nerve **(Fig. 2.2)**.

- The primary optic vesicles grow to the surface and touch its inner surface. As the primary optic vesicles touch the surface of the ectoderm, the neuroectoderm bends back, forming a cup with an opening towards the surface ectoderm. The primary optic vesicles are turned into a two-layered structure and are called secondary optic vesicles **(Fig. 2.3)**.

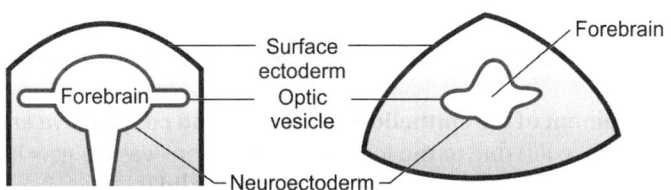

Fig. 2.1: Beginning of formation of optic vesicle.

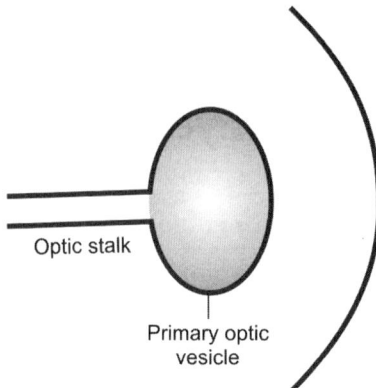

Fig. 2.2: Primary optic vesicle.

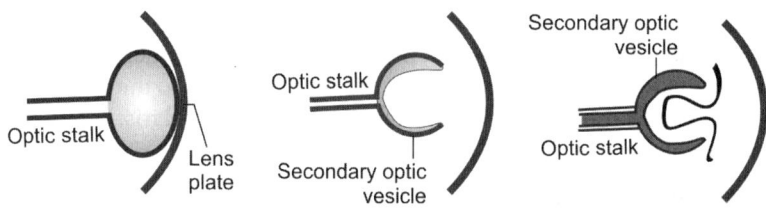

Fig. 2.3: Lens plate, optic stalk, and secondary optic vesicle.

❖ The secondary optic vesicle will develop the retina in two layers. The outer layer will develop the retinal pigment layer. The inner layer will develop the sensory retina. The two layers of the optic cup thus formed are continuous up to the rim of the optic cup. The tip of the cup will give rise to the epithelium of the ciliary body and iris.

Fate of the Surface Ectoderm

❖ The two ectoderms, i.e., neuro and surface, develop to gather.
❖ The contact of the neuroectoderm to the inner surface of the surface ectoderm starts many changes in the surface ectoderm. They are the development of the lens, the epithelium of the cornea, and the conjunctiva.

DEVELOPMENT OF THE LENS

The lens develops in the following stages:
1. The place on the surface ectoderm where it comes into contact with the surface neuroectoderm enlarges and thickens to from the lens plate (the future lens).
2. The enlarged lens plate bends back to form the lens pit.
3. The two edges of the lens plate come together to form a hollow spherical structure called the lens vesicle.
4. The lens vesicle gets detached from the surface ectoderm and shifts back to give rise to the lens **(Fig. 2.4)**.

The stages of development of the epithelium of the lens and conjunctiva are:
1. The gap on the surface left due to the formation of the lens vesicle gets bridged and forms the epithelia of the conjunctiva and cornea. It also forms lid folds.

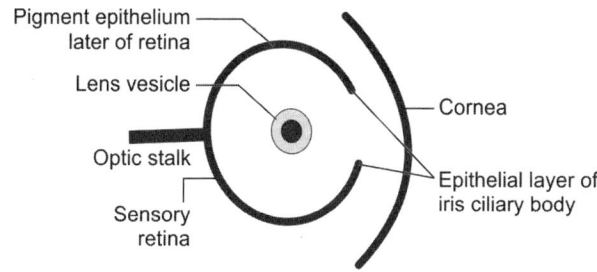

Fig. 2.4: The cornea, lens vesicle in the primary vitreous, and optic stalk.

2. The optic cup closes from above downward in a curved fashion, leaving a space that will be occupied by the lens and vitreous.
3. The gap between the two advancing edges of the optic cup is called the fetal fissure, through which the hyaloid artery will develop to supply nutrition to the developing lens until birth.

Structures Developing from the Mesoderm

❖ The vitreous develops from three sources. The surface and neuroectoderm plus mesoderm.
❖ The mesoderm surrounding the optic cup gives rise to the sclera, extraocular muscles, and lower part of the orbit.

CHAPTER 3

Physiology of the Eye

The physiology of the eye can be divided into the following parts:
- Metabolism
- Physiology of vision
- Binocular vision
- Aqueous humor and intraocular pressure (*see* **Chapter 1**)

METABOLISM

Metabolism of the Cornea

The cornea has a high rate of metabolism to keep it transparent, which is essential for vision. Cornea transmits 100% of visible rays (380–760 nm). It gets its nutrition from two sources: the tear in front, which is the main source of oxygen, and the aqueous behind. It is avascular, with scant blood supply from the periphery. The three factors that contribute to its transparency are anatomical, deturgescence, and intraocular pressure. The anatomical factors that keep the cornea transparent are its avascularity, absence of pigment, no visible nerves, arrangement of epithelial and endothelial cells, stromal fibrils, and normal tear film in front.

Metabolism of the Lens

The lens is nothing, but lens fibers contained in capsules. The lens fibers are proteins in nature; they are divided into two types: soluble (85%) and insoluble (15%). The lens is surrounded by aqueous, which is its sole source of nutrition through the capsule. An increased ratio of insoluble protein to soluble protein causes opacity. The lens epithelium creates energy similar to carbohydrates metabolism. **Most of the glucose metabolized in the lens is by anaerobic glycolysis.**

Metabolism of the Retina

As has been seen earlier, the retina is an outer pouch of the brain connected to the optic nerve. Hence, the metabolism of the retina is similar to that of the brain. The retina is the most metabolically active tissue; its nutrition comes via the retinal pigment epithelium of the choroidal circulation. The inner layers of the retina are supplied by the retinal vessels on its surface. The outer layer is supplied by choriocapillaris; if any of the two fail, the retinal cells die. The choroid is less delicate than the retina and suffers less if its blood supply is reduced.

PHYSIOLOGY OF VISION

The physiology of vision is further divided into:
- **Optics of the eye**
- **Visual sensation**:
  - Light sensation

- Form sensation
- Color sensation
❖ **Neurology of vision**:
  - Visual pathway
  - Accommodation
  - Convergence

Optics of the Eye

It is better to discuss the principles of optics before discussing the optics of the eye. Optics is the study of the behavior and properties of light. It is divided into two main groups: geometrical optics and physical optics. The former is based on the assumption that light moves as a straight ray. The latter is based on the theory of waves. The geometrical optic is mainly discussed under two heads, i.e., refraction and reflection.

Light

Light is an electromagnetic radiation that makes objects visible; it is made up of photons. The term photo means light. The light occurs over a wide range of wave lengths, from gamma rays that have the smallest wavelength to radio waves with the longest wave length measured in meters.

The electromagnetic radiation between 400 nm and 700 nm is visible to unaided human eyes. It is also referred to as white or natural light, which is ambient light (sunlight). It can also be artificially produced by electricity.

The following paragraphs will discuss visual optics, a study of white light that lies between ultraviolet and infrared. Though the natural light is called white light, infact it is a combination of seven colors called **VIBGYOR**. The ultraviolet rays have a wavelength of 397–400 nm and the infrared, 647 to 723. The light travels in a straight line; for all calculations, it is represented as a ray of light that is taken to be travelling from left to right.

When a ray of light meets a surface, it can pass through the object, be absorbed by the object, or be reflected by the object, depending on the brightness of the object. The brighter the object, the greater the reflection, as in a mirror. If all rays are absorbed, the object looks black and white when all rays are reflected back. The other colors are imparted by the wavelength of the reflected ray.

The reflected rays follow the law of reflection, while the rays that pass through the medium (the object) follow the law of refraction. The denser the medium, the greater the refraction.

The Law of Reflection

The law of reflection states that the incident ray, the reflected ray, and the normal to the surface of the mirror all lie in the same plane, and the angle of reflection is equal to the angle of incidence. The angles are measured in degrees in relation to the normal of the mirror **(Fig. 3.1)**.

There are two types of mirrors. They are plane and spherical; the latter can be either convex or concave.

The plane mirror is a flat surface without curvature. The spherical mirrors have a curve, an axis, and a center of curvature.

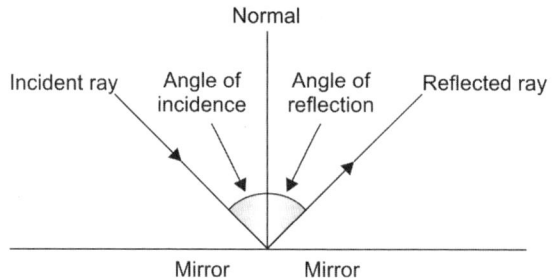

The angle of incidence and the angle of reflection are equal

Fig. 3.1: Reflection by a plane mirror.

Note: Incident ray: The ray falling on the plane mirror; Normal is A line perpendicular (90°) to the plane mirror. Reflected ray: The ray reflected by the plane mirror.

Image Made by a Plane Mirror

An object in front of a plane mirror forms an erect, virtual, laterally rotated image of the same size at an imaginary plane behind the mirror; the distance between the object and the image is the same. The image cannot be projected on a screen **(Fig. 3.2)** if the image is rotated at an angle. The image will move through the angle twice the previous angle, i.e., if the mirror is rotated by 20°, the image will move by 40°.

Image Formation by a Concave Mirror

The law of reflection in spherical mirrors is the same as in plane mirrors. Each spherical mirror has an arc, a center of curvature, a vortex, and an axis. The center of the arc of the mirror is situated on the principal axis of the mirror. At the point where the parallel rays meet the principal, the size of the image formed by a concave mirror depends on the focal length and distance of the object from the mirror **(Fig. 3.3)**.

Table 3.1 shows characteristics of images in a concave mirror.

Image Formation by a Convex Mirror

The image formed by a convex mirror is virtual, erect, and small when placed at any distance. The anterior surface of the cornea and the anterior surface of the lens act as convex reflecting surfaces, producing a virtual, erect, and small image that moves with the object (the source of light). This property has been utilized to produce the Purkinje image and is the basis for the Placido disc and keratometer.

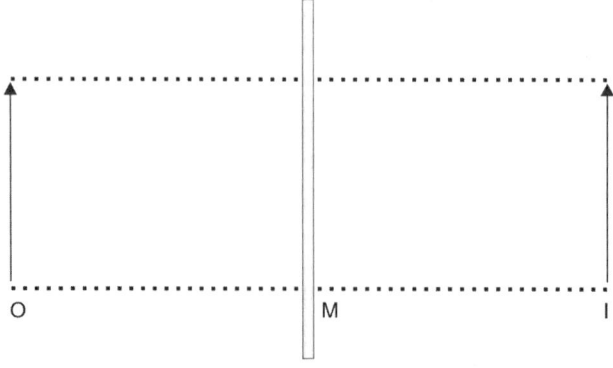

Fig. 3.2: Image formation by a plane mirror.
O = Object, M = Plane mirror, I = Image: OM = MI

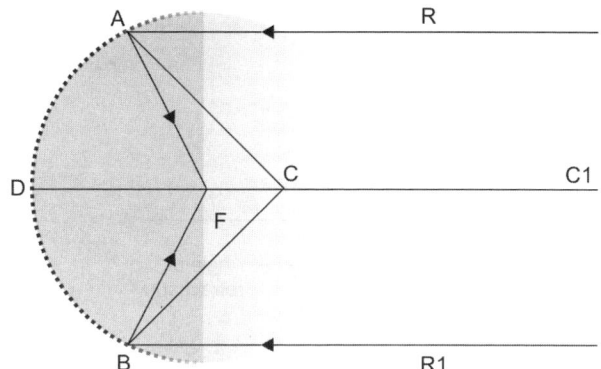

Fig. 3.3: Reflection by a concave mirror.

Note: ADB is a concave mirror; DCC1 is the principal axis of the mirror; AR and BR1 are the two parallel rays falling on the concave lens at A and B, respectively; AC and BC are two normal; F is the focal point, and FD is the focal length of the mirror.

Table 3.1: Characteristics of images in a concave mirror.		
Sl. No.	**Position of object**	**Characteristics of image**
1.	At infinity	At the focus, real and pinpoint
2.	Between the center of curvature and infinity	Between the mirror and center of curvature, real inverted and small
3.	Between focal point and mirror	Between center of curvature and infinity real inverted magnified
4.	At the center of curvature	At the center of curvature—real, inverted, of same size as the object
5.	At the focal point	At infinity, real inverted
6.	Between focal point and the mirror	The image is form behind the mirror it is virtual erect and magnified

Note: All the images are inverted and real in front of the mirror, except when they are between the focal point and the mirror.

The Law of Refraction

The law of refraction, also known as Snell's laws. Earlier, it was noted that when a ray travels through a uniform medium, it travels in a straight line. As it strikes a denser medium, it is partially reflected and passes through the denser medium, while it passes through the second medium, it deviates from its original path. This is called refraction, which follows the law of refraction **(Fig. 3.4).**

The law states that the incident ray, the refracted ray, and the normal at the point of incidence lie in the same plane. The incidence ray forms the angle of incidence, and the refracted ray forms the angle of refraction with the normal. The angle of refraction in such condition is less than angle of deviation. The ratio of the sine of the angle of incidence to the sine of the angle of refraction is a constant for the pair of given media.

If the already refracted ray passes from the denser medium to a rarer medium, it will deviate from the normal. As depicted in **Figure 3.5**, it consists of a rectangle of glass ABCD with air all around and a refractive index of 1.4.

The **Figures 3.6** and **3.7** are the basis of refraction through a prism, which in turn is the basis of the formation of optical lenses, both concave and convex.

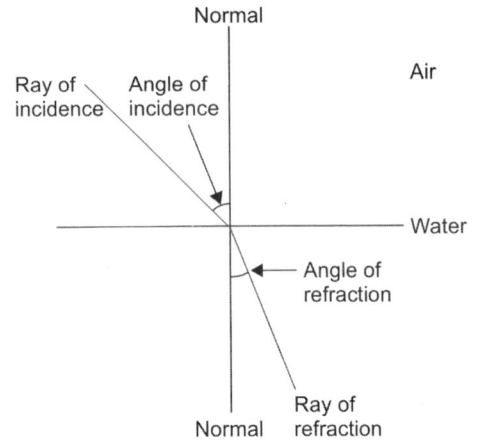

Fig. 3.4: Refraction.
Note: Refractive index of air is 1, refractive index of water is 1.33.

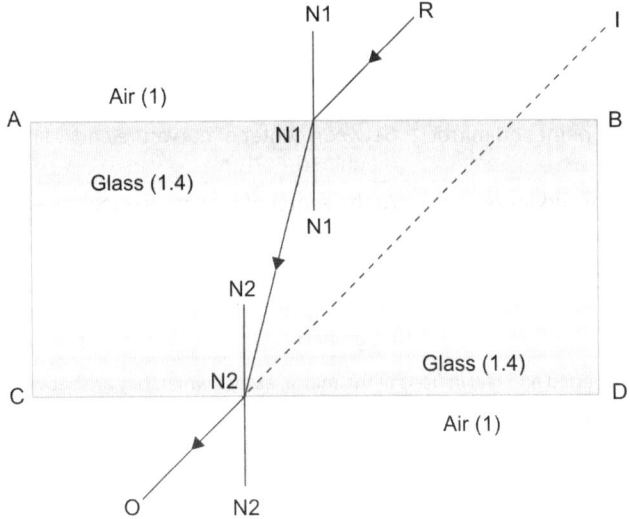

Fig. 3.5: Refraction through a plane glass slab.

Note: N1, N1, and N1 are normal on surfaces A and B between air (lighter) and glass (denser); N2, N2, and N2 are normal on the surfaces C and D between glass (denser) and air (lighter); R, N1, is the ray of incidence; N1, N2, is the ray as it travels through the glass; and N2, O, is the refracted ray; N1, N1, and N2 are the angles of refraction on surfaces A and B; angles O, N2, and N2 are the angles of refraction between glass (denser) and air (lighter); O, N2, when traced, becomes parallel to the line of incidence N1, R.

Prism

A prism is a triangular optical device that is bound by two inclined surfaces that meet at an apex. The surface on the third side, i.e., opposite the apex, is the base of the prism **(Fig. 3.6)**.

When a ray of light strikes any of the inclined surfaces of the prism, it is refracted twice, i.e., when it enters from the air to the glass and again when it leaves the glass to enter the air **(Fig. 3.7)**. **Figure 3.5** shows the behavior of rays in a prism.

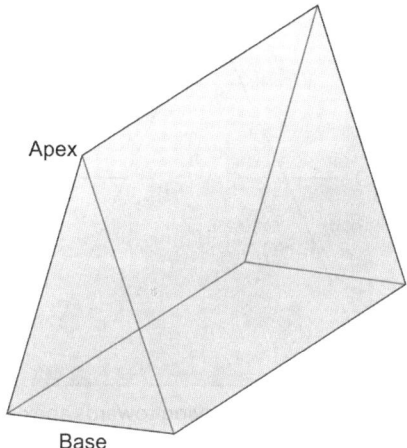

Fig. 3.6: Three-dimensional figure of a large glass prism.

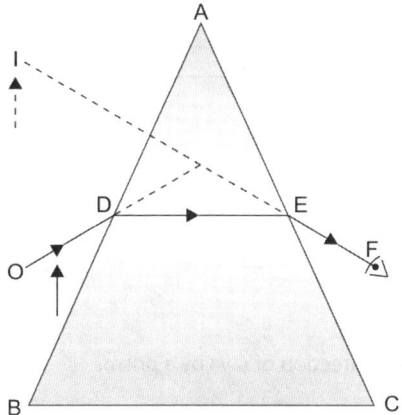

Fig. 3.7: Refraction through a prism.
(ABC = Glass prism; BC = Base; A=Apex; BAC= Angle of prism; O = Object;
DE = Refracted ray parallel to the base; I = Image of the object. Seen by F the observer)

The object O seems to be at position I when seen through the prism. The deviation depends on the refractive index of the prism and the refracting angle. The image moves only towards the apex and not otherwise **(Fig. 3.8)**.

The rays of light can be adjusted by changing the direction of the ray in relation to the prism. A ray can be rotated by 90° or may be reversed, as seen in **Figure 3.9**.

If two prisms of the same power and refractive index are put base to base, they will act as a slap and behave as such, i.e., the ray of incidence and refracted ray will be parallel to each other **(Fig. 3.10)**.

Identification of the prism: Identifying a large prism is not difficult; its shape and size are sufficient for its identification. Difficulty arises in identifying small prisms; it is more difficult to find out the presence of a prism incorporated in a spectacle glass because there are rarely more than six prism diopters. The prisms are made of glass or plastic. To find out the presence and power of a prism in a spectacle glass, hold the glass near the eye and look at a vertical line. If the two ends of the line outside the lens and the line inside are continuous, there is no prism in the glass. If the line inside the lens shifts towards one side, the lens under examination has a

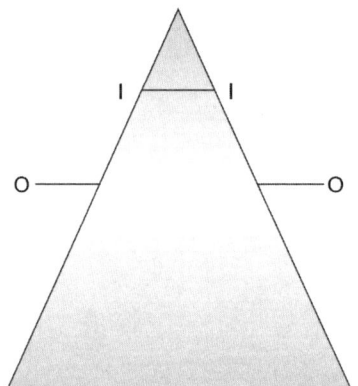

Fig. 3.8: Image moving towards apex.

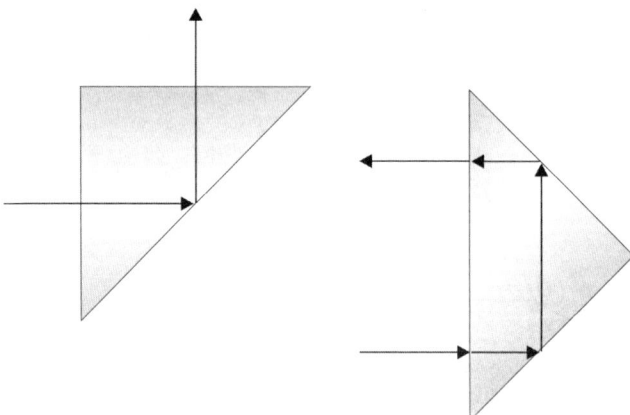

Fig. 3.9: Change of direction of rays by a prism.

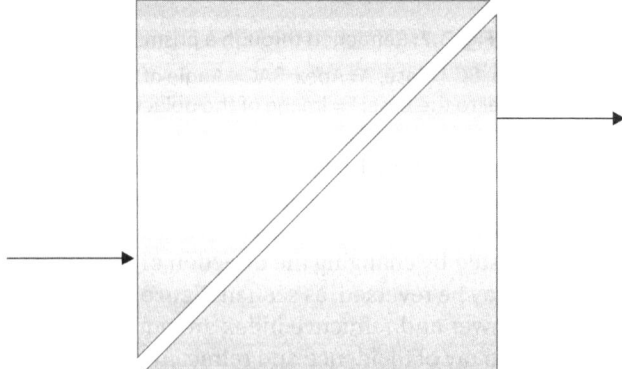

Fig. 3.10: Parallel rays.

prism **(Fig. 3.11)**. By flipping the lens, the line inside the lens will move towards the other side. The appropriate prism that will join the three lines will be the power of the prism.

The distance between the lines LL and L2L2/L3L3 denotes the power of the prism, which is measured by putting an appropriate prism with a base against the apex to align the lines L2L2/L3L3 with the line L1L1. The power of a prism is expressed in prism diopter PD according to the position of its base; for example, a prism of 4 PD will be prescribed as 4 PD base out or base in.

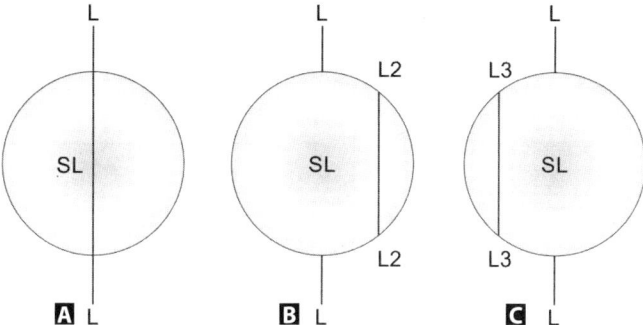

Figs. 3.11A to C: Identification of the prism in spectacle glass: (A) When the line LL is continuous across the spectacle lens SL, there is no prism in the spectacle lens; (B) When there is a prism in the spectacle lens, the line LL is shifted to position L2L2; (C) By flipping the spectacle lens SL, the line LL shifts to L3L3 by the same distance as in Figure B.

Uses of the prism: Prisms are used less commonly than spherical or cylindrical lenses. They may be used alone or incorporated into the spectacle lens to correct diplopia with an appropriate base. They are more frequently used to measure the angle of squint in the form of a prism bar. Prisms do not improve vision; they neither change the power of the lens nor the axis of the cylinder.

The prisms have replaced plane mirrors to reflect the rays in a variety of ophthalmic instruments.

Lenses

Lenses are transparent optical devices bound by two surfaces, one of which is a curved surface that could be spherical or cylindrical **(Fig. 3.12)**. There are three types of lenses: spherical **(Figs. 3.13 and 3.14)**, cylindrical, both of which may be concave or convex, and sphero-cylinder, which is a combination of both sphere and cylinder. According to the shape of the lens, lenses are called biconvex, planoconvex, or concavo-convex . Biconcave, plano concave, and convex concave. The convex lenses are thin on the periphery, and the concave lenses are thick at the periphery.

The convex lenses are called by various names, i.e., plus lenses, converging lenses, and positive lenses. They are thick in the center and thin on the periphery. The concave lenses are known

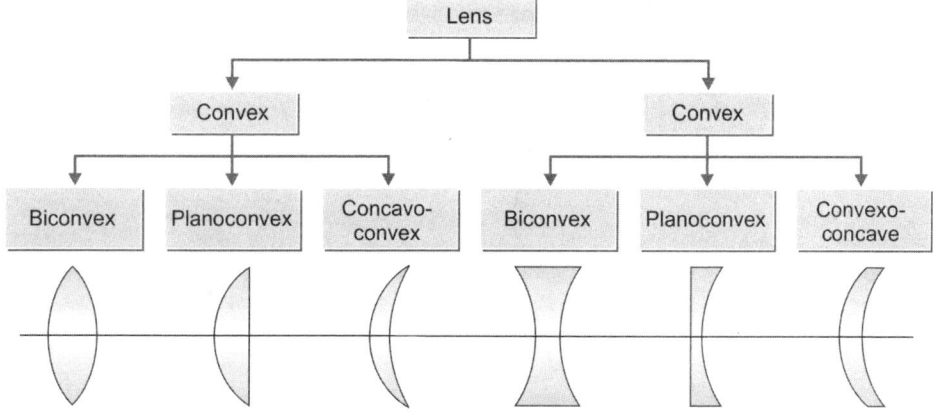

Fig. 3.12: Various shapes of lenses.

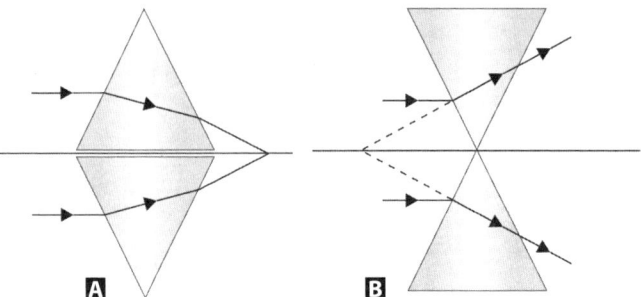

Figs. 3.13A and B: Basis of construction of spherical lenses.

1. Two prisms of the same power, put base to base, act as convex lenses;
2. Two prisms of the same power, put apex to apex, act as concave lenses.

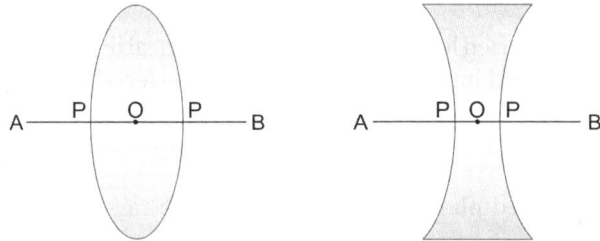

Fig. 3.14: Various parts of spherical lenses.

AB is the principal axis of a spherical lens. P is the pole of the spherical lens; It is the highest point in a convex lens and the lowest in a concave lens.

as minus lenses, diverging lenses, or minifying lenses. The convex lenses produce real inverted images, except when the object is very near the lens. The image moves against the movement of the lens **(Fig. 3.15)**.

The concave lenses produce a virtual, erect, minified image that moves with the movement of the lens to identify the lens **(Fig. 3.16)**.

The lens should be held between the index finger and thumb in front of the eye. If the object seems magnified, it is convex; if it is minified, it is concave. In the case of a lens without power

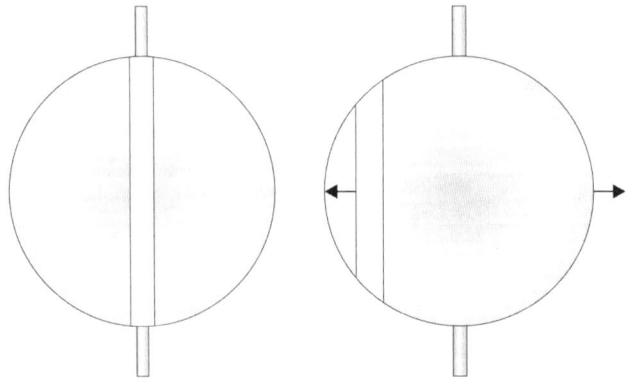

Fig. 3.15: Movement of the image in a convex sphere.

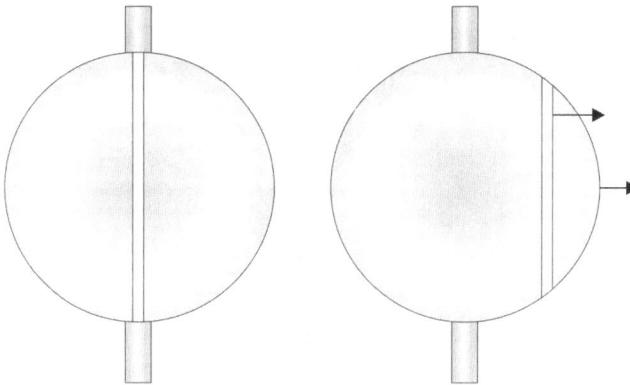

Fig. 3.16: Movement of the image in a concave sphere.

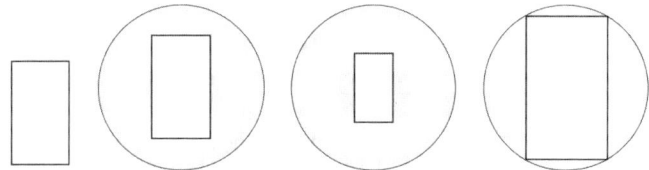

Fig. 3.17: Change in size of the same object O when seen through a plane glass A, a concave lens B, and a convex lens C.

(plane), there will be no change in the size of the object **(Fig. 3.17)**; in none of the cases, there will be a change in the shape of the object.

A change in object denotes the presence of a cylinder in the lens. The next step is to move the lens held between the thumb and index finger from side to side. If the image does not move, it is plain glass. If the image moves with the movement of the lens, it is concave. If the image moves against it is convex, difference in movement in the image in two axes denotes the presence of a cylinder.

Type, Power, and Presence of the Cylinder can be found by Two Methods

1. By putting glasses of the opposite sign against the lens being examined and looking for movement of the object, the process is continued until the image stops moving in all directions.
2. A **lensometer** is a handy tabletop telescope that looks more or less like an uniocular clinical microscope. It is used to find out the type, both spherical and cylindrical power, power of the cylinder and its axis, optical center of the glass, addition for near correction, presence of a prism, and its orientation **(Fig. 3.18)**. Modern digitalized lensometers give a printout as well.

The strength of a lens is the measurement of its convergence or divergence power, measured in diopters.

A diopter is a unit to measure the convergence or divergence of a lens; it is the reciprocal of the focal length in meters. Powerful lenses have a shorter focal length, and weaker lenses have a longer focal length. The diopter is denoted by the latter D. A spherical lens is written as D sphere (D Sph) and a cylinder as D Cyl with its axis.

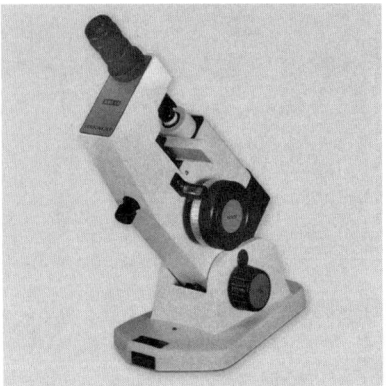

Fig. 3.18: Lensometer.
(*Courtesy:* Appasamy Associates)

The following chart shows the relationship between focal length and its power:

Diopter	Focal length
¼ D	4 m = 400 cm
½ D	2 m = 200 cm
1 D	1 m = 100 cm
2 D	½ m = 50 cm
4 D	¼ m = 25 cm
10 D	1/10 m =10 cm

The position and size of the image depend on the distance of the object from the lens and its converging or diverging power.

Points to Remember during the Formation of an Image by a Convex Lens

- If the distance of the object is greater than the focal length, the image will be formed on the other side, it will be real and inverted.
- If the distance between the objects is less than the focal length, the image will be virtual, erect, magnified, and formed on the same side of the object. This principle is used in a simple magnified corneal loupe*.
- If the object is at the focus, the image will be formed at infinity and magnified.
- If the object is at infinity, the image will be formed at focus. It will be real and pinpoint.

*Corneal Loupe

The corneal loupe can be uniocular or binocular (**Fig. 3.19**).

The image formed by a concave lens is always virtual, erect, and smaller than the object on the side of the object between the focus and the lens, irrespective of the distance of the object from the lens.

In contrast to the above, image formations by concave lenses are simple which is always erect virtual, smaller than the object, on the side of the object, between the focus and the lens, its character is not influenced by the distance between the object and the lens.

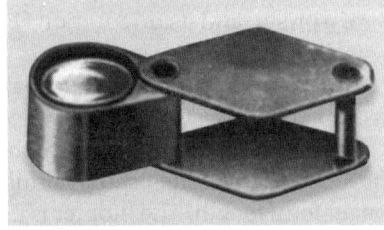

Fig. 3.19: Uniocular corneal loupe.

The magnification of uniocular loupe is much more than binocular infact it is 10 times. The magnification of a binocular loupe is only 1.5 times. The use of a uniocular loupe requires more practice. Otherwise, the corneal loupe is a versatile, simple, and handy gadget. The device consists of two plano-convex lenses of +20 D that make the power +40 D. The lenses are encased in a sturdy body **(Fig. 3.20)**.

The lenses are placed in such a way that the plane surfaces are parallel and face each other. There is a small gap between the two. The focal length of the corneal loupe is 2.5, with a magnification of 10 X. The object should be within the focal length of the loupe. The image formed by the loupe is erect, virtual magnified on the same side of the object. Image formation in a uniocular corneal loupe **(Fig. 3.21)**.

Binocular Corneal Loupe

A binocular loupe consists of two +6 D spheres mounted in a frame, i.e., hinged to a headband, so as to adjust the distance between the binoculars and the observer's eye. The distance between the binoculars and the observer's eye can be adjusted. Generally, two prisms of a four-prism diopter with a base are added to the spherical lenses to relax the convergence of the observer. The magnification of the binocular loupe is only 1.5 X. The binocular loupe has a longer working distance. The advantages of a binocular loupe are: Good stereopsis is a larger field with both hands of the observer that facilitates manipulation of the eyes **(Fig. 3.22)**.

The above have been replaced by spectacle-mounted binocular magnifiers and corneal telescopes, popularly known as operating telescopes **(Fig. 3.23)**.

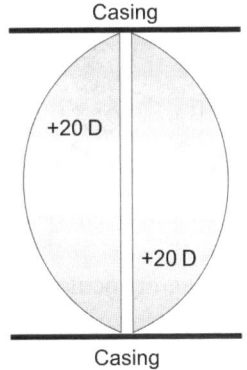

Fig. 3.20: Construction of a uniocular corneal loupe.

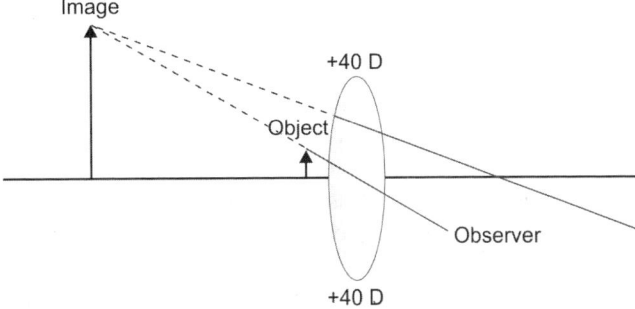

Fig. 3.21: Optics of a uniocular corneal loupe.

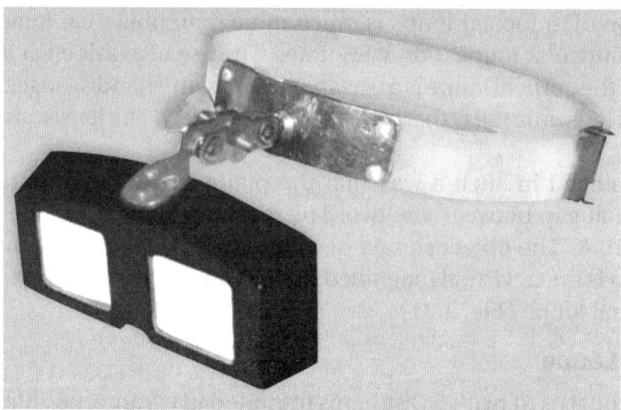

Fig. 3.22: Binocular corneal loupe (Binomag).

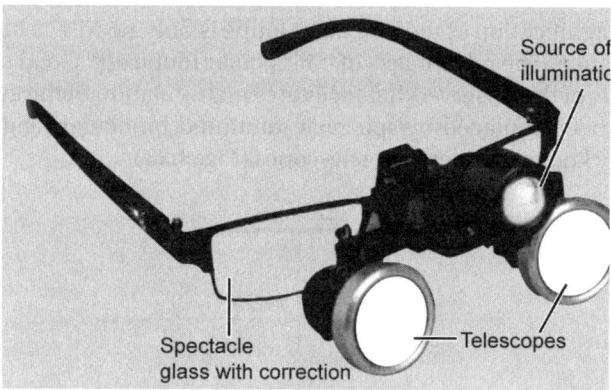

Fig. 3.23: Operating telescope.

The other two instruments used to magnify ocular structures are slit lamps and operating microscopes.

Power of the Combination of Two Lenses

The power of the two lenses will be additive if they are very close to each other and the power of the lens is small. The centers of the lenses are in the same line. The examples are shown in **Figure 3.24**.

Cylindrical Lenses

The cylindrical lenses are part of a cylinder; they can be convex or concave. The convex effect is from the outer surface, while the concave effect is from the inner surface **(Fig. 3.25)**.

The cylindrical lens has no power along its axis. The power is at right angles to the axis. The rays passing through a cylinder followed the rules of refraction similar to those of spherical lenses. A single cylinder forms a liner image in contrast to a spherical lens that forms a pinpoint image. When the cylinder is added to the sphere, the shape of the image is a combination of the two. When a cylindrical lens is added to a sphere, the combination is called a sphero-cylinder. The cylindrical power is added to the spherical power algebraically at right angles to the axis of the cylinder.

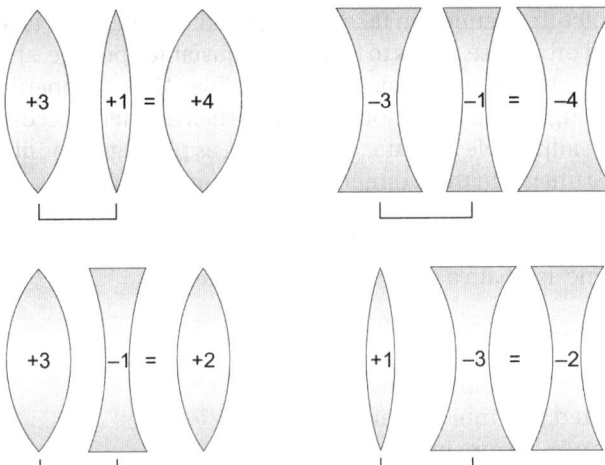

Fig. 3.24: Power of two lenses combined.

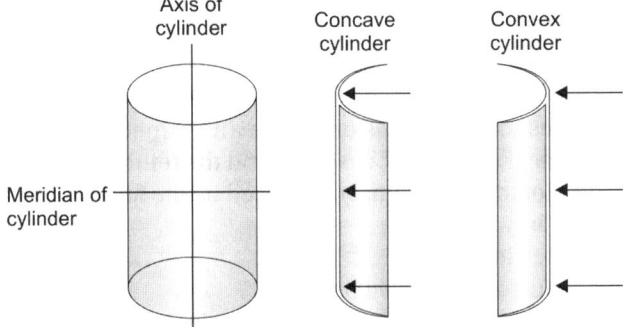

Fig. 3.25: Principle of cylindrical lenses.

CLINICAL OPTICS

The optics of a normal eye can be compared to those of a pinhole camera (**Fig. 3.26**).

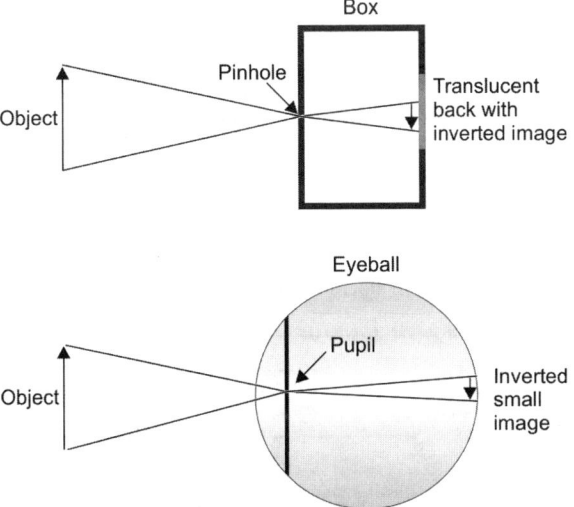

Fig. 3.26: Comparison of a pinhole camera with an eye.

It is obvious that pictures cannot be taken by a pinhole camera. To take a photograph, the camera requires a light proof case, a lens to focus, an adjustable aperture, and photographic film. The film needs to be treated photochemically to be visible. All the properties are present in the eye, which has a focusing device in the form of the cornea and lens, accommodation to adjust the focus, a pupil as an adjustable aperture, and a retina as photographic film that, when treated neurologically, creates images in three dimensions and natural color.

The eye at rest is supposed to have a single convex lens of +60 D with a focal length of 24.00 mm. The power has two components, i.e., the cornea with +43 D and the lens with +17 D. Both are situated on the same axis with a common optical center.

The Simplified System

- One principal plane is 2.00 mm behind the cornea.
- A nodal point situated 5.00 mm behind the plane
- Anterior focal point: 15.00 mm in front of the cornea
- Posterior focal point at 24.00 mm behind the cornea
- The total refractive power is +60 D = 43 D + 17 D.

Such a condition is hypothetical; deviation from such a position is more common, and an eye without an abnormality in the focusing system is called ametropia. In contrast to this, the eye with normal focus is called emmetropic, which is defined as a condition where parallel rays are brought to focus on the photosensitive layer of the retina **(Flowchart 3.1)**. In simple terms, an ametropic patient will require glasses for distant vision, while an emmetrope will not require glasses. Converging rays from the near point are focused behind the retina without accommodation.

The abnormal position of the retinal image is caused by the following factors, which may act alone or in combination. **They are:**

- **Abnormal length of the globe**
  - Length of the globe in an adult is 24.00 mm.
  - A change of 1.00 mm either way produces ametropia.
  - 1.00 mm of increase will produce myopia of 3 diopters.
  - 1.00 mm decrease will produce hypermetropia of 3 diopters.
- **Abnormal corneal curvature**
  - Curvature of a normal cornea is 8.00 mm.
  - If there is a change in corneal curvature, the image will not be formed on the retina.
  - 1.00 mm reduction in the curvature of the cornea will result in six diopters of hypermetropia.
  - 1.00 mm increment in the curvature of the cornea will result in six diopters of myopia.
  - Uneven curvature of the cornea will result in astigmatism.

Flowchart 3.1: Types of errors of refraction.

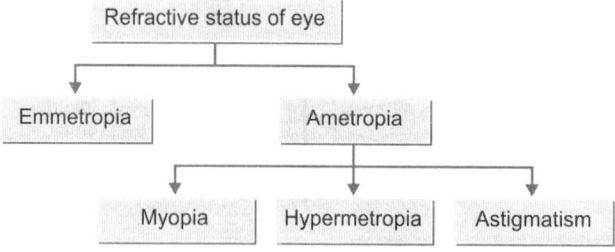

- ❖ **Abnormal lenticular curvature**
  - ◆ An increase in lenticular curvature causes myopia.
  - ◆ A decrease in lenticular curvature causes hypermetropia.
  - ◆ Irregular lenticular curvature causes astigmatism.
- ❖ **Refractive index of ocular media:** Increased refractive index causes myopia, while a decreased refractive index causes hypermetropia. The change in refractive index is more profound in lenses.

Abnormal Refraction

It has been noted that when parallel rays are focused on the retina with accommodation at rest, the condition is physiological and called emmetropia. In contrast to this, when parallel rays are not focused on the retina with accommodation at rest, it is called ametropia, which can be myopia, hypermetropia, or astigmatism.

Myopia

Myopia is defined as the refractive status where parallel rays are focused in front of the retina with accommodation at rest. Accommodation worsens myopia.

Myopia is the most common type of error of refraction in both sexes and is more frequent in children, with a tendency to increase in the first few years after onset. Thereafter, it stops increasing, easily corrected by glasses. A high degree of myopia has some complications that do not allow vision to reach a normal level. Myopia has a strong genetic link. However, it is possible to have myopia without a family history. Generally, myopia involves both eyes with similar power; however, cases of unilateral myopia are also reported. The increase in power in the eyes is generally equal; children developing myopia between 5 and 6 years have more chances of an increase in refractive error. The progress is gradual; it may be minus 1-3 per year. The increase in power stabilized after 20 years. Wearing glasses has no influence on the progression of myopia.

Uniocular myopia is often missed because the child may not be aware of it or consider it to be normally present in all children. The adult, too, may not complain of diminished vision even in presbyopia, as he uses the myopic eyes for near. In the case of uniocular myopia, an adult uses his myopic eye for near vision and his emmetropic or hypermetropic eye for distance vision. A child with uniocular myopia may present with a squint.

Clinical Types of Myopia

1. **Congenital myopia:** The child may be born with myopia, which is not detected at birth; it becomes obvious by 2-3 years when the parent realizes that the child has grossly diminished distant vision but very good near vision. The condition is mostly binocular; the power ranges between minus 8 and 10 D, almost equally in both eyes. The power does not increase with age, as seen in other childhood myopias. Children with congenital myopia may not develop nystagmus or squint but are prone to other complications of high myopia, mainly retinal detachment. This child should be periodically examined by indirect ophthalmoscope to detect peripheral degeneration; if found, the degeneration should be treated as per practice. These children are prone to developing lenticular opacity at an early age, worsening existing myopia.
2. **Simple myopia:** This is the most common myopia seen in children between 5-10 years. It is bilateral and begins with a low error, which is invariably spherical and equal in both eyes. The increment may be 0.5-1.0 D yearly; children with a higher rate of increment are likely to pass into the stage of progressive and degenerative myopia. The main complaint

is diminished distant vision; the child may not complain of it. The two common modes of presentation are the parents complain that the child watches the TV from very close proximity and resents being asked to watch from a distance like other children. The child keeps the book very close to his face. The second group comprises children who have difficulty seeing the words written on the board. Otherwise, the teacher may point out the defect to the parents and advise an ophthalmic checkup. The condition is easily corrected with glasses. That may not exceed >5–6 D by 12 years of age, after which the progression stops. The complications are few and mild; the condition is called school myopia. In contrast to another less frequent condition commonly known as college myopia, which too is bilateral and almost equal in both eyes and frequently associated with astigmatism, the power is rarely >1.00–1.5 D, which may progress to minus 2-3 in the next few years and remains stable. It is also corrected satisfactorily by glasses.

3. **Progressive myopia:** Progressive myopia is that type of myopia where the increment of power is fast, i.e., minus 3–10 D within 3–4 years. The vision can be improved to 6/6 with glasses; they do better with contact lenses, but they are prone to developing peripheral retinal degeneration and juvenile glaucoma. The children should be frequently checked for increased power.
4. **Degenerative (pathological) myopia:** Degenerative myopia, as the name suggests, is always associated with myopic degeneration, mostly in the posterior pole. The power of degenerative myopia is generally high. That cannot be corrected with glasses. Sometimes, a lower degree of myopia may also be associated with myopic degeneration of the posterior pole.

The degree of myopia may not have any visible signs except that the child squeezes the lids to produce the pinhole effect to increase vision, which is found to be diminished; it may be a loss of 2–3 lines on the vision chart. That improves to 6/6 by pinhole. Good near vision or diminished vision; on examination, there may be phoria or tropia. With a high degree of myopia, the eyes look larger than normal. The cornea is larger than in emmetropia. The AC is slightly deep without tremulousness of the iris; the pupil is larger but reacts briskly. The keratomitric readings are within normal limits, and the fundus does not show any pathology, which is a prominent feature in progressive and degenerative myopia, both of which are associated with liquefaction of the vitreous.

Treatment

There is no medical treatment for myopia. Improvement of diet, supplementation with vitamins and antioxidants, and eye exercises are not effective in preventing the progression of myopia, the lowering of power, or the removal of glasses. The use of atropine solution in concentrations of 0.01–0.05% has not been found to be effective. The definitive treatment is optical or surgical. The latter is not indicated for all patients. They are contraindicated for children under 20 years of age. The optical treatment consists of spectacles and contact lenses. The contact lenses could be any of the following: hard, semisoft, or soft. The most popular surgeries undergone by suitable patients are on the cornea, in the form of radial keratotomy and LASIK. The latter has mostly replaced the former in cases of high myopia where clear lens extraction or phakic IOLs are employed.

The spectacles are the best choice, especially for children. Who cannot manage contact lenses, and operations on the cornea and lens are contraindicated. The spectacles are the cheapest and easiest to handle; they should be prescribed underage matched cycloplegia. All children should be refracted under atropine as per practice in the institution. The refraction under complete cycloplegia unmasks the associated astigmatism and pseudomyopia.

Pseudomyopia

Children presenting with pseudomyopia really do not suffer from myopia; they are hypermetropic children who have been prescribed myopic glasses instead of hypermetropic with the wrong presumption that all children with diminished distant vision are myopic. These children, when prescribed minus glasses, initially improve only to deteriorate soon. The unsuspecting optician increases the power, worsening it more. These children should be asked not to use glasses for a few days and undergo refraction under cycloplegia, which reveals hidden hypermetropia. The child should be prescribed glasses after the effect of atropine has passed off, that may take as much as 10–15 days.

Hypermetropia

Hypermetropia is an error in refraction where parallel rays are brought to focus behind the photosensitive layer of the retina. The rays arising from the near point are still far away from the retina when accommodation is at rest. With accommodation, the rays that focus behind the retina can be brought on or near the retina.

Children are born with +2 to +3 D hypermetropia due to short axial length. As the child grows, the axial length increases; by 5 years, the child's eyes reach adult size with a 24.00 mm axial length, neutralizing the existing hypermetropia. As the size of the eye stabilizes, the eye remains emmetropic with normal near vision. If the axial length fails to increase, the eye remains hypermetropic by 2–3 diopters; if the eye is congenitally short, the hypermetropia is greater without increasing. If the increment in length overshoots the normal range, it becomes myopic. A person who has been emmetropic throughout his life may become hypermetropic after 30 years due to flattening of the cornea, which is corrected by suitable glasses. These people, left uncorrected, develop near-vision defects earlier than usual, at the age of 40. Hypermetropia is generally genetic; incidence of hypermetropia is less common than myopia. It is seen in both sexes worldwide, and bilateral or unilateral hypermetropia is less common. The power is generally equal in both eyes. If the power difference between the two eyes is considerably high, the eye with higher power is likely to develop esotropia and may be amblyopic. The hypermetropia may be corrected fully or partly by accommodation. Hypermetropia can be an axial curvature or index.

Axial Hypermetropia

This is the most common type of hypermetropia due to the short axial length generally associated with some degree of astigmatism.

Curvature Hypermetropia

One millimeter flattening of the cornea results in hypermetropia of +6 D. Thus, small eyes with small corneas generally suffer from curvature hypermetropia. A relatively flat lens induces curvature hypermetropia, which is common after 50 years of age.

A lens displaced backward causes hypermetropia. A minus glass placed in front of the emmetropic eye artificially causes hypermetropia. Similarly, a plus lens in front of an emmetropic eye produces myopia.

Index Hypermetropia

The refractive index of a clear lens is 1.34. If this is reduced, hypermetropia sets in. The most common example is the reduction of sugar in the blood generally seen following the start of antidiabetic drugs. A less common cause is systemic dehydration.

Accommodation in Hypermetropia (Flowchart 3.2)

When the power of a lens increases, its focal length decreases. This happens when the eye accommodates. The power of the lens at rest is +17 D with a focal length of 24.00 mm; when the eye is accommodated, it becomes about +20 D to +24 D. This forms the image in front of the retina. A normal ciliary body has some amount of natural accommodation that corrects +0.5 D to +1.0 D of hypermetropia. This is called latent hypermetropia, and the remaining part is called manifest hypermetropia. The manifest hypermetropia is divided into two parts, i.e., facultative and absolute hypermetropia. All the hypermetropias put together make up the total hypermetropia.

The other clinical classification of hypermetropia is as follows:
- **Low hypermetropia:** Refractive error is <+2.00 diopters (D).
- **Moderate hypermetropia:** The refractive error is between +2.00 D and +5.00 D.
- **High hypermetropia:** The refractive error is beyond +5.00 D.
- It is unusual to have hypermetropia higher than +6.00 D in the phakic eye, in contrast to myopia, where it may be as high as minus 20 D.

Symptoms of Hypermetropia
- Asymptomatic low-to moderate-level hypermetropia may not complain of diminished distant and near vision. In contrast to myopia, where myopia as low as minus 1.00 D will have diminished distant vision.
- Diminished near vision under 40 years. The patients come with complains of diminished near vision with fairly good distant vision. On cycloplegic refraction, it is found that he has facultative hypermetropia. Most of his accommodation is used to keep the distant vision at 6/6, leaving no accommodation for the near. His near vision will be corrected by correcting his distant vision with a plus lens.
- **Diminished distant vision:** This happens in absolute hypermetropia that is not corrected by accommodation.
- **Sudden blurring of distant vision:** This happens in children who use excessive accommodation for distant vision, causing pseudomyopia.
- **Asthenopia:** Constant use of accommodation to get good accommodation results in non-visual symptoms of watering, intolerance to light, headaches, and tiredness of the eye, for which the patient keeps rubbing the eyes. Introducing infection, leading to a low degree of conjunctivitis and recurrent stye, chalazion, and chronic blepharitis, making it mandatory

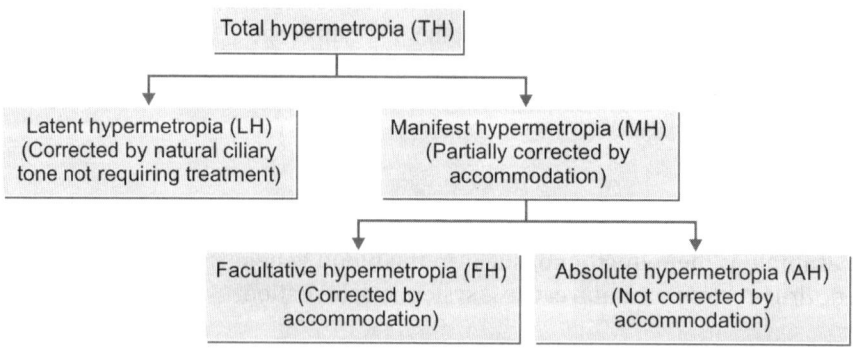

Flowchart 3.2: Various types of hypermetropia.

to refract all eyes under cycloplegia with the above symptoms. Even when distant vision is normal.
- **Convergent squint:** This is common in children who are brought with convergent squint and turn out to have hypermetropia under cycloplegia. A converging squint is more common in the eye with higher power.
- **Amblyopia:** This happens more in the eye with higher power in bilateral hypermetropia.

Treatment

Like myopia, there is no medical treatment for hypermetropia. The power of the plus lens may be reduced if the patient develops central nuclear sclerosis or has uncontrolled diabetes. The only treatment is optical, either by plus lens in spectacles or contact lenses. Surgery in hypermetropia is not as rewarding as in myopia **(Fig. 3.27)**.

All eyes should be refracted underage-matched cycloplegia. Only mydriatics have no role under 10 years. However, it may be used after 30 years.

Pathological Hypermetropia

This happens when parallel rays are focused 24.00 mm behind the cornea, but the retina has moved forward, as seen in central serous retinopathy, shallow retinal detachment at the posterior pole. The other common cause is reduction of refractive power of the eye due to the removal of lens from the pupillary area, the condition is called aphakia. Other causes of pathological hypermetropia are too short axial length as seen in microphthalmos and nanophthalmos*, soft eye, tumor pushing the sclera forward.

Nanophthalmos*

Nanophthalmos is a congenital anomaly of the globe where only defect is in its dimension without any other ocular or systemic disease. It is a rare disease.

A more common cause of pathological hypermetropia is aphakia.

Aphakia

Aphakia is the commonest cause of index hypermetropia that is absolute in nature. It is defined as the total or partial absence of the lens from the pupillary area, with the former being more common. The commonest cause of aphakia is the surgical removal of the lens, either completely or partially. The complete removal is called intracapsular lens extraction, while incomplete removal is called extracapsular lens extraction, i.e., performed by doing an anterior capsulotomy, removing the nucleus, and washing out as much cortex as possible, Leaving the

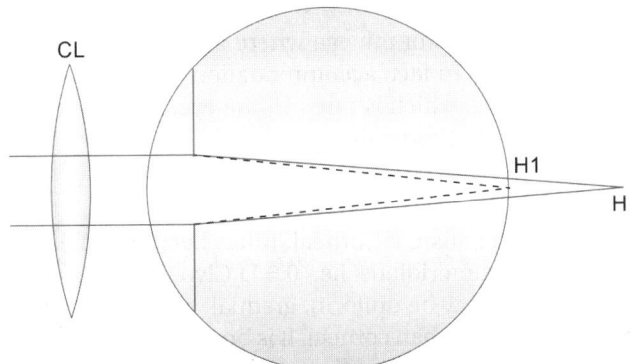

Fig. 3.27: Hypermetropia corrected by a convex lens.
(E = Hypermetropic eyeball; H = Hypermetropic image; H1 = is image brought on retina by convex lens; C = Convex lens)

posterior capsule intact, Intracapsular lens extraction has been given up in favor of intraocular lens (IOL) implants. An eye with an IOL is called pseudophakia. A well-performed IOL makes the eye almost emmetropic, unlike intracapsular and extracapsular lens extractions that require high-plus lenses in the anterior focal plane of a spectacle. The correction requires additional plus lenses, either in a separate glass or as a bifocal. Aphakia causes a reduction of the total dioptric condition from +60 D to +43 D. Focusing parallel rays 31.00 mm from the cornea, the image thus formed cannot be brought to focus due to the total absence of the lens. Thus, an uncorrected aphakic eye has neither distant nor near vision.

Signs of Aphakia

- Diminished distant and near vision.
- Scar of surgery (whenever applicable)
- Deep anterior chamber.
- Tremulousness of the iris
- Normal pupillary reaction.
- Visible iridectomy
- Absence of the third and fourth Purkinje images
- Jet-black pupil in the case of intracapsular lens extraction
- After cataracts following extracapsular lens extraction.

Management

Postoperative aphakia is corrected by +10 D to +11 D Sph with +1 D to +2 D Clyn. To this is added +2.5 D to +3 D Sph for near-correction.

Nonsurgical aphakia has all the signs of surgical aphakia without a scar and is corrected by a spherical lens with the usual near correction.

The power of aphakic correction depends on the pre-existing error of refraction. A myopic eye will require <+10 D, and a hypermetropic eye will require >+10 D.

A +10 D sphere in a spectacle is as effective as a +17 D sphere inside the eye.

The disadvantage of spectacle correction is the enlargement of the image by one-third. If the other eye is emmetropic or has a low error of refraction, this causes troublesome diplopia.

These disadvantages are partly overcome by contact lenses and fully abolished by IOLs. The aphakic eye corrected by contact lenses will still require near correction in the form of spectacles. An eye with a well-calculated and properly placed IOL will generally not require near correction. **Figure 3.28** show various types of correction for aphakia.

Astigmatism

Astigmatism is the refractive status of the eye where all the parallel rays are not focused in one plane with accommodation. In fact, accommodation worsens astigmatism. Eyes without astigmatism are called stigmatic, which is rare. All the eyes are astigmatic of low degree, not causing any symptoms or requiring correction.

Etiology

The commonest cause of astigmatism is corneal. It has been noted early that the cornea has different curvatures in different meridians, i.e., 0.5 D Clyn, which is within the physiological limit. The change in curvature may be uniform, gradual, smooth. The next cause is lenticular astigmatism, which is less common than corneal. It is brought about by tilting and displacement of the lens; a still rare cause is retinal astigmatism.

Various types of astigmatism depend on the smoothness of the corneal curvature.

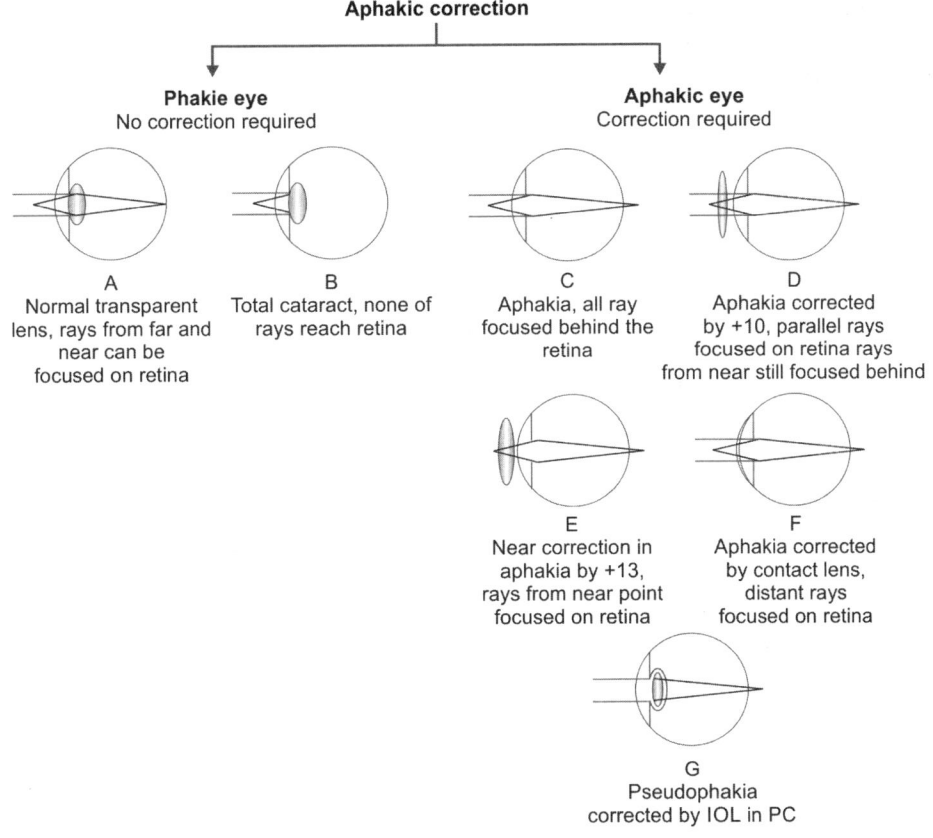

Fig. 3.28: Optics of aphakia and pseudophakia and their optical correction.

They are:
- **Regular astigmatism:** In this case, both meridians are at 90° to each other with the same power all along the axis. Regular astigmatism is divided into the following groups, depending on the curvature of the vertical meridian:
  i. *Astigmatism with the rule:* This is corrected either by a concave cylinder at 180° or a convex cylinder at 90°. The meridian may be aligned slightly on either side by 20°, but the angle between the two remains 90°.
  ii. *Astigmatism against the rule:* This is corrected by a convex cylinder at 180° or a concave cylinder at 90° to each other. There may be a slight variation in the axis on each side of the principal axis.
  iii. *Oblique astigmatism:* Here the principal axes are at right angles to each other. The axes are at 45° or 135°.
  iv. *Bi-oblique astigmatism:* In this case, the angles between the two axes are no more at right angles but have equal power all through the axis.
- **Irregular astigmatism:** Here, the two meridians are neither at right angles to each other, nor is the power the same all along a meridian.
- According to the position of the image in relation to the retina, the astigmatism can be classified as follows:
  1. Simple
     - Myopic
     - Hypermetropic

2. Compound
   - Myopic
   - Hypermetropic
3. Mixed

Various types of astigmatism is shown in **Flowchart 3.3**.

Simple Astigmatism

Is that astigmatism with one meridian emmetropic and the other focusing either in front or behind the retina. The first is simple myopic astigmatism, which is corrected by a single minus cylinder. The other is simple hypermetropic astigmatism corrected by a single hypermetropic cylinder; none of the conditions require spherical addition.

Compound Astigmatism

Compound astigmatism is astigmatism in which an image is not formed on the retina in any meridian, i.e., both meridians are ametropic. If both meridians are focused in front of the retina, the condition is called compound myopic astigmatism. In contrast to this, if both meridians are focused behind the retina, the condition is called compound hypermetropic astigmatism. Both conditions require a sphere of the same sign at an appropriate angle. The power of the cylinder does not exceed the power of the sphere.

Mixed Astigmatism

Mixed astigmatism is a type of astigmatism where one meridian is myopic and the other is hypermetropic. The condition is corrected by spheres and cylinders of opposite signs. The value

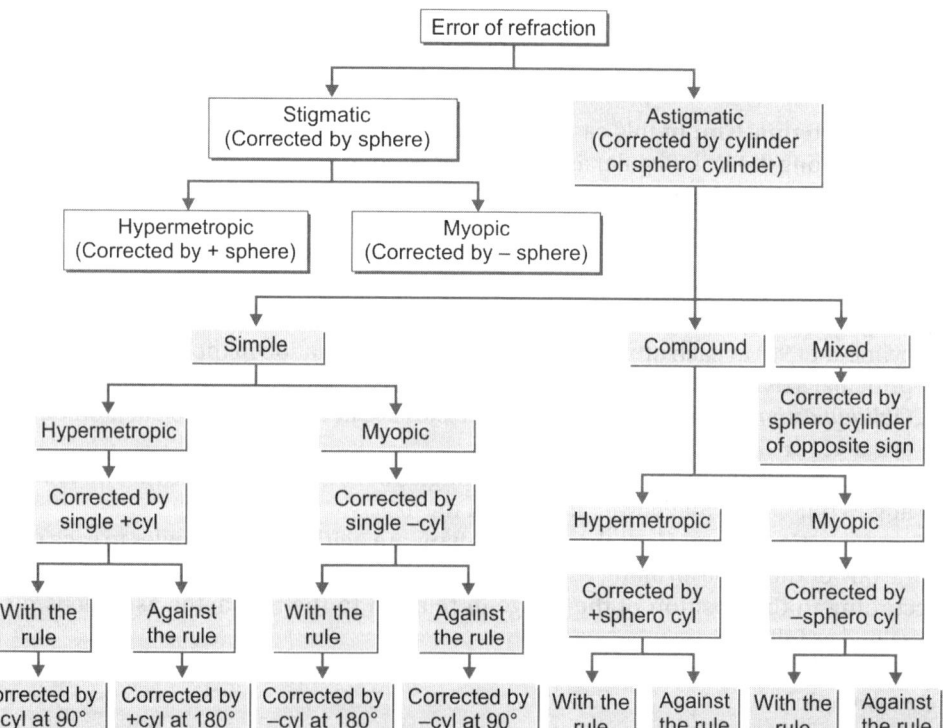

Flowchart 3.3: Various types of astigmatism.

of the cylinder is always greater than the value of the sphere. For example, an eye with mixed astigmatism will improve following both conditions, that is, plus one sphere with minus two cylinders at 180° will be as effective as minus one sphere with +2 D Clyn at 90°.

Irregular Astigmatism

Irregular astigmatism, where the dioptric value changes not only in two meridians but in the same meridian.

The common causes are corneal opacity, pterygium, keratoconus, and growth at the limbus. Vision cannot be corrected by spectacles. Contact lenses give better results; the best results are seen in keratoplasty.

Symptoms of Astigmatism

Low degree of astigmatism is better tolerated in young persons but may be troublesome in adults. The symptoms may be any of the following or in combination: Diminished distant vision, distorted image, and difficulty in near work because the accommodation required for near work worsens astigmatism; if the patient is under 40 years old (pre-presbyopic) and complains of diminished near vision, he will improve with astigmatic correction without near addition.

Signs

There are no signs that can be co-related to the astigmatism except diminished vision. A patient with high astigmatism may tilt the head to compensate for the astigmatism.

Diagnosis

- Unsatisfactory improvement of vision with pinhole
- Better improvement with a stenopaeic slit in comparison to a pinhole
- Retinoscope under cycloplegia under 40 years of age, retinoscopy is the gold standard in the diagnosis of astigmatism.
- Autorefractometer. This is suitable for nonverbal people who do not communicate in the language of the examiner. It is also handy for mass refraction in large surveys.
- Keratometer for corneal astigmatism
- Computerized keratoscopy

The glasses are prescribed after at least 48 hours of retinoscopy to allow the accommodation to return to its precycloplegic state. The following are the methods to confirm the axis and level of astigmatism:

- Autorefractometry
- Cross-cylinder
- Astigmatic dial
- Astigmatic fan
- Duochrome test
- Friend test

Management

All cases of astigmatism do not require treatment; mild degrees of astigmatism are generally without symptoms, and the condition becomes obvious on retinoscopy. The first line of treatment is spectacle. The axis and degree of astigmatism should always be determined per retinoscopy finding under cycloplegia; the subjective method may be off the mark. The next choice is a contact lens, which corrects only the spherical part of compound astigmatism. The remaining part may be corrected by spectacles. Toric lenses correct both spherical and cylindrical components. Irregular astigmatism is best treated with contact lenses.

Presbyopia

Presbyopia is not an error of refraction; it is a physiological process of diminished near vision seen after 40 years of age, universally and equally among both sexes in emmetropic eyes. It develops early in hypermetropies and is delayed in myopes. It is a wrong assumption that myopes do not develop presbyopia.

A person who could read at 30 cm finds it difficult to read at this distance but can do so either by moving the object away from the eyes or by increasing illumination. Once these fail to achieve a satisfactory result, he seeks an ophthalmic consultation. Those who have to work at a fixed near point, like tailors and goldsmiths, require near correction early. Persons with poor health or on parasympatholytic drugs also require presbyopic correction. The other causes of diminished near vision are uncorrected or undercorrected hypermetropia or overcorrected myopia. Myopes without presbyopic correction can do near work without glasses because their far point falls within their near point. The hypermetropes use most of the accommodation for clear distant vision; hence, they have less accommodation available for near vision. The following conditions are also associated with difficulty in near vision at any age: aphakia, pseudophakia, and internal ophthalmoplegia.

Management

Management of presbyopia involves a simple prescription of age-matched plus lenses over distant correction. Before prescribing a near correction, the following should be noted:

1. **Distant vision:** A patient with presbyopia may resent examination of distant vision, which he considers as unnecessary. Even when vision is 6/6 in both eyes, it is better to exclude facultative hypermetropia by adding plus lenses until the eyes have 6/6 vision. Correction of diminished distant vision should precede presbyopic correction.
2. **Working distance:** The next point is to find out the near working distance of the person and compare physiological distance for age; find out the near point of accommodation and convergence; and exclude opacities in the medial macular lesion, phoria, tropia, amblyopia, and anisometropia.
3. **Exclude anisometropia:** A patient with myopia in one eye and hypermetropia or emmetropia in the other eye may not seek near vision correction as he uses the myopic eye for near vision and the other eye for distant vision.

The near-vision defect is corrected by substituting loss accommodation with various methods. The commonest method consists of near-vision glasses. The power of addition is equal in both eyes, and the near-vision spectacle can be unifocal or multifocal. The latter can be bifocal or trifocal. The bifocals have power added at the lower part of the lens. The trifocals have an intermediate addition in between far and near vision. Besides these lenses, the lenses may be progressive, where power increases from above downward.

Low Vision

Low vision is not a complete loss of vision; it is better to call patients with low vision as partially sighted or partially blind.

It is better to know the definition of blindness as designated by the WHO. It is the total absence of light in both eyes, and visual acuity not exceeding 6/60 in the better eye with the best correction, and a limitation of the field of vision of <20° all-round. As per the guidelines of WHO 1977, low vision falls into the various categories shown in **Table 3.2**.

Characteristics of Low Vision

1. It is not blindness.

Table 3.2: Types of impairment.

Category	Type of impairment	Visual acuity (best corrected)
1.	Low vision	6/18 to 6/60
2.	Low vision	< 6/60 to 3/60
3.	Blindness	< 3/60 to 1/60 or count fingers (CF 3 m – CF 1 m) OR Field of vision between 5° and 10°
4.	Blindness	< CF 1 m to light perception or Field of vision less than 5°
5.	Blindness	No light perception

2. It is bilateral.
3. Color blindness is not a type of low vision.
4. Low vision has some salvageable vision that is not better than 6/18 in a better eye.
5. It can be a central or peripheral loss.
6. It can be stationary or progressive.
7. A color vision defect is not blindness or low vision.
8. All people with low vision do not improve with low-vision aids.

Flowchart 3.4 shows various types of low-vision aids.

Low Vision Aids

Low vision aids (LVA) are devices that help visually handicapped people use their residual vision by making objects bigger, brighter, and blacker with good contrast.

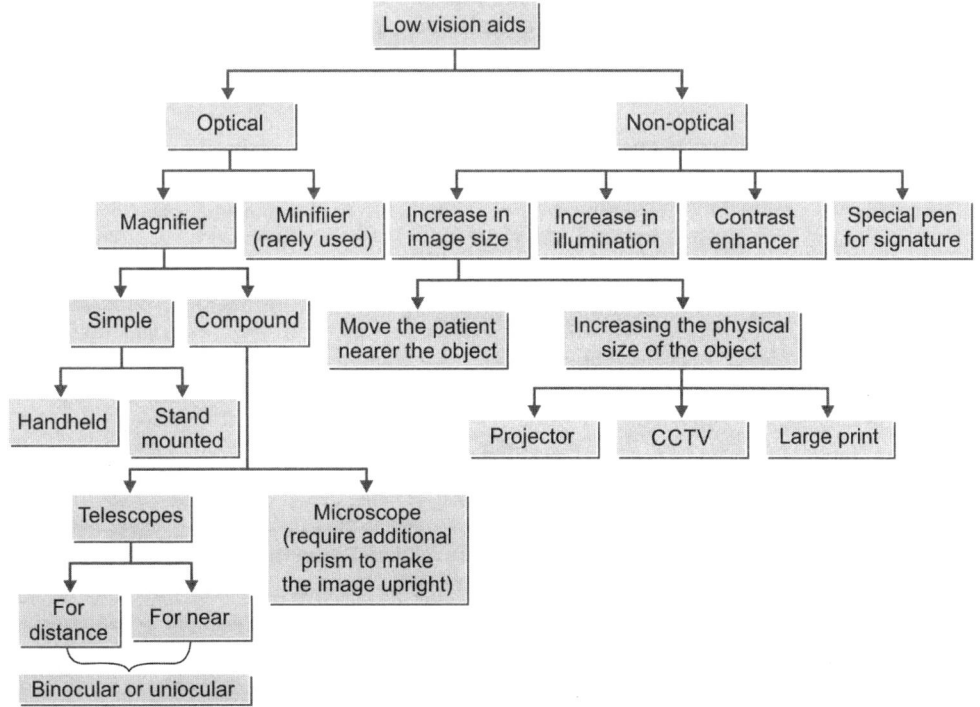

Flowchart 3.4: Classification of low vision aids.

Braille

Knowledge of low-vision aids is incomplete without reference to a Braille book. Braille is a system of raised dots, the same as the morse codes used in the telegraph. They can be in single sheets or in book form, and they are available in various languages. A Braille letter consists of a set of raised dots arranged in two parallel rows, each having three dots. The total number of Braille sets is 26. The following are the English alphabets in Braille **(Fig. 3.29)**.

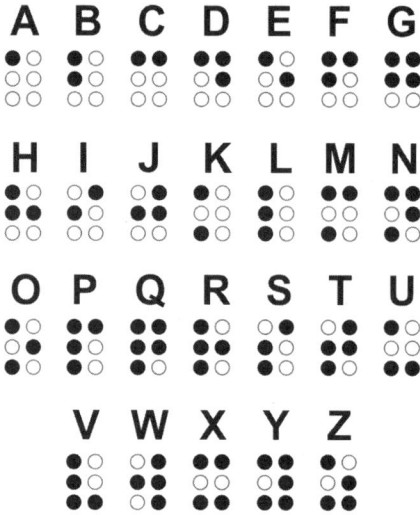

Fig. 3.29: Example of Braille letter in English.

Note: The numbers and geometric figures can also be expressed in Braille.

CHAPTER 4

Symptomatology

Symptoms are the complaints of the person pertaining to the disease or discomfort, like pain, diminished vision, redness, etc. While signs represent the features that the examiner elicits in a person complaining, like diminished vision, pupillary changes, squinting, etc., some of the symptoms are signs as well, and vice versa, like ptosis, lagophthalmos, etc. Many of the symptoms lead directly to a diagnosis, like diminished near vision after 40 years of age as presbyopia. Diminished night vision of long time may lead to the diagnosis of retinitis pigmentosa, while subacute loss of night vision can be easily diagnosed as vitamin A deficiency.

The symptoms in ophthalmology can be divided into two main groups: ocular and nonocular. The ocular symptoms may be visual or nonvisual.

Visual Symptoms

The common visual symptoms are diminished distant vision, diminished near vision, or a combination of the two; night blindness; color blindness; diplopia; colored haloes; diminished field; frequent changes of power; black spots in front of the eye and a curtain in front of the eye. The visual symptoms are binocular more often.

Less common causes are:
- Polyopia (one object looks more than two)
- Metamorphopsia (the shape of the object looks distorted)
- Glare (dislike of light)
- Photophobia (intolerance to light)
- Blepharospasm
- Photopsia (flashes of light)
- Chromatopsia (changes in the color of the object)

A person may have more than one symptoms in both eyes or may have different symptoms in two eyes.

Causes of visual symptoms are:
- Patient requires glasses for distant (error of refraction).
- Patient requires glasses for near (presbyopia).
- Opacities in the media (cataract, corneal opacity)
- Diseases of the inner layers of the eye and optic nerve
- Disorders of the visual path
- Amblyopia

Amblyopia

Amblyopia is a state of diminished, uncorrectable distant vision of long time. The most frequent age to develop amblyopia is 6 months when the macula is developing; it rarely develops after 6 years of age. Once developed, it lasts for the rest of life unless corrected before the age of 8 years. The condition goes undetected unless examined specifically. The condition is generally unilateral, and the loss of vision is rarely more than 2–3 lines. The condition is more common in children with squints. The other causes are unequal power in two eyes and opacities in the media. The causes of amblyopia are congenital and infantile cataracts, ptosis, and corneal opacity, unilateral error of refraction, anisometropia, and squint. The amblyopia in squint persists even after successful surgery if not treated before surgery. The gold standard of treatment of amblyopia is occlusion of the better eye completely or partially. The occlusion should be given by a specially trained person. For the best results, amblyopia should be detected before 6 years of age and continued until vision has improved to a satisfactory level. It is mandatory to remove the causes of amblyopia before initiating occlusion therapy. The conditions are anisometropia, lenticular opacity, and ptosis.

Diminished Distant Vision

Diminished vision may be the only symptom or may be associated with other ocular or nonocular causes. It is generally bilateral but may vary in degree; one eye may be more affected than the other. Unilaterally diminished distant vision is less frequent and may go undetected or be discovered by chance. Diminished distant vision can be acute or gradual; acute loss draws attention early, and it could be painful or painless.

The causes of gradual, painless, diminished distant vision are mostly errors of refraction, gradually developing opacity in the media, and chronic disorders of the macula, uvea, and optic nerve.

Causes of Sudden and Painless Diminished Vision

Methyl alcohol poisoning, quinine toxicity, transient ischemic attack, and cortical blindness and malingering.

Transient Ischemic Attack

Amaurosis fugax is a mostly bilateral, sudden, transient loss of vision that is commonly bilateral but may be unilateral. It is due to diminished blood supply to the central retinal artery. It is a disease of old age compounded by hypertension and diabetes.

Cortical Blindness

Cortical blindness is a sudden, profound loss of vision that is permanent. The patients may not realize the absence of vision and deny the presence of blindness; it is due to loss of blood supply to the cerebral cortex or injury to the back of the head.

Methyl Alcohol Poisoning

Methyl alcohol poisoning is a sudden, painless loss of bilateral vision following the consumption of spurious alcohol. It generally occurs in clusters of persons with a common source of spurious alcohol. Most of the persons die of alcohol poisoning; the remaining develop optic atrophy, leading to diminished vision ranging from hand movement to no perception. Both pupils are dilated and sluggish.

Causes of Sudden Unilateral Loss of Vision

The causes can be divided into vascular and nonvascular. The vascular causes are central retinal artery obstruction, central retinal vein occlusion, vitreous hemorrhage, central serous retinopathy, acute ischemic optic neuropathy, amaurosis fugax, and malinger. Nonvascular causes are acute optic neuritis and retinal detachment.

Diminished Near Vision

The most common cause of diminished near vision is presbyopia, which is universal after age 40. It is so slowly progressive that the person does not realize its presence unless he is unable to do his near work at a comfortable distance. It is a physiological condition that develops early in hypermetropes and is corrected by adding plus lenses to distant correction. The other causes are uncorrected hypermetropia, posterior polar, and capsular opacity macular degeneration. Causes of sudden diminished near vision are: the installation of cycloplegics (atropine, etc.), internal and external ophthalmoplegia, aphakia, under correction of hypermetropia, and overcorrection of myopia.

Causes of Diminished Near as well as Far Vision

- Uncorrected aphakia and pseudophakia
- Uncorrected errors of refraction
- Advance cataract
- Macular degeneration

Causes of Diminished Vision in Bright Light

The patient has comfortable vision in the room, but as he steps out in bright light or as bright light falls on his eyes, his vision is greatly reduced. The most common causes are dilatations of the pupil for examination. The other causes are central nuclear sclerosis, posterior polar cataract, and macular degeneration.

Diminished Vision in Dim Light (Night Blindness)

The most common cause is vitamin A deficiency followed by retinal dystrophy (retinitis pigmentosa) and, less commonly, choroidal dystrophy. Out of this, only vitamin A deficiency is fully preventable and treatable.

Diminished Color Vision

This is commonly referred to as color blindness, which it is not. It does not fit the definition of blindness. It is a genetic disorder seen in 8% of healthy males, present from birth. The person may not be aware of it unless tested specifically, for it is not a treatable condition.

There are two types of color blindness: congenital and acquired. The former is more common; it is an X-linked recessive anomaly. The only visual disturbance is defective color sense, which does not cause diminish vision or the field of vision. Patients with diminished vision too may have diminished color sense. The above symptoms, when present, are independent of color sense. The defect is present at birth and does not progress. The congenital color defect has been divided into the following groups: protanopia, which has a defective red sensation; Deuteranopia, where green sensation is absent; and tritanopia, where blue sensation is absent. The red-green defect is most common; the term achromatopsia is used to denote severe loss of color sense with the absence of all three colors. Visual acuity is diminished, associated with nystagmus in achromatopsia. It is not treatable by optical devices or medicine; different-colored glasses are of no use. The color defect is diagnosed by Ishihara's chart. It is the most widely used test, best for red-green defects, and is a screening test. For an accurate diagnosis, the following tests are performed: the Farnsworth-Munsell 100 hue test, the Edridge-Green lantern test, and the Holmgren's wools test.

Acquired color defects are far less frequent and are caused by diseases of the macula, optic nerve, and lens. Some of the drugs taken for long periods of time may also result in diminished color sense.

Rainbow-round Artificial Light

This is called halo; it may be unilateral or bilateral. The cause is generally edema of the cornea; less common is early immature cataract. The most common cause is the early stage of narrow-angle glaucoma, where it may terminate in a few hours, only to recur. It may be followed by an acute attack of narrow-angle glaucoma.

Double Vision (Diplopia)

To a person suffering from diplopia, everything looks double. That may disappear by closing any eye; this is the most common type of diplopia, the most common cause being paralysis of the extra ocular muscle. In less common situations, the diplopia disappears upon closing the affected eye. This is called unilateral diplopia. The second image in diplopia is called a false image. The false image is generally fainter. The distance between two images varies greatly according to the severity of the squint. The common separation is horizontal, as seen in the paralysis of horizontal muscles. Less common are vertical deviations; still rarer are tilts of the images. The causes of binocular diplopia other than paralytic squint are restrictive squint, tumors of the orbit, thyroid disorder, and myasthenia.

The diplopia can be crossed or uncrossed. In the case of a crossed diplopia, the image is formed on the opposite side of the object; in the case of an uncrossed diplopia, the object and the image are on the same side.

The image seen by the left eye will be perceived as being on the right side, and that seen by the right eye will be perceived as being on the left side in crossed diplopia. In contrast to this, the image and the object will be on the same side, i.e., the image of the right eye will be formed on the right side in uncrossed diplopia. If the patient has exotropia, the images appear crossed. In the case of esotropia, the diplopia will be uncrossed. The diplopia is tested by moving a vertical object in the field of vision of the patient with both eyes open and his head straight. The patient moves the eyes in various directions without moving the head. The diplopia is charted by putting diplopia goggles in front of the eyes. The red glass is in front of the right eye, and the green glass is in front of the left eye.

Diminished Field of Vision

The loss of field is called a scotoma. It could be central or peripheral, unilateral or bilateral, of the same or different grades, positive or negative. If the patient is aware of the scotoma, it is called positive, and if the patient is not aware of the scotoma, it is called negative. An example of a negative scotoma is blind spot. The positive scotomas are acute in onset; the positive scotomas in the long run become negative. The causes of acute scotomas are optic neuritis, ischemic optic neuropathy, central serous retinopathy, and retinal detachment. The scotomas, as per their location, can be central, centrocecal, scattered, arcuate, hemianopia, or quadrinopic. There can be an enlargement of the blind spot and constrictions of peripheral fields **(Fig. 4.1)**.

Frequent Changes in Power of Glasses

Frequent changes in the power of glasses can be seen in the following situations:
- Progressive myopia
- Hypermetropia shifting towards absolute hypermetropia
- Central nuclear cataract
- Hyperglycemia

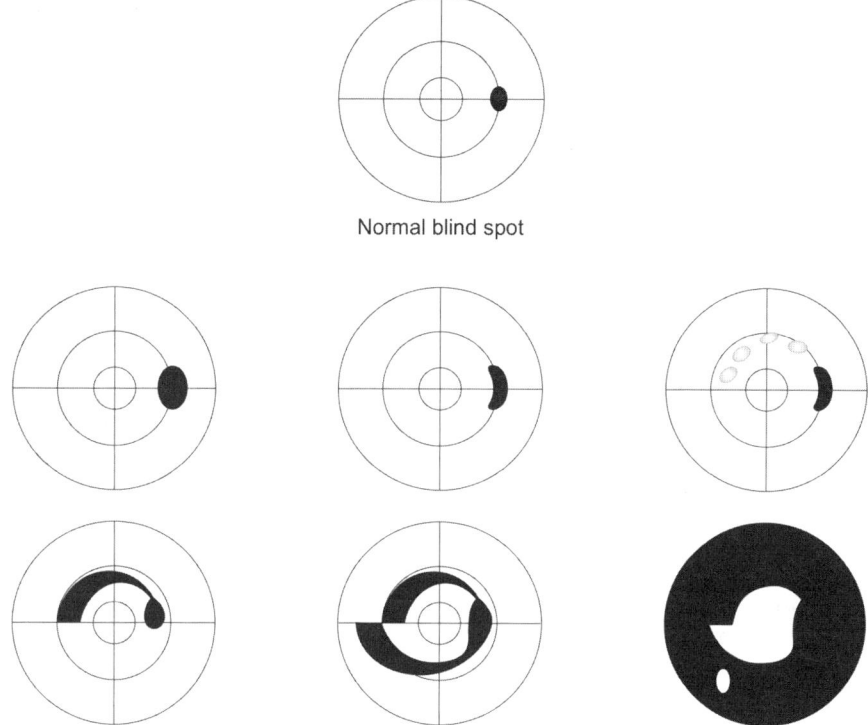

Fig. 4.1: Various types of field defects due to involvement of the optic nerve and neuroretinal defect.

- Hypoglycemia
- Drugs taken orally
- Drugs instilled locally
- Chronic simple glaucoma

Asthenopia

This is a vague tiredness of both eyes that the person describes variously as dull pain in the eyes and a pulling sensation of the eyes, generally associated with mild redness of the eyes and frequent watering. The common causes are uncorrected errors of refraction and latent squints.

Less Common Visual Symptoms

- **Polyopia:** Everything looks more than two (diplopia). The most common cause is the early stage of immature cataracts.
- **Metamorphopsia:** The outline of the object looks distorted. The straight lines look curved. The most common cause is macular degeneration.
- **Glare:** The patient does not like bright light.
  The common causes are: Pupillary size is larger than normal, caused by the ingestion of some drugs, myopia, and albinism. The symptoms are relieved by dark glasses.
- **Photophobia and blepharospasm:** The first is intolerance of light, generally associated with forceful closure of the lids and moving the eyes from light. The forceful closure of lids, along with photophobia, is called blepharospasm. Both conditions are associated with watering and pain in the eye. Blepharospasm can be relieved shortly by instillation or anesthetic

agents, but not by dark glasses. The symptoms are more marked in children. The common causes are phlyctenular keratoconjunctivitis, acute iritis, foreign bodies in the cornea, congenital glaucoma, and exposure to ultraviolet rays.
- **Photopsia:** The patient complains of seeing flashes of light even with closed lids. This is a serious symptom requiring prompt attention by way of indirect ophthalmoscopy because this may be the warning sign of retinal detachment.
- **Black spots in the field of vision:** This is very common in myopes. The patient complains of either a single black spot or a string of spots, generally single, in the field of vision. The opacities may or may not move with the movement of the eyes. They are generally permanent and harmless but may herald vitreous detachment or shallow retinal detachment. A sudden increase in the number of opacities and the association of flashes of light require prompt examination by an indirect ophthalmoscope.
- **Chromatopsia:** Patients feel that light-colored objects are tinged by other colors. To them, a white wall may have a light blue or pink tinge. This happens frequently following lens extraction in jaundice, making the object look yellow. There is no condition where white will look black or red will look green. The condition is short-lived, not requiring treatment.

NONVISUAL OCULAR SYMPTOMS

They may be alone, in combination, along with visual symptoms, acute, chronic, unilateral, bilateral, equal in both eyes, or otherwise.
- Redness, watering, and discharge from the eyes; sticking of the lids
- Pain in the eye that may radiate
- Drooping of lids or inability to close the lids
- Deviation of the eyes (squint)
- Whiteness in the eyes: corneal opacity, cataract
- Bulging of the eye (proptosis/exophthalmos), sinking of the eyes (enophthalmos)

Redness of the Eyes

Redness of the eyes is a very common sign and symptom that brings patients for consultation. The watering may be associated with discharge; it may be painful or painless; it may be associated with diminished vision.

The common causes of redness of the eyes are:
- Injury
- Acute infection: Bacterial/viral
- Allergy
- Acute iridocyclitis
- Acute glaucoma
- Episcleritis and scleritis
- Phlycten
- Pterygium
- New growths

The redness could be localized or generalized, more around the limbus, prominent in the fornices. The localized causes of conjunctival congestion are shown in **Figure 4.2.**
- Subconjunctival hemorrhage
- Pterygium
- Phlycten
- Episcleritis

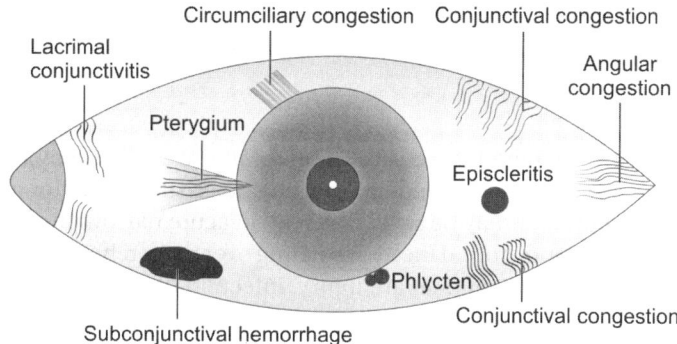

Fig. 4.2: Localized conjunctival congestion.

- Scleritis
- Angular conjunctivitis
- Multiple phlyctens
- Circumciliary congestion.

Watering from the Eyes

Normal eyes are always wet due to normal tears, but without overflow of the tears. A person is not aware of this wetness. Awareness of wetness is called watering of the eyes. It may be slight or may be copious and may be associated with discharge.

There are two types of watering:
1. **Active watering:** This is called lacrimation, where there is overproduction of tears with normal drainage.
2. **Passive watering:** This is called epiphora. This is an overflow of tears with normal production. In rare instances, both may be present.

Causes of Lacrimation

- Corneal foreign body
- Injury to the eye
- Keratitis, superficial or deep, with or without infection
- Phlyctenular keratoconjunctivitis
- Acute anterior uveitis
- Panuveitis
- Acute glaucoma
- Acute conjunctivitis: bacterial, viral, or allergic
- Reflex lacrimation

Causes of Epiphora

Chronic nasolacrimal duct block, either congenital or acquired, Absence of the sac, ectropion of the lower lid, small or absent lower puncta.

Discharge from the Eyes

Normal eyes do not produce any discharge. Discharge from the eye means disease of the conjunctiva due either to infection or allergy. The discharge consists of tears, mucus, and microorganisms; it could be watering in viral conjunctivitis or trauma, mucopurulent due to mild bacterial conjunctivitis, or purulent due to a severe conjunctival infection like ophthalmia neonatorum. Spring catarrh produces thread-like discharge.

Pain in the Eyes

It may be in the eyeball or in the lids or sac. The pain in the eyeball may be associated with tenderness that is referred to as ciliary tenderness, a characteristic of anterior uveitis. The pain in the eye may be dull and mild or may be severe, as seen in acute narrow angle glaucoma. One of the causes of severe pain in and around the eye radiating over the forehead is due to herpes zoster ophthalmicus (HZO). The causes of pain are injury, infection of the cornea, acute iridocyclitis, and acute congestive glaucoma. The causes of pain in the lids are stye infected chalazion and cellulitis lids. Acute pain is associated with acute dacryocystitis.

Drooping of the Upper Eyelid

The normal lid covers 2.00 mm of the upper cornea. If it covers more than 2.00 mm, it is considered to be real drooping and is called ptosis.

The causes of ptosis are divided into two groups:
1. True ptosis where the levator is involved. The causes can be congenital (commonest), neurological (paralysis of the third nerve), myological (myasthenia), or senile.
2. Pseudoptosis is a condition where the action of the levator is present, but the lid comes down due to other causes. The other cause is edema of the lid, either due to infection or allergy. A large growth also brings down the upper lid. Absence or softening of the globe also causes pseudoptosis.

The lower lid is not capable of developing ptosis. In contrast to drooping, it goes up in certain neurological conditions, and the condition is called reverse or upside-down ptosis.

Inability to Close the Lids

The lids are closed due to the action of the orbicularis oculi, supplied by the seventh cranial nerve. Underaction of the orbicularis is the most common cause of the inability to close the lids and is called lagophthalmos. That can be complete when there is no action of the orbicularis or partial when some action of the muscle is retained. Lagophthalmos is generally unilateral but can be bilateral; the most common cause of bilateral lagophthalmos is leprosy. The other cause of the inability to close the lids is mechanical due to the protrusion of the globe. Due to exophthalmos proptosis, a large ciliary staphyloma, or a large growth on the anterior part of the globe.

Deviation of the Eyeball

Normally, when a person fixes a distant object, the eyes are straight, and the distance between the cornea and medial canthus is equal in both eyes. The image of a bright light held at 33.00 cm in midline in front of the face forms a bright shadow in the center of the cornea. This image is called the Hirschberg test. A deviation of the image medially is caused by divergent squint (exotropia). A shift laterally is caused by a convergent squint (esotropia). The two eyes are parallel when moving horizontally or vertically **(Fig. 4.3)**.

The two eyes are no more parallel when looking at a near point. They converge towards the nose. Any deviation of one eye in relation to the other while both eyes are looking at a distant object is called a squint. The squint may be present at birth, may develop in childhood, or may

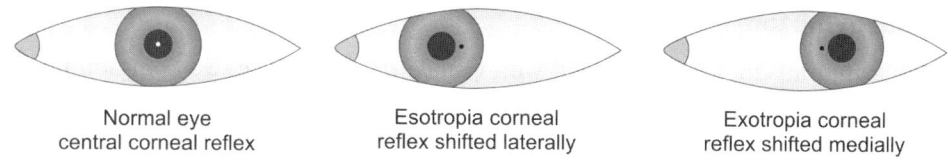

Fig. 4.3: Horizontal deviation of the eye.

be delayed until adulthood. Squint has been broadly divided into two groups, i.e., concomitant (nonparalytic) and paralytic. The former is more common; the other classification is true and false. Squint here again; the former is more common.

Swinging of the Eyeball (Nystagmus)

Presence of oscillation in the eyes is always abnormal. The swinging of the eye is called nystagmus. It generally starts in childhood and lingers throughout life. The patient is unaware of this abnormal movement, which may be noticed by an onlooker. The movements could be horizontal, vertical, or torsional. It is a bilateral phenomenon; the horizontal nystagmus is most frequent. The nystagmus may become worse when occluding one eye.

Change in the Color of the Cornea and Pupil

People generally call the cornea the black of the eye; in fact, the cornea is colorless and transparent. The color imparted to it is due to the dark iris behind it, which is generally black; the still-black circular area in the center of the iris is the pupil. The opacities may either be in the cornea or in the pupil.

Both types of opacities are white. The opacities in the pupil can either be an exudative membrane in the pupil or an opacity in the lens called a cataract. Lighter opacities may go undetected. A person becomes aware of corneal opacity when the opacity is dense.

Prominent Eyeballs

Sometimes people may have eyes that are more prominent than others; this may be familial or due to a large eyeball, as seen in high myopia or large ciliary staphyloma, with a normal position of the globe in relation to the rim of the orbit. Otherwise, the eye wall may be pushed forward; such conditions are called proptosis or exophthalmos. Proptosis generally has growth behind it, pushing it forward. In exophthalmos, the process is more complicated because a substance called exophthalmos produces substances. Seen in thyroid orbitopathy in the past, the two conditions were called by separate names; now, both are referred to as exophthalmos. The bulge is measured by an instrument called an exophthalmometer.

Sinking of the Eyeballs

The vertex of the eyeball lies in the plane of the orbital margin, giving a normal appearance to the lids. In cases where the eyeballs are soft or small, the interpalpebral fissure becomes narrow and the eyeball sinks in the orbit. The condition is called enophthalmos, and the causes are microphthalmos, phthisis, and factures of the orbit.

Proptosis is more commonly unilateral, while exophthalmos is bilateral more often.

Note: The term anophthalmos denotes the total absence of the eyeball, as happens following enucleation; in rare instances, the eyeball may be totally absent congenitally.

Nonvisual Symptoms

Nonvisual symptoms may be associated with visual symptoms. The two common nonvisual symptoms are headaches and vertigo. Out of the two, headaches are more common. The headaches are broadly divided into two groups. They are migraineous (due to migraine) and nonmigraineous. The nonmigraineous causes of headache are uncorrected errors of refraction, overcorrection of errors of refraction, latent squint, chronic raised intraocular tension, and chronic anterior uveitis. The most common nonocular cause of headache is raised intracranial tension.

CHAPTER 5

Examination of the Eye

Examination of the eyes consists broadly of two parts: history and eliciting signs. History should precede examination. Both eyes should always be examined, even when one eye seems to be normal.

HISTORY
While taking history, the following points should be elicited:
- Purpose of the visit
- Complaints: Ocular, nonocular, combined
- Patients may have single or multiple symptoms. The common isolated symptoms are diminished distant vision, diminished near vision, squint, ptosis, and inability to close the eye. The multiple symptoms may be diminished near as well as distant vision. Redness of the eye with diminished vision or combination of redness, watering, and diminished vision.
- Find out if the symptoms are unilateral, bilateral, simultaneous, or if the other eye developed symptoms after the first eye, time lapse between the two recurrences.
- Properly taken history may many a time lead to the diagnosis directly. The most common examples are:
    - A school going child complains of an inability to see the writing on the board in the school.
    - The mother complains that the child sits too near the TV.
    - The parents complain that the child keeps his book too close to his face. The above symptoms directly lead to the diagnosis of diminished distant vision.
    - An elderly person who was comfortable with his near correction for years finds the glasses less comfortable and has better vision without them. Though his distant vision has diminished during the same period, he is most probably suffering from an immature cataract or has undiagnosed raised blood sugar.
    - A child from below the poverty line is brought with complains of diminished night vision for the last few weeks. The diagnosis is that the child suffers from vitamin A deficiency.
    - In contrast to the above, a young man complains of increasing night blindness and is suffering from retinitis pigmentosa.
    - A person around 40 years of age who complains of discomfort in near vision is suffering from presbyopia.
    - A person complaining of diplopia of recent origin has a case of paralytic squint.
    - A person complaining of drooping of the upper lid and diplopia after physical excretion is suffering from myasthenia.
    - Inability to close the eye for a short duration is Bell's palsy.

History should be taken under the following headings:
- History of the present disorder
- Past history

- Personal history
- Family history

History of the Present Disorder

It should include duration, time of onset, acute or chronic, unilateral or bilateral, associated with redness, watering, pain in the eyes, diminished vision, diplopia, inability to close the eyes, inability to open the eyes, and disfigurement.

Past History

A history of past illnesses may directly be associated with the present illness. The most common examples are injuries from the past, which may be related to many ocular disorders years later. The most common examples are traumatic cataracts, glaucoma, corneal opacity, sympathetic uveitis, and retinal detachment. A history suggesting anterior uveitis in the past may be responsible for complicated cataracts, secondary glaucoma, and cystoid macular edema. Scars over the lids and forehead may suggest herpes zoster ophthalmicus (HZO) in the past. A history of prolonged use of strong steroids, such as in spring catarrh chronic, uveitis, and IOL in children, may be responsible for glaucoma and the early onset of cataract. The past histories of diseases that are not relevant to the present disorders are acute conjunctivitis, stye chalazion, and dacryocystitis. They cannot be blamed for age-related cataracts, glaucoma, detachment, and many more conditions. Histories of past surgery on the eye are more relevant. The examples are squint surgery in childhood, IOL in childhood glaucoma, and retinal detachment surgery in all ages.

Personal History

About visual requirements should be noted.

Family History

Disorders present at birth or in childhood are likely to have a genetic background. The conditions should be noted. The common conditions are errors of refraction, corneal degeneration, retinal degeneration, glaucoma, retinoblastoma, and congenital anomalies. The family members include parents, siblings, grandparents, and blood relatives. Family history is important for counselling.

EXAMINATION OF THE EYE

Both eyes must be examined; even when the patient resents the examination of the other eye, he considers it normal. The examination of the eyes consists of recording vision, external and internal examination, and special investigation.

Recording of Vision

The recording of vision is the most important examination and should precede other examinations. It consists of distant vision, near vision, field of vision, and color vision. All the tests should be done for each eye separately.

Distant Vision

There are various methods of noting distant vision, with a fixed order in which they should be taken.

Chapter 5: Examination of the Eye

The universal practice is to examine the right eye first, followed by the left, and then the two eyes together. The vision is tested first without spectacles, then with spectacles. The power of the spectacle, along with the near correction, should be noted. The following terms indicate the side examined: RE = right eye; LE = left eye; BE = both eyes; the other methods employed are OD, OS, and OU, respectively.

Testing of distant vision is done by various methods at 6 or 3 meters. The charts used at 3 meters are half the size of the charts used at 6 meters. If 6 meters of space is not available, a plane mirror is placed in front of the vision charts/drum at 3 meters, and the letters on the chart are revered. Some of the English letters look the same when looked at through the mirror **(Fig. 5.1)**.

The revered chart is kept a little behind, up, and above the head of the patient. The charts can be self-illuminated, as in a vision drum, or illuminated from outside.

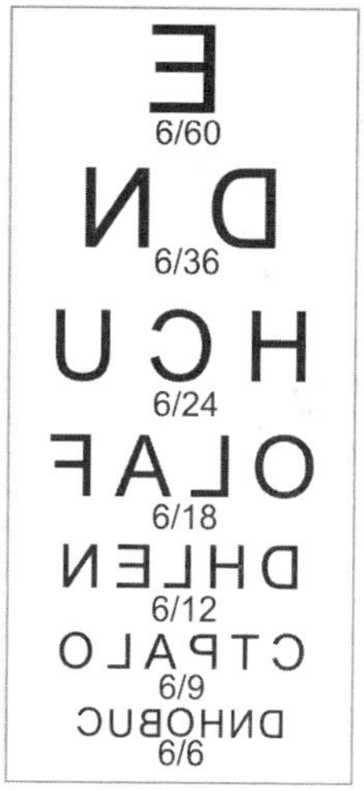

Fig. 5.1: Snellen's chart reversed.

The most common chart is Snellen's chart:
- Letters in various languages and number **(Fig. 5.2)**.
- E-chart **(Fig. 5.3A)**
- C-chart (Landolt) **(Fig. 5.3B)**

There are seven lines of letters in Snellen's chart. The top line has a single letter, and the number of letters increases but decreases in size in successive lines. The seventh line has seven letters. The Snellen vision charts are used at a distance of 6 meters (20 feet) **(Fig. 5.2)**. If the space is <6 meters, some modifications are required. The first is to reduce the size by half using 3 meters of space **(Fig. 5.4)**.

The other method is to use a plane mirror kept at 3 meters in front of a reversed Snellen's chart as shown in **Figures 5.1 and 5.2**.

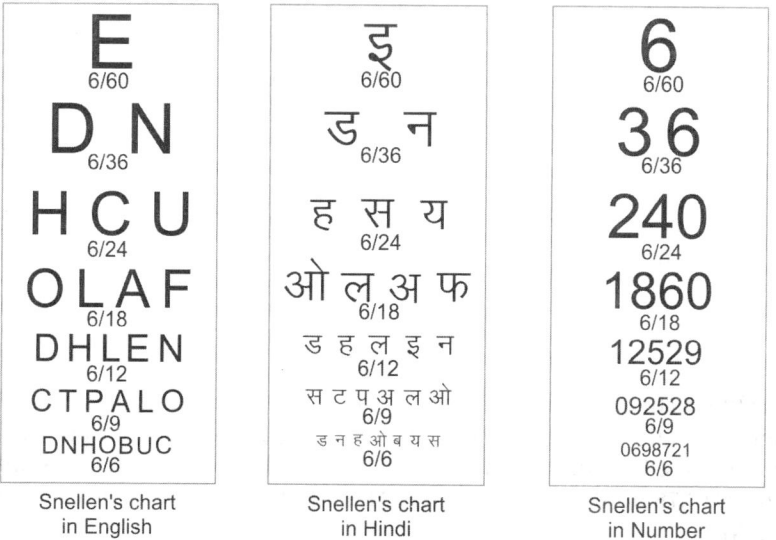

Fig. 5.2: Various types of Snellen's charts.

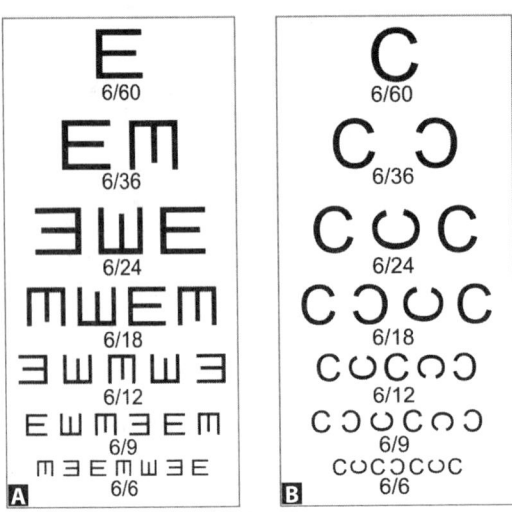

Figs. 5.3A and B: E and C charts.

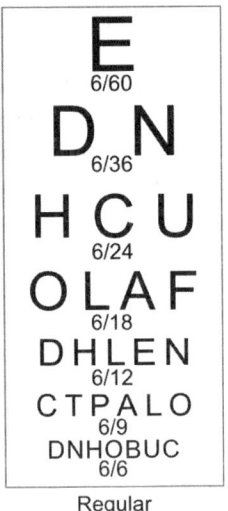

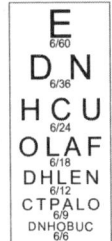

Fig. 5.4: Figure showing comparison between regular Snellen chart and its reduced counterpart.

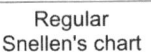

Fig. 5.5: Log-MAR chart.

- **Log MAR chart:** The log-MAR chart has ten lines with five letters in each line. It is read at four meters away; the reading is noted in a number prefixed by the sign + or –. The vision of 6/60 on the Snellen chart is equivalent to +1 on the log MAR scale. Similarly, 6/36 is equivalent to +0.78 on the log MAR scale. The numbers are gradually reduced to 0.00 for 6/6 **(Fig. 5.5)**.

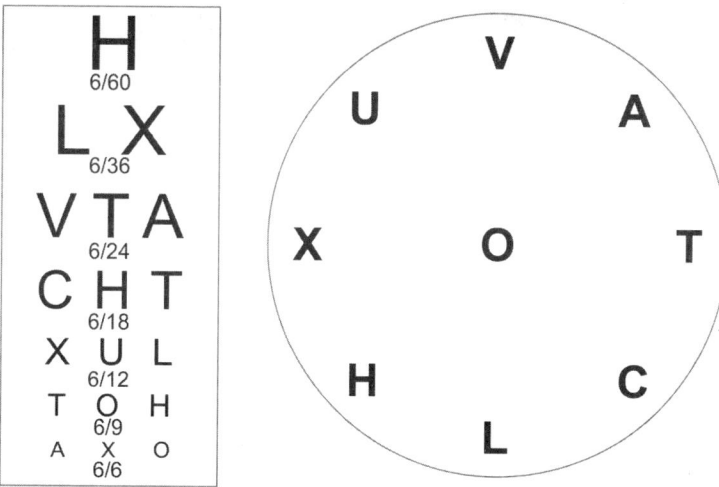

Fig. 5.6: Two charts of STYCAR.

- **STYCAR chart:** The term STYCAR stands for Snellen's test for young children and retarded. It is used at 6 meters, and a small card with similar letters is provided to the child. Who points to the corresponding letter shown in the main chart **(Fig. 5.6)**.
- **Early treatment diabetic retinopathy study (ETDRS):** Is tested on log-MAR. It is designed to eliminate inaccuracies of Snellen test.
- **Digital:** This is an advanced form of test used when the testing distance is <3 meters, the size of the optotypes (letters) can be adjusted as per distant available.
- There are many more vision charts used in various countries.

Some of the English letters look the same when seen through the plane mirror; hence, they need not be reversed in the vision drum. The letters are A I O M H V X Y T U.

Recording of Distant Vision

- The patient sits at a distance of 6 meters from the regular chart, at 3 meters when the size of the charts is reduced to half or using a reversible plane mirror with reversed **(Fig. 5.1)** and at 4 meters from a log MAR chart.
- One eye is tested at a time, and the other eye is covered without pressing over the globe. It is convention that the right eye is tested first. Once two eyes have been tested, the vision in both eyes together is noted. The vision of two eyes together is better than that of a single eye, provided the other eye is fixing. The advantages of binocular vision are that the vision by both eyes is better than single, depth of focus increases giving better stereopsis, and the binocular field is larger than uniocular.

The Process of Testing Distant Vision

- The patient is asked to read the chart from above downwards, and the number of lines read is noted. If the patient can read all the letters up to the seventh line, his vision is noted as 6/6 or 20/20. His inability to read all the lines indicates diminished distant vision.

Table 5.1 gives the lines read and corresponding vision.

Table 5.1: Line read and corresponding vision.	
Line read	**Vision**
Seven	6/6 or 20/20
Six	6/9
Five	6/12
Four	6/18
Three	6/24
Two	6/36
One	6/60

❖ If the patient is unable to read the topmost letter (6/60), he is moved towards the chart by one meter at a time, vision is noted at every meter from which the patient can read. If he can read the top letters from 5 meters, his vision is noted as 5/60; similarly, it is noted as 4/60, 3/60, 2/60, and 1/60 at successive distances.
❖ If the patient cannot recognize the letter at 1 meter, the effort to examine the vision on chart is given up.
❖ The patient is brought back to his seat and asked to count the fingers of the examiner at various gradual decreasing distances, i.e., one meter, half a meter, and near the face. The findings are designated as counting fingers (CF) and noted as CF 1 meter, CF 1/2 meter, and CF close to face.
❖ If the patient fails to count the fingers close to his face, the examiner moves his hand in front of the eye. If the patient can see the moving hand, the vision is noted as hand movement (HM).
❖ If the patient cannot see the moving hand, the test is changed to the ability to perceive light. To perform this test, a bright torch is focused in front of his eye, and he is asked to indicate if he can see the light. Ability to see the light is noted as perception of light (PL), and absence of light is noted as no perception of light (No PL).
❖ If the patient has PL, the torch is focused from four directions, i.e., temporal, nasal, upper, and Lower. Appreciation of light is denoted as plus mark at each quadrant.

Causes of the Absence of Light Perception

Anophthalmos, absence of eyeball (enucleated eye), eviscerated eye, central retinal artery occlusion, total retinal detachment, optic atrophy (primary, secondary, or glaucomatous), and transaction of the optic nerve.

Causes of Faulty Projection of Light

Advanced glaucoma, large retinal detachment, advanced retinal dystrophy, and bitemporal hemianopia.

Any amount of corneal opacity, lenticular opacity, high error of refraction, or large macular lesion will not cause loss of perception. Perception of light once lost is not correctable. In the absence of light, there is no need to test the projection of light.

The recording of distant vision without glasses is followed by finding out if the person uses glasses; if so, it is for near, distance, or both. If the patient is using near correction, the spectacle is unifocal, bifocal, trifocal, or progressive **(Fig. 5.7)**.

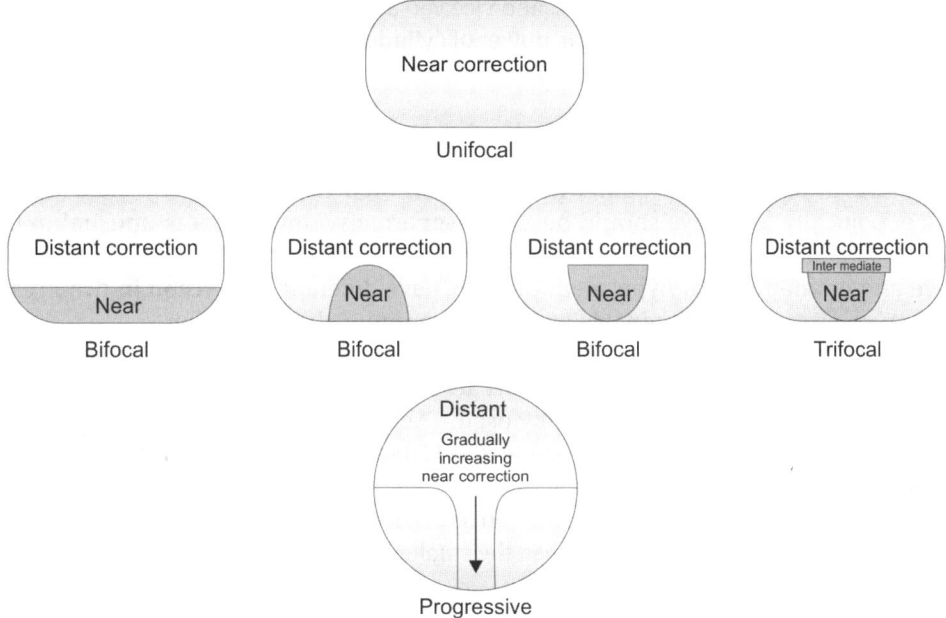

Fig. 5.7: Various types of near addition.

The next step is to find out the type of glasses.
The commonly used procedure is as follows:
1. Hold the spectacle by the frame between your thumb and index finger (do not touch the lens).
2. Bring the spectacle near the eye (examiner) with side bars away from the eye.
3. Examine one lens at a time.
4. Look at a distant object.
5. Holding the spectacle away from the eye and seeing a near object is wrong.
6. Move the lens from side to side, up and down, and rotate.
7. Note:
   i. The movement of the object, i.e., with or against
   ii. Size of the object enlarged or reduced
   iii. Look for distortion in rotation.
8. i. If there is no movement of the object, no change in size, and no distortion, the glass under examination is plain glass (without power).
   ii. If the image moves with the movement of the glass, the image is smaller, there is no change in shape, no distortion on rotation, move movement is equal in all meridians. The glass is a myopic (negative) sphere.
   iii. If the image moves against the movement of the glass, enlarged, not distorted, with equal movement in all the meridians, the lens is hypermetropic (positive).
   iv. Change in shape, distortion on rotation, and unequal movement in different meridians mean the presence of a cylinder.

Methods of Finding Out the Power of the Glasses

There are two methods of finding out the power of the glasses. The first is mechanical, by putting lenses of opposite signs successively until there is no movement in the combination. For example, a plus lens is neutralized by a minus lens, and vice versa. The second is by lensometer that gives not only distant power, addition for near, power of cylinder, its axis, presence of prism, direction of its base and center of the glass **(Fig. 5.8)**.

Examination of Near Vision

Near vision is tested in normal light, with light falling on the reading material held at reading distance. Logically, each eye should be tested separately. However, it is unusual to find a difference in near vision in two eyes except in high anisometropia; a person with myopia in one eye and emmetropia or hypermetropia may have different near vision in two eyes. It is mandatory to examine the distant vision before examining the near vision.

Like vision charts for distance, there are charts for near vision. They are smaller than the distant charts and are hand-held. The common charts are Snellen's near vision chart and Jaeger's near vision chart; the former is more frequently used. The illiterates are tested on proportionately smaller E and C charts or charts with multiple dots **(Figs. 5.9 and 5.10)**.

The size of letters ranges between 5 and 48 points, where 5 is the smallest and 48 is the largest. A point is 1/72 of an inch. The results are noted as N (near), followed by a point, i.e., N5 to N48. The former denotes that the person can read the smallest letter in the chart, and N48 denotes the largest letter read at 30 cm.

Examination of Color Vision

Eight percent of the male population suffers from some type of color vision defect. The defect is never complete (achromatopsia). The commonest color vision defect is red-green deficiency. The color deficiency is equal in both eyes. It is not possible to have two types of color deficiency in two eyes. The most common type of chart used to screen color defects is the Ishihara plate **(Fig. 5.11)**.

They are generally available in book form; the other device used is the Edridge green lantern **(Fig. 5.12)**.

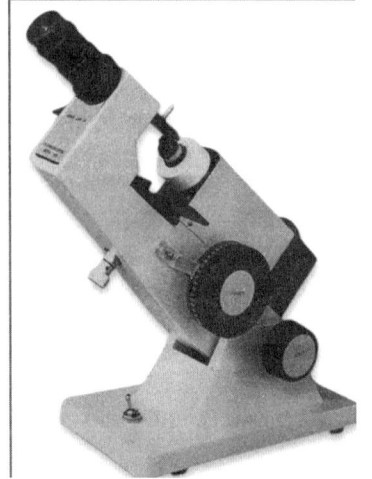

Fig. 5.8: Lensometer.
(*Courtesy:* Appasamy associates)

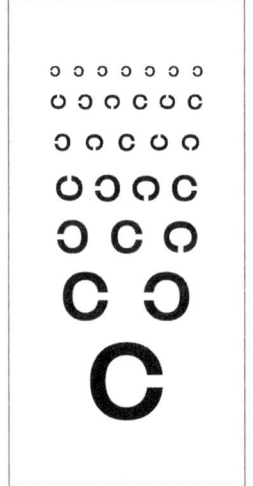

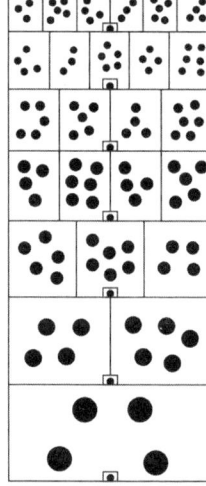

Fig. 5.9: Near vision chart for illiterates.

Chapter 5: Examination of the Eye

N6

It was an old tree. Asced had been carried to the island by a strong wind some fifty years back. It had found shelter between two rocks and had taken root there. A tree had sprung up to give shade and shelter to a small family. An old man sat beneath the tree.

Ponder magic window loving search

N8

He was mending a fishing-net. He had fished in the river for ten years, and he was a good fishermen. He knew where to find good fish. He knew where the river was deep and where it was shallow, he knew which baits to use which fish liked worms and which liked gram

Power sight foolish game point small

N10

He had taught his son to fish, but his son had gone to work in a factory in a city, nearly a hundred miles away. He had no grand-son, but he had a grand-daughter, Sita.

delight story vision create wonder

N12

She could do all the things a boy could do, and sometime she could do them better. She had lost her mother when She was very small.

Mirror cinema sister value perfect

N14

She was taught, all the things a girl should know, and she could do these as well as most girls would do.

Pattern years growth style

N18

Her grandparents could not read or write. There was a school in the village.

Feast noble temple

N24

But poor Sita never went to school.

love plan take

N36

Work at home kept her busy
Life was always a joy.

Fig. 5.10: Near vision chart in English.

This is used specifically for pilots, loco pilots, railway guards, and long-distance truck drivers. The color vision tests are done in room illumination.

Examination of the Field of Vision

When an eye fixes an object at a distance, it not only sees the object of interest but also things round it. The visible area seen round the point of fixation (subject of interest) is called the field of vision of the eye. The visual field has been defined as "an island of vision in a sea of blindness."

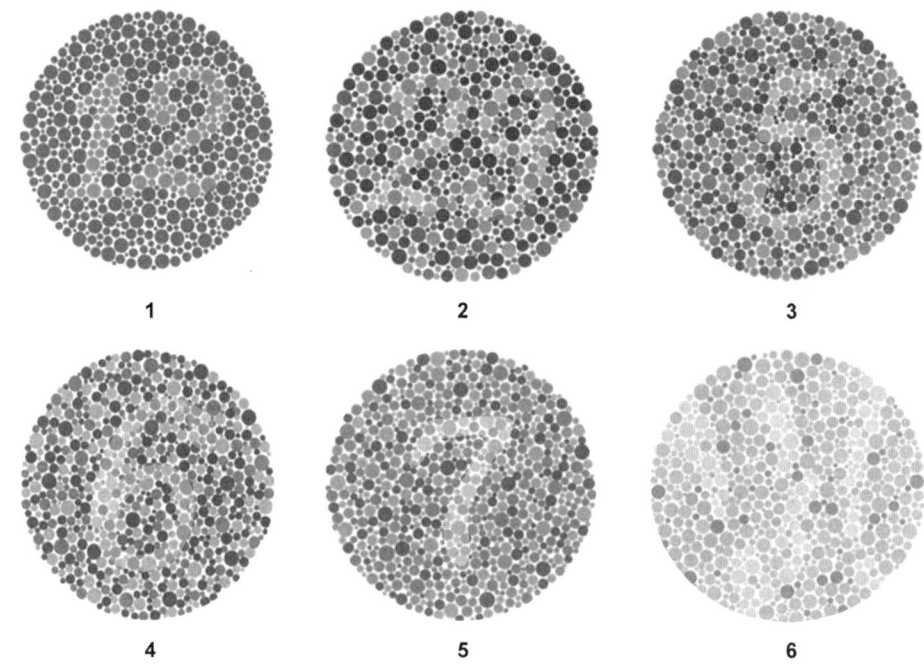

Fig. 5.11: Ishihara plates. (*For color version, see Plate 1*)

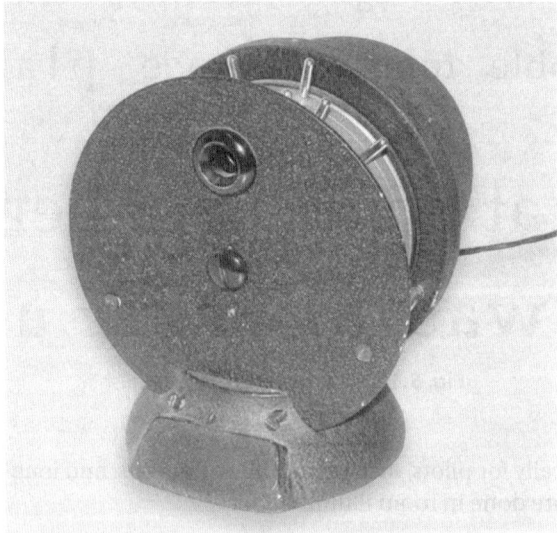

Fig. 5.12: Edridge green lantern.

The fields of clinical vision have been divided into two types, i.e., peripheral and central **(Fig. 5.13)**.

The peripheral field is not circular but follows the contour of the orbit. It is maximum on the temporal side and smaller in the superonasal and inferonasal areas. The center of vision corresponds to the macula and is called the point of fixation. The blind spot represents

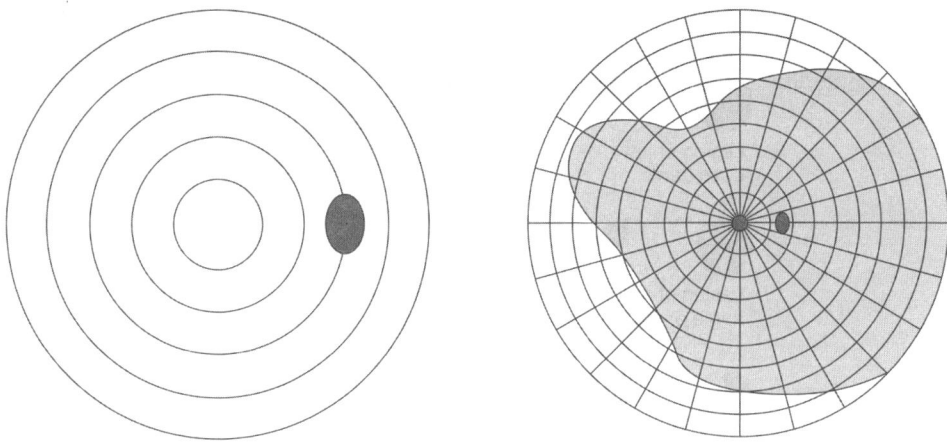

Fig. 5.13: Example of peripheral field (right eye) and central field.

the optic nerve head. The fields of two eyes, when added, are larger than those of a single eye. The central field is far smaller than the peripheral and is circular, extending 30° all around the point of fixation. The normal shapes of the fields are mirror images of each other. The defects in the field are called scotomas, the shape of which differs at different levels **(Figs. 5.14 and 5.15).**

The field defects can be unilateral or bilateral. They are called homonymous or heteronymous. **Flowchart 5.1** shows various types of bilateral field defects.

The central field is tested on the Amsler grid and Bjerrum screen is shown in **Figures 5.16** and **5.17.**

The Amsler grid is a small hand-held chart (10 × 10 cm) used for reading distances and is most useful in macular lesions. The Bjerrum screen is a large figure drawn on a black background used at a distance of one meter.

The **Flowchart 5.2** shows various types of field examinations.

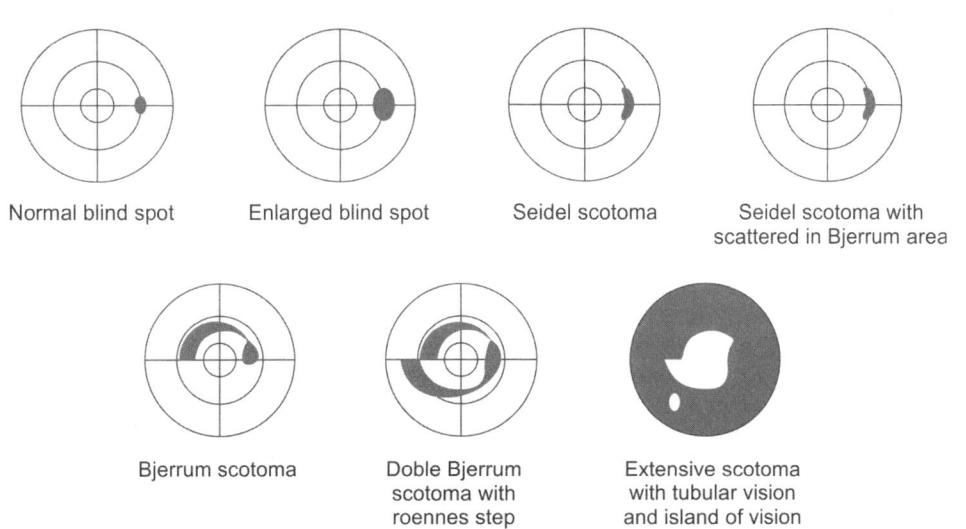

Fig. 5.14: Various types of central field defects.

Scotomas in lesion of visual path from papilla to optic radiation

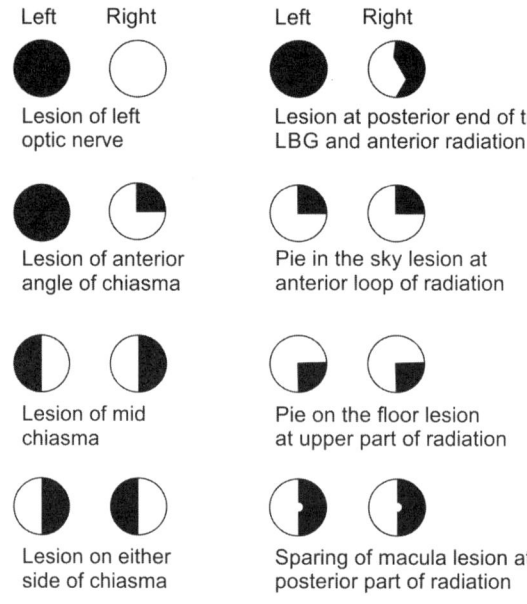

Fig. 5.15: Various types of peripheral fields.

Flowchart 5.1: Various types of bilateral field defects.

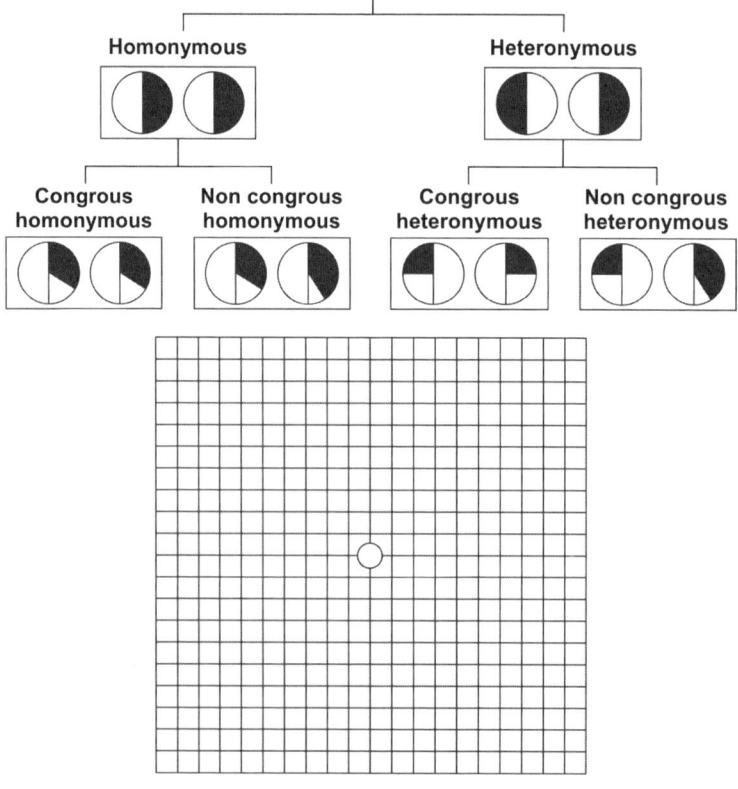

Fig. 5.16: Amsler grid.

Chapter 5: Examination of the Eye

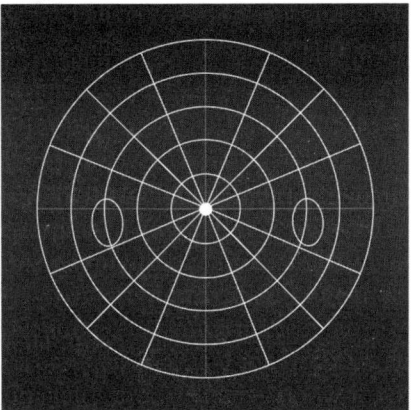

Fig. 5.17: Bjerrum screen.

Flowchart 5.2: Various types of field examinations.

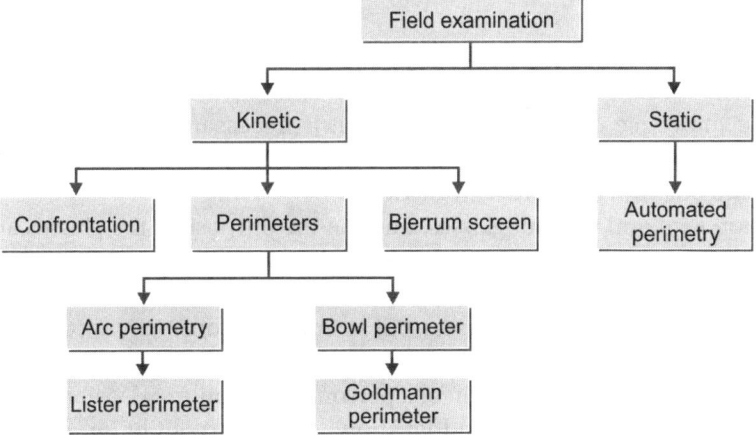

Note:
1. Kinetic methods are those where the target moves from the periphery towards the center, with the patient fixing a central point. The size and color of the targets can be changed.
2. **Static methods:** The visual fields are charted by using a stationary target, the illumination of which can be adjusted either for bright or dim light, with the size of the target remaining constant. The static perimeter has mostly eliminated the kinetic perimeters from clinical practice.
3. The confrontation method is an outdoor procedure, not requiring any equipment, hence cheap and handy. The disadvantage of the procedure is that it can only locate large field defects like advanced glaucoma and hemianopsia.
4. The Lister perimeter is made up of a rotating arc; the target can be moved on the arc. The radius of the arc is 330.00 mm, with a central fixation point at 33.00 cm from the cornea **(Fig. 5.18)**.
5. **Goldmann perimeter:** Here the arc is replaced by a hemispherical bowl, on which the target is moved mechanically, and the size of the targets can be adjusted. It can chart both central and peripheral fields. It can pick up early glaucomatous changes. The inside of the bowl is dimly illuminated **(Fig. 5.19)**.
6. **Automated perimeters:** The automated perimeters are better than other methods and are capable of reproducing the findings that are important to note in the progression of glaucoma. The instrument has an electronic fixation control with an automatic recording of missed points. The instrument is electronically operated. The disadvantages of the instruments are their cost and the prolonged learning time of the operator. The operator observes the illuminated points on the screen at the back of the instrument, invisible to the patients. The perimetry should be done in each eye separately.

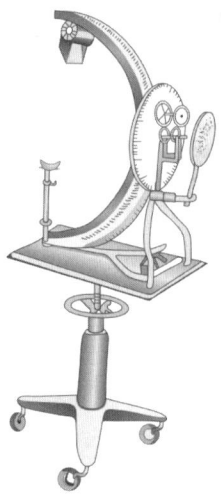

Fig. 5.18: An early modal of Lister perimeter.

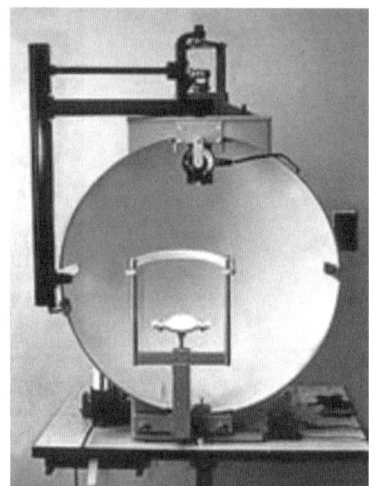

Fig. 5.19: Goldmann perimetry.

Examination of the Eye with Subnormal Vision

❖ To find out the cause of diminished vision, it is necessary to find out the duration of diminished vision—was it sudden, gradual, or recurrent. Sudden loss of vision is generally unilateral and does not improve with glasses.

❖ Record vision with and without glasses, find out the purpose of the glasses and the power of the glasses, and also find out if the vision can be improved by modifying the power of the glasses.

❖ If the vision is subnormal without glasses, put a pinhole in front of the eye under examination, keeping the other eye closed by the occluder, and ask the patients to read the chart from the largest letter downwards. If the vision of a person with subnormal vision improves, the eye has a correctable error of refraction that should be confirmed by subjective or objective methods. Subjective methods consist of putting lenses that improve the vision. Find out the power of the lens that gives the best vision. The subjective method is not an ideal solution; it fails to find out correct power and axis of a cylinder. It may not be possible to diagnose hidden hypermetropia in a child with active accommodation, resulting in the production of pseudomyopia. The best is an objective examination that can be done either with a normal or dilated pupil. The procedure is called refraction of the eye. The eyes with diminished vision are best refracted under cycloplegia. The cycloplegics commonly used are atropine drop 1%, home atropine 2%, cyclopentolate 0.5% to 1%, tropicamide 0.5%, and phenylephrine 10%. The last drug is used in persons above 40 years. The drug is mydriatic without cycloplegic action.

❖ Refraction can be done by any of the following instruments, i.e., a retinoscope and an autorefractometer. Refraction is an optical procedure to find out if the eye has an error in refraction. It can be done without or with cycloplegia; the former is called dynamic retinoscopy, and the latter is called static retinoscopy. The former can be done by a plane mirror retinoscope **(Fig. 5.20)**, a streak retinoscope **(Fig. 5.21)** that can be linear or circular, and an autorefractometer.

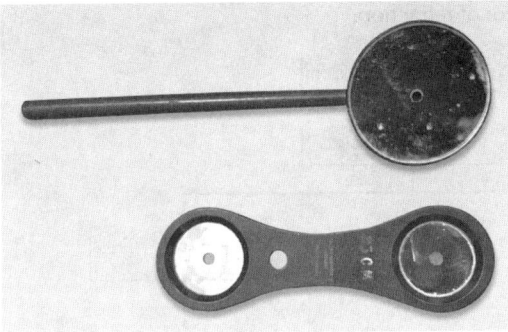

Fig. 5.20: Mirror retinoscopes.

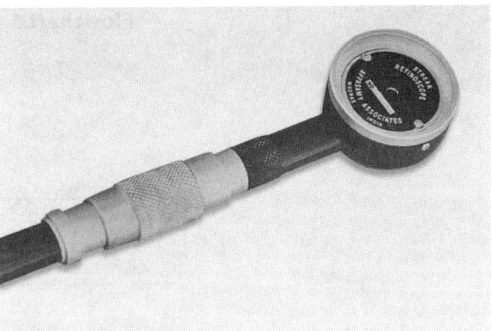

Fig. 5.21: Streak retinoscope.
(*Courtesy*: Appasamy associates)

- Static retinoscopy is the gold standard, commonly done by a plane mirror retinoscope, that consists of a circular plane mirror mounted in a frame with a handle. The mirror has a circular deficiency in the center for the examiner to look into the dilated pupil of the patient **(Fig. 5.20)**. The light is reflected by the mirror into the dilated pupils of the patients. The retinoscope can have either a plane mirror or a concave mirror on two ends. The presence of a plane mirror is indicated by a white dot at the bottom of the plane mirror. The plain mirror throws parallel rays into the dilated pupil. The concave mirror at the other end has a curvature of 25.00 cm and throws a converging ray. The peephole in the center, or the concave mirror, has a +2D lens to relax the accommodation of the examiner. The concave mirror is rarely used except in high myopia.
- To perform retinoscopy, the patient sits with a dilated pupil (static retinoscopy) at a distance of 1.00 meter in front of the examiner. The source of illumination comes from a bulb kept behind the head of the patient, slightly shifted to one side. This keeps the face of the patient in the dark; the light, when thrown into the dilated pupil of the patient from a mirror, illuminates the pupil as a circular pink spot. That can be moved horizontally or vertically. The pink spot looks uniformly pink in the absence of any opacity in the media (cornea lens and vitreous). The opacity, when present, looks black; an opacity in the posterior part of the lens is stationary.

The following are noted regarding the movement of the glow:
- If the glow moves with the movement of the mirror, the eye is emmetrope, hypermetrope, or myopic <1 diopter.
- If there is no movement, the eye is myopic by 1D. If the image moves against the movement, the eye is myopic more than 1D.
- The next step is to put a +1.5D lens in front of the eye, and the resulting movement is noted. If the movement is stopped by the +1.5D lens, the eye is emmetrope.
- If the image still moves with; add plus lenses in a gradual increment until the movement is abolished. The eye is hypermetropic.
- If the image starts moving against with +1.5D the patient has myopia <1 D, gradually reduce the power towards the minus side till the movement is abolished. The lens that abolishes the movement is myopic refraction.
- If the image moves with +1.5D, keep on adding plus lenses until the movement is abolished. The eye is hypermetrope.
- Note down the retinoscopic values and add –1.5D to the retinoscopic finding.

Chapter 5: Examination of the Eye

Flowchart 5.3: Error of refraction.

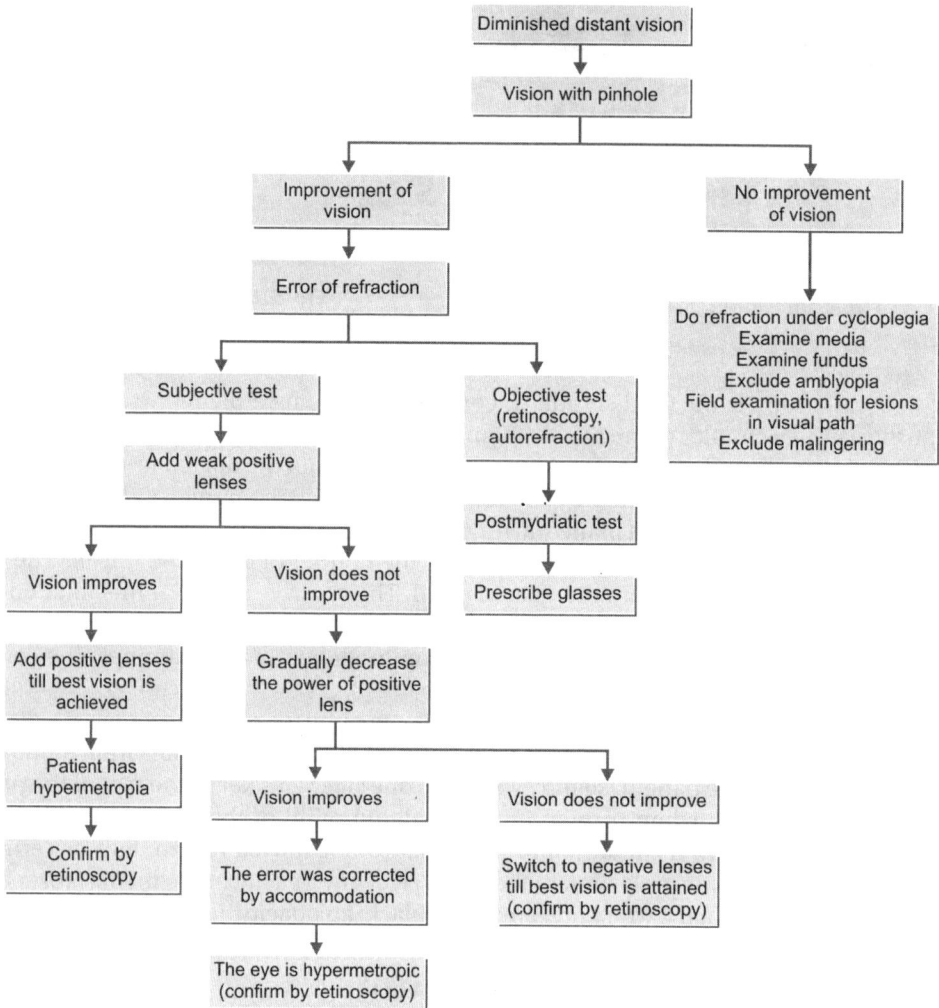

The resultant power will be the power of the glass the patient will require, i.e., if a patient has +2D in two meridians and adds −1.5D, the value left will be +0.5D. This will be the hypermetropic value of the eye. The other example is that if the retinoscopy finding is−2D, adding−1.5D will make the total sum−3.5D. This will be the myopic number that the patients will require **(Fig. 5.22)**.

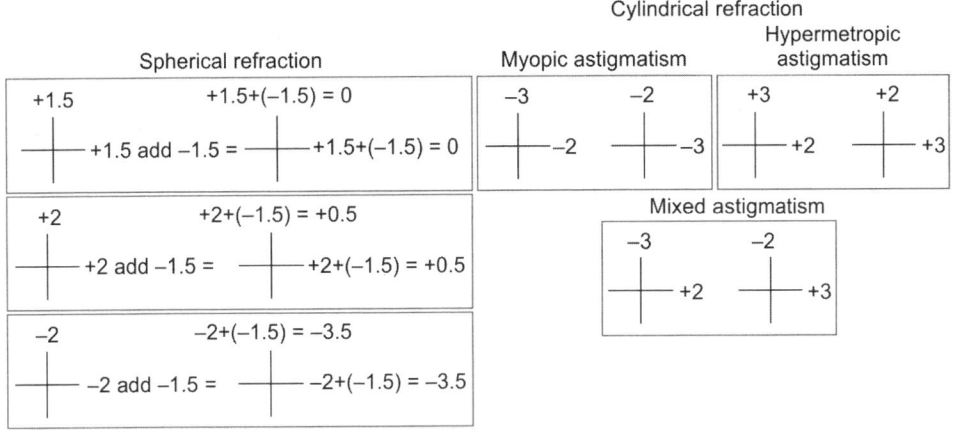

Fig. 5.22: Various types of retinoscopy.

CLINICAL EXAMINATION OF THE EYE

Clinical examination of the eye is broadly divided into two parts, i.e., external examination and internal examination. The external examination is divided into two parts, i.e., examination in diffuse light and in focal illumination. The internal examination requires specialized equipment.

EXAMINATION UNDER DIFFUSE LIGHT

The examination under diffuse light consists of the following:
- Head posture
  - Position of chin;
  - Turning of head to the left or right side;
  - Tilting of head
- Symmetry of the face
- Position of eyebrow
  - Raised
  - Flat
- Loss of eyebrows
- Interpalpebral aperture (distance between upper and lower lid)
- Deviation of eye-squint
- Oscillation of the eye (abnormal movement of the eye=nystagmus)
- Bulging of the eyeball (proptosis/exophthalmos)
- Sunken eyeball

Head Posture

- **Position of the chin:**
  - It may be elevated. The causes are:
    - Ptosis (drooping of the upper lid)
    - Paralysis of elevators (superior rectus and inferior oblique)
    - High errors of refraction
    - Loss of upper field of vision.

- Causes of depression of the chin are:
  - Paralysis of depressors (inferior rectus and superior oblique)
  - Loss of lower field of vision
- **Turning of the head:** The head may be turned towards right or left.
  - The causes of turning of head towards right are paralysis of the right lateral rectus or paralysis of the left medial rectus.
  - Causes of turning of head towards left are paralysis of the left lateral rectus or right medial rectus.
- Tilting of the head is seen in paralysis of cyclovertical muscles, i.e., superior rectus, inferior rectus, superior oblique, and inferior oblique in any eye.
- **Symmetry of the face**
  For all practical purposes, the two sides of the face are symmetrical. The conditions when the symmetry is lost are:
  - Congenital (present from birth)
  - Trauma (injury to face)
  - Facial palsy (paralysis of the seventh nerve)
- **Position of the eyebrows**
  - The brows are symmetrically arched in the lower part of the forehead.
  - It may be raised in cases of ptosis and pseudoptosis.
  - It becomes flat in facial palsy.
- **Loss of eyebrow**
  The eyebrows may become scanty (less) or may become absent in:
  - Old age
  - Thermal burn
  - Leprosy
  - Hypothyroidism
  - Chemotherapy.

Changes in Interpalpebral Aperture

The space between the two lids is called the interpalpebral aperture (fissure). It is roughly 8.00 mm in the middle, and the interpalpebral aperture is narrow in newborns. Its length is 30.00 mm in adults. When the eyes look at a distant object, the upper eyelid covers 2.00 mm of the upper cornea. If it covers more than that, the condition is called ptosis: true/pseudo. The lower lid touches the lowest parts of the cornea. If there is a bare space between the upper lid and cornea and or cornea and lower lid, the condition is called lagophthalmos, or lid retraction. The interpalpebral aperture becomes narrow in ptosis, pseudoptosis, soft eye, and microphthalmos. The same happens if the globe is completely or partially removed. The former is called enucleation, and the latter is called evisceration. The causes of the widening of IPA are lagophthalmos, proptosis, and exophthalmos.

Squint (Strabismus)

The eye is said to be squinting when it loses its parallelism and instead of being straight, look at different points (*For details, see Chapter 17*).

Nystagmus

Normally, the eyes do not show any oscillation in their primary position or in any direction. The movement of the eyes in various directions is equal and smooth, without jerks. The oscillation of the eye is called nystagmus (*For details, see Chapter 17*).

Bulging of the Eyeballs

The normal eyeball under the lid is in the same plane as the rim of the orbit, and the interpalpebral aperture is normal. If the eye protrudes beyond the orbital rim and the IPA is widened, the condition is called proptosis/exophthalmos. Previously, the two conditions were dealt with separately. Now a day they are thought to be synonyms. In the past, proptosis was defined as active protrusion due to intra orbital mass or reduced volume of the orbit. It can be unilateral or bilateral. In contrast to this, exophthalmos is supposed to be due to thickening of the extraocular muscles, specifically in thyroid disease. Both conditions are measured by an exophthalmometer.

Sinking of the Eyeball

In this condition, the eyeball sags behind the rim of the orbit, producing narrow palpebral aperture, flattening of the lid curvature, flattening of the cornea and small soft eye.

EXAMINATION UNDER FOCAL ILLUMINATION

To examine the eye under focal illumination the two things required are: Source of illumination and a magnifier. The former can be either a handheld battery-operated torch, an electrically operated lamp, or incorporated into the magnifier (biomicroscope). The magnifiers can be simple handheld magnifiers, uniocular or binocular corneal loupes, or operating telescopes and operating microscopes. The corneal loupes and operating telescope have been discussed earlier.

Slit Lamp

The instrument is basically a microscope that is placed horizontally rather than a clinical microscope that is used vertically. The source of illumination in a clinical microscope is from under a transparent slide, while in a slit lamp, the object is opaque, and illumination is focused from above the part examine. The slit lamps can be table-mounted or handheld. The parts of the slit lamp can be divided into an adjustable table, an optical part comprising a microscope, and an illuminating system. The microscope is binocular; with two eyepieces, the images from both are converted to a single image in the optics. The distance between the two eye pieces is adjustable. The power in the eye pieces is also changeable; the microscope can be moved horizontally to change the distance between the eye and the objective. The magnification of a slit lamp ranges from 5x to 50x; the commonly used magnification is 10x to 20x. The microscope retains stereopsis due to its binocularity **(Fig. 5.23)**.

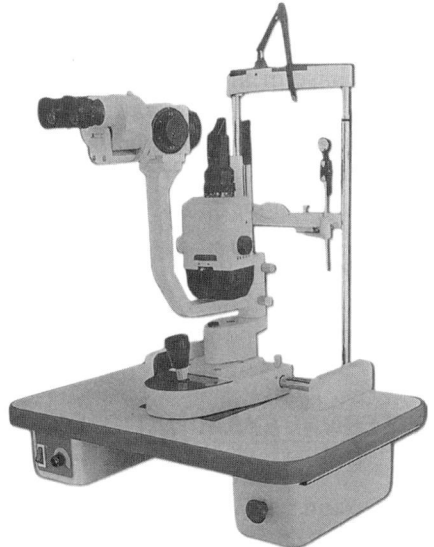

Fig. 5.23: Slit lamp (biomicroscope). (*Courtesy*: Appasamy Associates)

The illumination system comprises of an electrically operated low-voltage bulb that works on mains through a rheostat. The light from the bulb, after passing through a series of plus lenses and prisms, is converted into a circular spot. The width of the illuminated spot can be narrowed to a slit that imparts the name to the instrument "slit lamp". The height of the slit is also adjustable, and there are filters attached to the system that can change the color; the commonly used colors are white, cobalt blue, and green. By reducing the height and width, the slit can be converted into a pinpoint spot of 1.00 mm × 1.00 mm size. The cobalt blue filter is used to see the fluorescein staining of the cornea, applanation tonometry **(Fig. 5.24)**, contact lens fitting, and tear film break-up time.

The slit lamp microscope without attachments can be used to examine up to the anterior vitreous face. To examine the structures beyond this, it requires the following attachments: They are either plus lenses or minus lenses mounted on a slit lamp by suitable attachment or handheld. The various types of plus lenses are El Bayadi and Volk. The power of the plus lenses ranges from +60 D to +90 D. The power of the minus lens commonly used is –55 D. The plus lenses give an enlarged view, while the minus lenses give a minified image of the central part of the posterior segment. They cannot be used to visualize the periphery, for which a 3-mirror gonioscope is required. The angle of the anterior chamber is best seen by a 1-mirror gonioscope. The other attachment available to measure the intraocular tension is an applanation tonometer; in advanced slit lamps, a keratometer can also be attached. There are various types of cameras to take photographs of both the anterior and posterior segments.

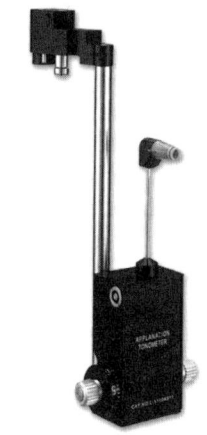

Fig. 5.24: Applanation tonometry. (*Courtesy:* Appasamy Associates)

The mechanical part consists of the following:
- Adjustable table
- The base of the slit lamp, which can be moved smoothly on the table to and fro in all directions. To the base are attached the following that help to adjust the following:
  - Height of the illumination system
  - Height and width of the beam
  - Angulations between the microscope and illumination
  - Chin rest
  - Headband
  - Fixation light

The microscope can be moved from one eye to the other. It can be moved towards or away from the eye.

EXTERNAL EXAMINATION OF THE SPECIFIC STRUCTURE OF THE EYE

The external examination consists of examinations of the lids, lacrimal system, orbit, conjunctiva, cornea, and sclera.

Examination of the Lid

- The lid is examined for its position
- Mobility
- Swelling
- Pain and tenderness
- Growth
- Blepharospasm

Position of the Lid

The common anomalies of the lid are congenital anomalies, drooping of the upper lid, retraction of the lids, and the inability to close the lids. The first may either be due to ptosis or pseudoptosis. The retraction is commonly seen in sympathetic over activity. The most common cause of the inability to close the lids is paralysis of the orbicularis or mechanical protrusion of the globe.

Mobility

Mobility of the lid is affected in two situations, i.e., the inability to lift the lid from its drooping position. This is seen in the ptosis of the lid. The other condition is the inability to close the lids that is seen in paralysis of orbicularis, i.e., lagophthalmos.

Swelling

Swelling of the lid can be unilateral or bilateral, with pain or without pain. The painful conditions are inflammation and infection of the subcutaneous tissue of the lid.
   The painless causes are allergies and new growths such as neurofibromatosis and hemangioma.

Pain and Tenderness

Pain in the lids is always secondary to infection, while tenderness, especially in the lid margin, is seen in stye and infected chalazion. The other causes are cellulitis of the lids and herpes zoster ophthalmicus.

Growth

Growths of the lid may be nonmalignant, like neurofibromatosis or hemangioma. The common malignant growths of the lid are epidermoid carcinoma, basal cell carcinoma, and adenocarcinoma of the tarsal glands.

Blepharospasm

This is the forceful closure of the lids on both sides, more common in children and generally associated with photophobia. This is a reflex, involuntary movement of all the lids. The causes are corneal foreign bodies, corneal injury, superficial keratitis, phlyctenular keratoconjunctivitis, and welding light injury (photo ophthalmia).
Note: The closure of lids is associated with another reflex called Bell's phenomenon. This is a protective mechanism to save the cornea from external invasion by foreign material. The reflex consists of the uprolling of the eyeball in an attempt to close the eyes. It is lost in paralysis of the third nerve but retained in facial palsy.

The lid is also examined under following heads:
(1) Skin of the lid; (2) Lid margin; (3) Action of: i. Levator; ii. Orbicularis; (4) Examination of IPA: i. Height; ii. Length
1. **Skin of the lid:** The skin of the lid is very loose and can be lifted from the underline orbicularis. The space under the skin is a common site for the accumulation of blood and exudate. The color of the skin changes in vitiligo, leprosy, ecchymosis of the lid, and hemangioma. The common causes of involvement are boils, furunculosis, rashes, ulcers, hematomas, and growths.
2. **Lid margin:** The lid margin extends from the skin of the lid to the posterior border of the lid. The anterior border is rounded, while the posterior border is sharp. The space between the two is the intramarginal strip on the anterior border, open the sebaceous glands along the lashes. The styes develop in the sebaceous, and the skin of the lid is examined for rashes and

swelling. The most common rashes are chickenpox, measles, and allergies. The most painful rashes are caused due to herpes zoster ophthalmicus, which developed in the distribution of the first part of the trigeminal. More common are the boils, which can be single or multiple.

The lid margin is examined for abnormalities in its position in the form of entropion and ectropion. The former is the inturning of the lid margin, and the other is the outturning of the lid margin. Absence of lashes is called madarosis, and rounding of the lid margin is called tylosis. Generally, madarosis is associated with tylosis.

The turning of the lashes is called trichiasis; the number of lashes turning in may be single, or all the lashes may be involved. The common causes of trichiasis are late stages of trachoma, leprosy, blepharitis, and acid and alkali burns.

The congenital anomalies of the lids are coloboma and adhesion, i.e., ankyloblepharon. The colobomas can be either in the upper or lower lid. They can be congenital or traumatic. Both types of coloboma may be present at any location on the lid margin. The congenital colobomas are generally on the medial side of the upper lid and deeper. The congenital colobomas of the lower lids are less frequent; they are broad and shallow. The surgical colobomas may be anywhere on the lid margin, may be partial or full-thickness, and the size may vary from a notch coloboma to a total avulsion.

Infection of the lid margin

The lid margin may be involved in infection, inflammation, infestation, and allergy. The above conditions are known broadly as blepharitis. The common infective disease of the lid margin is stye, the chalazion do not develop in the lid margin. The blepharitis can be ulcerative, squamous, or a combination of the two. Blepharitis is generally seen in two eyes. The upper lid is more involved. The two are differentiated by removing the crust on them; the ulcerative blepharitis develops fine hemorrhagic spots, while the squamous type does not show any blood.

3. **Action of: Levator and orbicularis**

    The levator is involved in the widening of the interpalpebral aperture; its ability to open the lids results in the drooping of the upper lid. Either due to true or pseudoptosis, the function of the orbicularis is to narrow the IPA. The ability to widen the IPA is called lagophthalmos.

4. **Examination of IPA: Height and length**

    The normal IPA in adults is 8.00 mm vertically in front of the cornea and 30.00 mm from canthus to canthus. The height is diminished in ptosis and pseudoptosis. The IPA is widened in lid retraction and lagophthalmos. The length is diminished in blepharophimosis, tarsorrhaphy, and ankyloblepharon. In blepharophimosis, both the width and length of the IPA are reduced.

EXAMINATION OF THE LACRIMAL SYSTEM

The lacrimal system is examined under the following heads: examination of the secretion systems and drainage system. The former requires examination less commonly than the latter. The examination of the drainage system consists of the examination of the puncta, canaliculi, and sac. Derangement of any kind leads to watering (epiphora). That is a prominent feature of the disorder of the lacrimal system. The other sign that requires examination is swelling of the sac.

EXAMINATION OF THE EYE WITH WATERING

The eyes are always wet due to the presence of normal tear film. A person is not aware of this wetness; when the person becomes aware of the tear, the condition is called watering from the eyes, that could be unilateral or bilateral, of short duration or chronic. Clinically, watering from the eyes has been divided into two groups, i.e., lacrimation and epiphora.

Lacrimation

Lacrimation is an active process of producing excess tears in the presence of normal drainage. Anything that irritates the fifth nerve supplying the eye will result in lacrimation. It can be unilateral or bilateral and is generally acute. The common causes are trauma to the cornea, corneal foreign bodies, superficial and deep keratitis, acute glaucoma, and photokeratitis.

Epiphora

Epiphora is a passive phenomenon due to a fault in the drainage system from the puncta to the nasolacrimal duct in the presence of normal tear production. Superadded lacrimation worsens epiphora. It is chronic in nature; the causes can be: ectropion of the lower lid, lagophthalmos, pinpoint lower puncta, obstruction in canaliculi, chronic inflammation of the sac, absence of the sac, and obstruction of the nasolacrimal duct.

Examination Case of Inflamed Sac (Dacryocystitis)

Dacryocystitis can be congenital or acquired; congenital dacryocystitis is less commonly acute. Chronic dacryocystitis is far more common than acute. Acute dacryocystitis is, in fact, a stage of pericystitis. Secondary to the chronic dacryocystitis, congenital dacryocystitis does not manifest before 2–3 weeks after birth. It is generally unilateral without acute signs; there is watering from the eye and supper-added infection results in mucopurulent discharge. The sac may be visibly enlarged, pressure over which causes regurgitation or discharge from both the puncta. The condition should be differentiated from ophthalmia neonatorum, which is hyperacute, bilateral conjunctivitis associated with purulent discharge manifesting within the first 10 days of life.

Chronic Dacryocystitis

It is seen in the third decade, more common in females, and may be bilateral without pain, swelling, or redness over the sac. The presence of the above points towards peridacryocystitis, for which the patient comes with pain and tenderness over the inflamed sac. Chronic dacryocystitis may complain of only watering from the eye. Sometimes the sac may be visibly distended, which, under pressure, produces mucopurulent discharge from the puncta. This is called regurgitation from the sac; the regurgitation is generally from both the puncta unless one of the canaliculi is also obstructed; obstruction of both canaliculi results in nonregurgitation. Regurgitation, if associated with a block in the nasolacrimal duct, the condition is called an encysted sac. The best way to find out the patency of the lacrimal passage is to put a bitter solution in the conjunctiva of the effected side. The best available drop is Chloromycetin drop. A person with a patent passage will feel a bitter taste at the back of the throat. Absence of bitter taste indicates obstruction in lacrimal passage from puncta to nasolacrimal duct. The other test is to inject saline in the lower puncta; in a patent passage, the person will immediately feel the saline in the throat. Non-passage of saline results in the regurgitation of saline from the puncta. The process of injecting saline into the lacrimal passage is called lacrimal syringing.

EXAMINATION OF THE ORBIT

The orbit is examined for two disorders: protrusion of the globe and retraction of the globe. The protrusion can be proptosis or exophthalmos. The retraction of the globe is called enophthalmos.

EXAMINATION OF A CASE OF PROPTOSIS

Proptosis is generally unilateral but may be bilateral. The common causes of bilateral proptosis are craniosynostosis, cavernous sinusitis, and bilateral orbital retinoblastoma.

Fully developed proptosis is easy to diagnose, the lids are retracted, the eye seems to be prominent, even to the extent of protrusion. The patient can close the lids over the prominent eyeball. Unless there is too much protrusion preventing lid closure, the protrusion can be examined clinically by the examiner standing behind the extended head of the patient and looking down at the eyebrows over closed lids. If the apex of the closed lid is visible beyond the eyebrows, it is a case of protrusion. Proptosis is measured by an instrument called an exophthalmometer. The causes of acquired proptosis are any mass in the orbit. The common masses that produce proptosis are new growths that may be malignant or nonmalignant, pus, blood, foreign bodies, and parasitic cysts.

Exophthalmos

The term exophthalmos is commonly used to denote the protrusion of the globe in thyroid diseases. It is a passive process due to the enlargement of extraocular muscles. The condition may develop on one side, only to involve the other side. The protrusion may not be equal on both sides; the protrusion is also measured by an exophthalmometer. Exophthalmos is more common after the second decade. It is more common in females. The earliest sign being lid retraction, mostly in the upper lid. Giving a staring look to the patient, the patient may complain of diplopia on examination. The extraocular muscle shows under action. The most common and earliest muscle to be involved is the inferior rectus. The conjunctiva is chemosed and congested.

EXAMINATION OF THE CONJUNCTIVA

The bulbar conjunctiva is the most prominent visible part of the three segments of the conjunctiva, the other two being the fornices and tarsal conjunctiva. The most common visible sign of conjunctival disorders is redness. The bulbar conjunctiva is examined by separating the lids between the index finger and thumb of the examiner with one hand and throwing the light with the other hand. The lower fornix is examined by pulling it down. This will also make the lower tarsal conjunctiva visible. The upper fornix is difficult to examine; the upper tarsal conjunctiva is examined by everting it. The normal conjunctiva is glossy, bright, transparent, and flush with the globe without any fluid or air underneath. The conjunctival vessels are few and visible; an increase in the number of vessels and dilated vessels constitutes congestion, which could be active; as in infection and inflammation, it may be generalized or localized. In passive congestion, the vessels are more dilated and fewer, as seen in raised venous pressure, thyroid orbitopathy, and absolute glaucoma. The conjunctiva is examined for discharge, congestion, discoloration, scars, papillae, follicles, foreign bodies, growths, fluid, and air under the conjunctiva. Fluid under the conjunctiva is called chemosis and air under the conjunctiva is called emphysema, membrane, and nodules.

Discharge

The causes of discharge from the eyes are: infective conjunctivitis, bacterial viral allergy, or chemical. The discharge in bacterial conjunctivitis is mucoid; it becomes mucopurulent and purulent if the infection is severe. The discharge in viral conjunctivitis without a superadded bacterial infection is watery; in allergic conjunctivitis, the discharge is watery; and in spring catarrh, it is ropy as well.

Congestion

A red eye is an indication of conjunctival congestion. The two types of congestion are conjunctival and circumciliary. The circumciliary congestion is always seen round the limbus due to inflammation of the cornea or anterior uvea. The conjunctival congestion can be generalized, which is more often than localized. The causes of generalized congestion are acute and chronic conjunctivitis. The causes of localized congestion are circumciliary, local injury, phlycten, episcleritis, scleritis, pterygium and growth.

Discoloration

The normal conjunctiva is transparent with few blood vessels; it can be moved over the sclera. The common causes of discoloration are: conjunctival melanosis (black), jaundice (yellow), subconjunctival hemorrhage (red), Bitot's spots (white), and xerosis (dirty white). The commonest cause of discoloration is subconjunctival hemorrhage.

Subconjunctival Hemorrhage

The subconjunctival hemorrhage is most alarming as it stands out prominently against the white background of the sclera. The subconjunctival hemorrhage is always acute and painless. Hemorrhage under the lids may not be visible. The subconjunctival hemorrhage can be generalized or localized. The generalized subconjunctival hemorrhage is divided into two types, i.e., when its outer border is visible. This is caused due to localized trauma; if the outer border is not visible, the cause is either in the skull or orbit in the form of injury.

The other cause of subconjunctival congestion is the sudden rise of intrathoracic pressure, as in whooping cough in children, and sudden compression of the chest. The subconjunctival hemorrhage is not likely to be infectious. Simple subconjunctival hemorrhage passes of without any treatment.

Scar

The conjunctiva, due to its good blood supply, heals promptly without scarring. However, if the edges of the wound are turned in, the conjunctiva develops a scar. This is common in bulbar conjunctiva. The scar in the tarsal conjunctiva is a combination of fibrous tissue of the conjunctiva and subconjunctival tissue of the tarsal plate. It cannot be moved over the tarsal plate. The commonest cause is trachoma, it has an irregular shape. The meibomian glands are visible under unscared conjunctiva.

Papillae

Papillae are large, polygonal, flat-toped structures consisting mainly of fine blood vessels encased in conjunctival epithelium. They are more numerous and larger in the upper tarsus, varying in number. They are diagnostics of spring catarrh and giant papillary conjunctivitis.

Follicles

Follicles are collections of lymphoid tissue under the conjunctival epithelium surrounded by capillaries; they are round bodies 0.5–2.00 mm in diameter. They are seen in follicular conjunctivitis, trachoma, and chemical conjunctivitis. Follicles are not seen in children under three months due to the absence of lymphoid tissues.

Membrane

In some cases of conjunctivitis, a thin layer of fibrinous material develops on the surface of the conjunctiva. This is called the conjunctival membrane, and it generally develops in severe conjunctivitis. However, it may develop in mild bacterial conjunctivitis. The common bacteria that cause membranous conjunctivitis are Corynebacterium diphtheria, beta-hemolytic streptococci, staphylococcus aureus, Neisseria gonorrhoeae, pneumococci, chlamydia, and adenovirus. Even noninfectious conditions like spring catarrh can produce membranes. The membrane generally develops in the lower fornix. Clinically, conjunctival membranes have been divided into two types, i.e., true and pseudomembrane. True membranes develop when exudate penetrates the superficial layer of the conjunctival epithelium. If this membrane is tried to be removed, the surface under the membrane bleeds. This differentiates it from pseudomembrane, where coagulated material develops over the conjunctival membrane without penetrating it and can be removed easily.

Nodules

The nodules on the conjunctiva can be infective, inflammatory, allergic, degenerative, or neoplastic.

The following are the common nodules seen on the conjunctiva: phlycten, episcleritis, scleritis, pinguecula, foreign body granuloma, infective granuloma, and adenocarcinoma.

Characteristics of Conjunctival Congestion

The conjunctival congestion develops from the fornix towards the cornea, bright red in color; the vessels are dilated, numerous, and irregular; there is no pain in pressing the globe. It is seen in conjunctivitis of all types. Generally associated with discharge.

Circumciliary Congestion

Is a localized congestion that develops round the cornea. It starts from the limbus, spreading towards the periphery without reaching the periphery. Circumciliary congestion may be all-round the limbus or in a sector. It is associated with ciliary tenderness and keratic precipitate (KP). It is seen in keratitis, acute and chronic iridocyclitis, but not in posterior uveitis. It is also seen in acute congestive glaucoma.

Episcleral Congestion

The third type of congestion of the eye is episcleral congestion due to the involvement of episcleral vessels. The congestion starting from the periphery, proceeding towards the limbus, not reaching it, and branches on either side, anastomosing with the vessels on each side, thus forming a circle called caput medusae.

Bitot's Spots

Bitot's spots are noninflammatory degeneration of the superficial layer of conjunctiva in the form of a white, raised, triangular area with the apex away from the limbus. They develop between the limbus and the canthus, more commonly on the lateral side. They are foamy raised spots; the foam can be wiped off with a swab only to reappear at the same place. They are composed of keratin and the gas-forming bacteria Corynebacterium xerosis. They are mostly associated with vitamin A deficiency and are rarely seen in conditions without vitamin A deficiency. The bitot spot developing in vitamin A deficiency disappears with the administration of vitamin A. The other type is not cured by vitamin A deficiency.

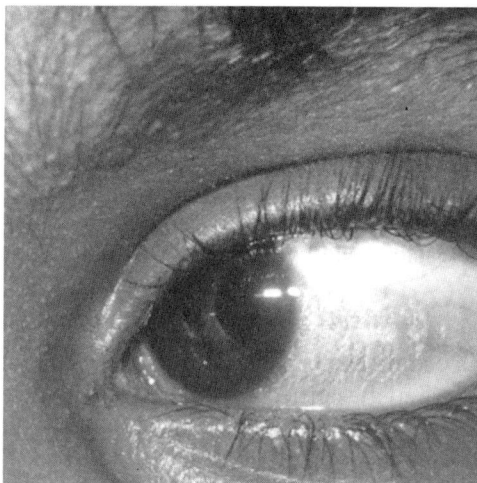

Fig. 5.25: Xerosis of conjunctiva. *(For color version, see Plate 1)*

Xerosis of Conjunctiva

Xerosis, or dryness conjunctiva, is mostly due to vitamin A deficiency. Otherwise, they are seen in milder form in dry eye syndrome or exposure of the conjunctiva in the large coloboma of the upper lid.

Mostly seen on the lateral side. The conjunctiva loses its lustre and wetness. It has a dirty white appearance with vertical lines in the conjunctiva. Xerosis is caused by diminished mucin secretion following the loss of goblet cells **(Fig. 5.25)**.

EXAMINATION OF THE GLOBE AND SCLERA

The globe consists of the cornea and the sclera. The cornea is a transparent, colorless, and nonvascular optical part of the globe with the primary function of converging rays; its second function is protection of intraocular structures. The sclera is a larger part of the globe; it is opaque without any optical function. The function of the sclera is protective and acts as an attachment for extraocular muscles. The blood vessels and nerves pass through the sclera without supplying it. Due to its opaqueness, it keeps the inside of the eye dark. The junction between the cornea and the sclera is the limbus. The globe is covered by the conjunctiva anteriorly and Tenon's capsules behind. The globe is surrounded by orbital fat; the optic nerve enters the globe at the posterior part. The globe is examined for its size, shape, color, and protrusion of intraocular structures (staphyloma).

Size

The adult globe (eyeball) has a diameter of 24.00 mm; the size at birth is 16.00 mm. Eyeballs smaller than 16.00 mm at birth are called microphthalmos; a globe smaller than 24.00 mm in adults is called an enophthalmos; and a small, soft, irregular eyeball is called phthisis bulbi. The large globe is called megalophthalmos; the other cause of the large globe is buphthalmos, which may be congenital or acquired.

Shape

The globe is spherical in shape. The globe loses its shape when it becomes soft or when intraocular structures protrude through it. The protrusion is called scleral staphyloma. The soft eye loses its spherical shape and becomes quadrilateral with an oval cornea of proportionate size.

Colors

The normal color of the sclera is marble white; at birth, due to its thinness, it has a blue tinge. The sclera sometimes has black patches scattered. The black patches are called melanosis bulbi. That can be congenital or acquired. They are noninfective and non-neoplastic. The other cause of the change in color in the sclera is scleral staphyloma.

Staphyloma

Staphylomas are defined as ectatic cicatrization of the outer coat of the globe with the uvea incarcerated. It is called total when the cornea and sclera are both involved. Otherwise, it can be corneal or scleral. The scleral staphylomas are black in color and covered by conjunctiva.

EXAMINATION OF CORNEA

The cornea is examined under the following heads:

Shape

The cornea looks circular when seen from the front. It becomes horizontally elliptical in a soft eye and quadrilateral in phthisis.

Size

Adult cornea is 10.63 mm vertically and 11.35 mm horizontally. In newborns, it is 10.00 mm in both meridians. Cornea smaller than 10.00 mm is called microcornea, generally seen in microphthalmos; a diameter more than 11.5 mm is called megalocornea, seen as a congenital anomaly, and in buphthalmos. Any cornea larger than 13.00 mm is abnormal and should be investigated.

Curvature

The average curvature of the cornea is 8.00 mm. The vertical curvature is slightly more. The corneal curvature is increased in keratoconus, megalocornea, and buphthalmos. The corneal curvature is flattened in phthisis and microcornea. The corneal curvature is roughly examined by oblique illumination; for finer changes in corneal curvature, it should be measured by a keratometer.

Surface

The anterior surface of the cornea is bright and smooth. It acts as a convex mirror, forming an erect, small virtual image in front of the cornea. The image moves with the movement of the object. The cornea becomes irregular in pterygium, keratoconus, corneal opacity, limbal dermoid, iris prolapse, keratoplasty, keratectasia, staphyloma, and soft eye. The irregularity of the surface can be seen on a Placido disc ophthalmoscope mounted with a Placido disc-like attachment.

Transparency

The cornea should be transparent to form a sharp focus; diminished transparency reduces vision. The loss of transparency is called corneal opacity that may develop at any layer of the cornea.

More than one layer may be involved; sometimes all the layers are affected with or without iris incarceration. Incarceration of the iris to the opacity is called leucoma adherence. Depending on the layer of cornea involved, the opacities are called: nebula, macula, and leucoma. The nebula is the faintest, not visible without magnification. The macular is denser than the nebula visible on focal illumination. Leucoma is the densest and most visible, not only in oblique illumination but also in normal light. It is possible that an eye under examination has more than one type of opacity. The opacities do not stain. The sensation over the opacity is reduced; the corneal opacities generally do not change in size. The corneal opacities may be unilateral or bilateral, when bilateral need not be symmetrical.

Topographic Recording of Corneal Opacity

It is better to draw a diagram of the corneal opacity under the following heads: number of opacities, position, size, grade, staining, vascularization, pigment in the opacity, and incarceration of the iris in the opacity.

Sensation

Cornea is one of the most sensitive parts of the body. The only sensation that a cornea has is pain. That can be abolished by a local anesthetic agent; there is no condition where the cornea is hypersensitive. The cornea is richly supplied by pain-sensitive nerves, which are terminal branches of the fifth nerve. The corneal sensation is tested by a wisp of cotton brought from the lateral side. In a cornea with normal sensation, the touch will cause the lids to close.

Staining

Normal cornea is shining and does not stain with any vital stain. The common stains used are: Fluorescein, Rose Bengal, and Lissamine green. The most commonly used stain is fluorescein, and Lissamine green is the least commonly used. Fluorescein for staining is available as an impregnated, autoclaved strip in a sterile pack **(Fig. 5.26)** for single use. To stain the cornea, the stained end of the strip is put in the lower fornix, and the patient is asked to close the eye for a few seconds. After that, the strip is removed, and the conjunctival sac is washed. The cornea is examined under oblique illumination; large stained areas are visible under simple torch light. However, faint stains require examination under a slit lamp with a cobalt blue filter.

Rose Bengal

Rose Bengal is another stain used to stain not only the cornea but also the conjunctiva. The stain causes severe burning; hence, it requires the installation of a local anesthetic agent before putting on the strip. The stain does not require any filter; it is examined under white light. It stains mucus as well. It is frequently used in dry eye syndrome. Staining with a combination of Rose Bengal and fluorescein is called differential staining.

Lissamine Green

Lissamine green is used less frequently. It stains the ulcer light green; it is difficult to see under white or cobalt blue light. It is best appreciated against a dark iris. It is frequently used in dry eye syndrome.

Thickness

The curvature of the cornea is not equal for both surfaces; the posterior surface is more curved. This causes an unequal thickness of the cornea. The cornea is thinnest at the center and thickest

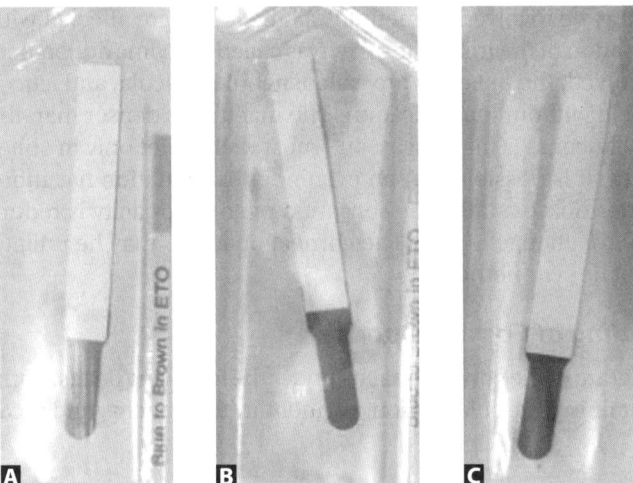

Figs. 5.26A to C: Various types of staining strip: (A) Fluorescein; (B) Rose Bengal; (C) Lissamine green.

at the limbus. The simple method of measuring the unequal thickness is to throw a thin, bright beam of light from the slit lamp and compare the illuminated thickness with the depth of the anterior chamber at the periphery. The accurate measurement is done on an instrument called a pachometer that can be optical or ultrasonic.

Vascularization

For all practical purposes, the cornea is nonvascular except at the limbus. The vascularization of the cornea is always pathological. The vascularization has been divided into three groups, i.e., superficial, deep, and retrocorneal. The superficial vascularization is the most common out of the three, and the last is the least frequent. The superficial congestion is caused by the extension of conjunctival vessels on the surface of the cornea; the vessels are large, thick, and tortuous. They may anastomos with each other. The deep vessels are from ciliary vessels, hence not visible at the limbus. They are thin and parallel to each other without anastomosing. They develop at the level of stroma in sectors. They are best seen under the magnification of slit lamps generally associated with KPs.

The retrocorneal vascularization may be corneal (intracorneal) or retinal. The retrocorneal vessels are in fact either conjunctival or retinal and have found their way in or behind the cornea following an injury to the limbus. The retinal vessels are ciliary in nature; they grow from the ciliary body to the back surface of the iris, passing the pupil, and upon the anterior surface of the iris, terminating at the angle.

Deposits

The corneal deposit can be superficial, deep, or on the back of the cornea. The common superficial deposits are foreign bodies, band keratopathy, marks of keratoplastic, and tattoos. The deep opacities are caused by foreign bodies: Krukenberg spindle, Hudson-Stahli line, Fleischer ring, Kayser-Fleischer ring, siderosis, and chalcosis. The commonest deposits on the posterior surface are KPs and blood (blood staining of the cornea).

EXAMINATION OF THE ANTERIOR CHAMBER

The anterior chamber is a space between the posterior surface of the cornea in front and the anterior surface of the iris and lens posteriorly in a normal eye. In pseudophakia, the lens is replaced by IOL, and vitreous in aphakia. The junction of the periphery of the cornea and iris is called the angle of the anterior chamber. The depth of the anterior chamber is maximum in front of the pupil. The anterior chamber is shallow in newborns. The normal depth is 3.5 mm in the emmetropic eye. The anterior chamber is examined for its depth and contents. The anterior chamber is shallow with narrow-angle glaucoma, swollen lenses, and microphthalmos. The anterior chamber is deep in aphakia, keratoconus, and buphthalmos. The anterior chamber depth is irregular in adherent leucoma, iris bombe, iris prolapse, and tumors of the iris. The angle of the anterior chamber is measured by an instrument called a gonioscope. The angle is said to be normal if it is 45° wide; if it is >45°, it is called wide; and an angle less than 45 degrees is called narrow.

The normal content of the anterior chamber is aqueous. The abnormal contents are blood (hyphema), pus (hypopyon), dislocated lens, cortical matter, ACIOL, dislocated PCIOL, gas, silicone oil, malignant cells, parasites, and foreign bodies. White material other than pus is called pseudohypopyon.

EXAMINATION OF THE UVEA

Out of the three layers of the uvea, only the iris is visible for direct inspection. The other parts are examined by special instruments like a direct and indirect ophthalmoscope, three mirror gonioscopes, and +70D to +90D lenses. The examination of the iris consists of an examination of the iris and pupil. The iris is examined for its color, surface defect (coloboma), vessels on the surface, and nodules.

The color of the iris ranges between brown and black. The iris is light-colored in albinos. There may be atrophic patches on the iris that look white. The difference in color of the iris is called heterochromia, which can be a complete heterochromia called heterochromia iridis. Sectorial heterochromia is called heterochromia iridum. The surface of the iris is rough; this is called the rugosity of the iris. The iris loses its roughness when swollen, as in acute iritis and acute glaucoma.

Coloboma of the Iris

The term coloboma denotes the absence of tissue in the iris. The coloboma may be partial, i.e., in the substance of the iris, or it may involve the iris from the pupillary margin to the root. **Figure 5.27** shows different types of coloboma iris.

Vessels on the Surface of the Iris

The surface of the iris has no visible blood vessels. The presence of blood vessels on the surface and at the angle is pathological. The blood vessels on the iris are in fact retinal blood vessels that travel over the choroid and ciliary, reaching the posterior surface of the iris, then passing through the pupillary margin and travelling over the surface to and in the angle. The neovascularization of the iris is an indication of severe retinopathy and a cause of nontraumatic hyphema.

Nodules on the Iris

The nodules on the iris can be inflammatory, commonly seen in leprosy, tuberculosis, and syphilis. It may develop on a foreign body or maybe a new growth.

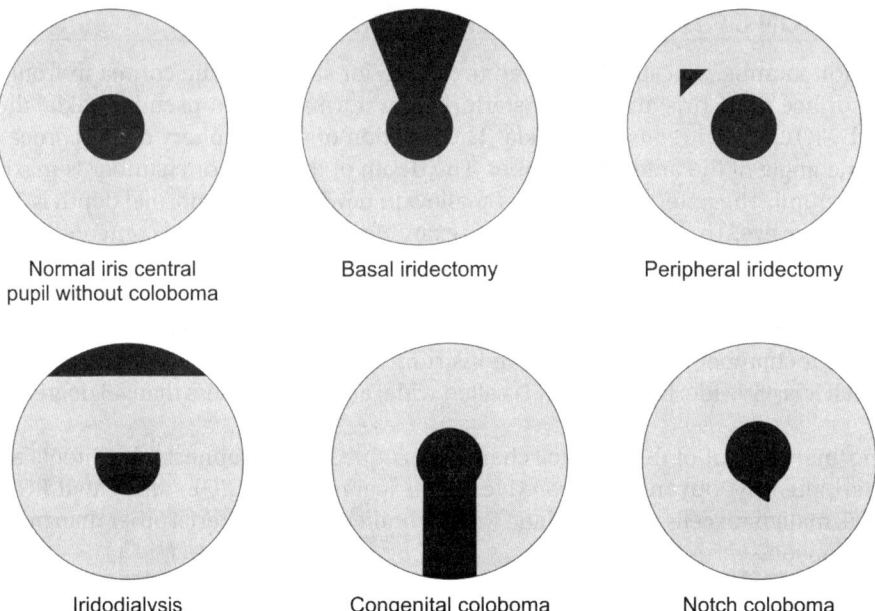

Fig. 5.27: Different types of coloboma iris.

EXAMINATION OF THE PUPILLARY MARGIN

The examination of the iris is incomplete without the examination of the pupil. The normal pupil is central, circular, and reacts briskly to light and accommodation. The pupil is examined for position, number, size, shape, color, and reaction.

Position

The change in position of the pupil may be congenital or acquired. The congenital shift of the pupil is called correctopia. The acquired causes are trauma and infection. The other causes are chronic iridocyclitis, prolapse of the iris, and adherent leukoma.

Number

Under normal conditions, there is only one pupil in each eye. The number may be more than one in a congenital anomaly called polycoria. The congenital polycoria has its own independent constrictor and dilator muscles and reacts to light. The acquired colobomas may be surgical or traumatic and are labelled as pseudopolycoria.

Size

The normal size of the pupil in adults is about 2.5 mm in diameter. It is small for newborns and old pupils. A pupil smaller than 2.5 mm is called miotic, and a larger pupil is called mydriatic. The commonest cause of miotic pupils is the instillation of miotic drugs; the commonest cause of mydriatic pupils is the instillation of mydriatic. The pupil is small in iritis and iridocyclitis and large in optic atrophy and chronic glaucoma.

Shape

The normal pupil is circular; it becomes irregular in diseases of the iris. The common cause of irregular pupils is the development of adhesion between the posterior surface iris and lens. Such adhesions are called posterior synechiae; the adhesion between the anterior surface of the iris and the posterior surface of the cornea is called anterior synechia, which can be peripheral when the adhesion is at an angle. Otherwise called central when away from the angle, generally posterior synechiae cause constriction of the pupil; when mydriatic is applied, the pupil becomes festooned **(Figs. 5.27 and 5.28)**, with the iris still attached to the lens.

The number of synechiae may vary from single to multiple. If the adhesion is all-round, the condition is called ring synechiae, which does not dilate with strong mydriatic. The ring synechiae prevent the passage of aqueous from the posterior to the anterior chamber. Thus, it is called seclusio pupillae; the entrapped aqueous pushes the iris forward in a bow shape. The condition is called iris bombe, causing the anterior chamber to be of irregular depth. If the constricted, nondilating pupil is covered by a layer of exudate, the condition is called occlusio pupillae. The other causes of irregular pupils are traumatic miosis, coloboma of the iris, and persistent pupillary membranes. The causes of anterior synechiae are chronic iridocyclitis, chronic secondary glaucoma, soft eye, and adherent leukoma.

Color

The black color of the eye is due to the color of the iris; the pupil, which is the center of the iris, is still darker. The normal pupil shows third and fourth Purkinje images and looks bright; the color of the pupil changes in various disorders. It is faint white in immature cataracts, pearly white in immature cataracts, and jet black in complete lens removal. The other cause of white pupils is retinoblastoma, which is called leukocoria.

Reaction

The normal pupil becomes small in bright light and large in dim light. The constriction of the pupil on which light has been directed is called a direct reaction. The constriction of the other simultaneously and equally is called an indirect reaction. In normal eyes, both direct and indirect reactions should be present and brisk. In a normal person, the pupil should constrict to 1.00 mm in the presence of bright light and remain so until the light is present. As soon as the light is removed, the pupil dilates to its original position. This is called a brisk pupillary reaction. If the pupil constricts slowly, it is called a sluggish pupil. The causes of sluggish pupils are dull light, recent use of mydriatic, ingestion of drugs that dilate the pupil, optic atrophy, and advanced glaucoma.

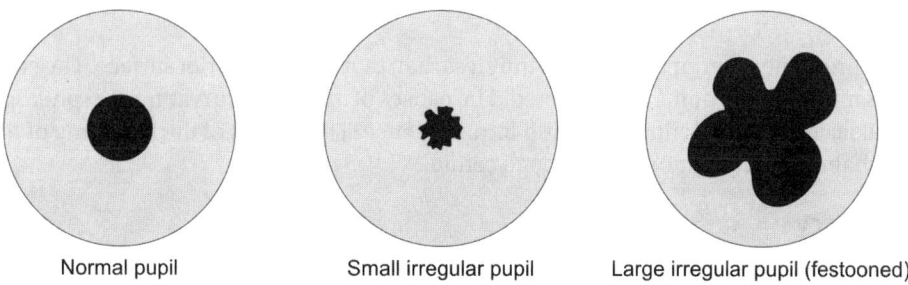

Fig. 5.28: Constricted irregular and dilated irregular pupil.

EXAMINATION OF THE LENS

Lens is one of the converging systems of the eye. It is placed behind the iris in front of the vitreous, suspended by a suspensory ligament (zonule) all around, which are attached to the ciliary body, contraction, and relaxation of the ciliary body result in a change in the curvature of the lens. The lens at birth is almost spherical, which gradually flattens to become ellipsoid in adulthood. The normal lens is transparent, but its transparency decreases as the person ages. The front surface of the lens acts as a convex mirror, forming a virtual, small, erect image. The back surface acts as a concave mirror, forming a real inverted image. These images are called Purkinje third and fourth images, which are abolished in the absence of a lens from the pupillary area. The iris casts a shadow on the anterior surface of the lens, which is best seen in immature cataracts but is absent in immature cataracts. The iris shadow is also absent in aphakia. Any opacity in the substance of the lens is called a cataract. The opacities in the lens are white. If the opacity extends from capsule to capsule all-round, it is called mature cataract; otherwise, it is referred to as immature cataract.

The only function of the lens is visual, which is examined under distant vision, near vision, color vision, and contrast. Diminished distant vision is the most common symptom of cataract. A central nuclear opacity causes myopia. The patients may present with increasing diminished distant vision and improved near vision. A patient of presbyopic age may say that he can see better without his reading glasses in spite of diminished distant vision.

Posterior polar opacities are most troublesome. It becomes worse in bright light; it does not improve with PH. The lens is examined under the following headings: presence, position, curvature, and transparency.

Presence

Present or absent, the former is called phakia, and later aphakia. The phakic eye may be transparent or opaque (cataract), which could be complete and called mature cataract, or incomplete when partially called immature cataract. Similarly, the lens may be totally absent in the pupillary area or partially. The examples are subluxated lenses and cataracts.

Position

Normal, dislocated, subluxated, and absent. A lens is called dislocated when it is totally absent from the pupillary area but not from the eye. A lens is called subluxated when it is partially present in the pupillary area.

Curvature

The curvature of the anterior surface is slightly less than that of the posterior surface. The curvature of the lens may increase or may be flattened. The causes of increased curvature are spherophakia, microphakia, lenticonus, lentiglobus, and intumescence. The causes of the flattening of the lens are buphthalmos, dehydration, and hypoglycemia.

Transparency

The normal lens is transparent. The presence of opacity is always abnormal; it could be congenital or acquired. The commonest acquired cause of lenticular opacity is age-related cataract. The cataract may be localized or generalized **(Fig. 5.29)**.

The opacities in the lens look white on oblique illumination; they look black on retinoscopy. The immature cataract is an opacity that does not extend from capsule to capsule in all directions. Its two main types are nuclear and cortical; the former develops in the center, and the latter spreads from the periphery towards the center in advanced stages. Both merge, and the condition is called mature cataract. The mature cataract, if not removed, passes on to the hypermature stage, assuming a pearly white color.

Table 5.2 shows the difference between immature and mature cataracts.

One condition that requires differentiation from immature cataracts is chronic simple glaucoma.

The difference between the two is given at **Table 5.3**.

The cataracts can be unilateral or bilateral and not symmetrical. In cases of unilateral, the other eye may show little change or may be normal; in such cases, the eye with cataracts should be investigated for the possibility of injury or uveitis in the past. The cataract can be simple or complicated. A cataract is said to be complicated when it has evidence of other diseases, like injury, uveitis, and glaucoma. A cataract is labelled as hypermature when the cortex is liquefied and the nucleus sinks below. The sunken nucleus has a brown tinge. The condition is also called Morgagnian cataract (MC).

Subluxation and Dislocation of the Lens

The lens is suspended by the zonules behind the iris, in front of the vitreous. The function of the zonules is to keep the lens in place. If some of the zonules are absent, the lens shifts from its position away from the absent zonules; this condition is called subluxation of the lens. If all the zonules are absent, the lens falls either back in the vitreous or in the aqueous; this condition is called dislocation of the lens. Shifting of the lens from its normal position is called ectopia lentis and can be congenital or acquired. The common causes of acquired ectopia are blunt injury,

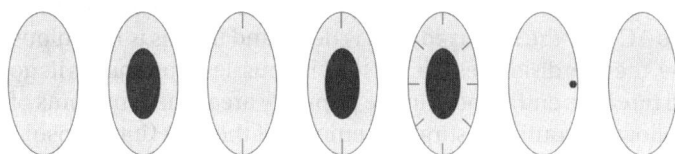

Various types of lenticular opacities seen from side

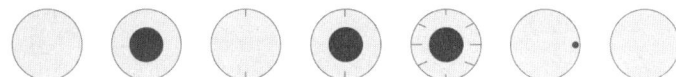

The same opacities seen from front

Fig. 5.29: Cataract.

Table 5.2: Difference between immature and mature cataracts.		
Feature	Immature cataract	Mature cataract
Vision	6/60 to CF and good projection	HM to PL and good projection
Color of pupil	Grey	Pearly white
Iris shadow	Present	Absent
Retinoscope	Pink glow from side of the opacity	No glow

Table 5.3: Difference between immature cataracts and chronic simple glaucoma.

Feature	Immature cataract	Chronic simple glaucoma
Age	Generally past fifty years	Generally past fifty years
Laterality	Bilateral	Bilateral
Vision	Diminished	Diminished
Cornea	Bright	Bright
AC	Normal	Normal
Pupillary reaction	Brisk	Sluggish
Pupil	Central circular, normal in size	Central circular, large
Lens	Opaque	May be opaque
Fundus	Normal when visible	Glaucomatous change
Tension	Normal	Raised
Diurnal variation	Negative	Positive
Water drinking test	Negative	Positive
Difference in tension between the two eyes	Not more than 5.00 mm	More than 7.00 mm
Field changes	No change	Typical change

long-standing uveitis, and buphthalmos. The place in the pupil without a lens is called aphakia. The lens, when grossly displaced, can be diagnosed by oblique illumination. A minor subluxation requires complete dilation of the pupil. In subluxation of the lens, the aphakic area gives a pink glow on retinoscopy. The pupil looks jet black in oblique illumination. The edge of the lens gives a bright reflex. The AC over the subluxed area is deep, and the iris is tremulous.

Most of the time, the lens dislocates back in the vitreous; less common is its going in the anterior chamber; and still rare is its entrapment in the pupillary area. The symptoms of dislocated lenses are the same as following complete surgical removal of the lens (intracapsular lens extraction); they are diminished distant vision less than CF 3 feet, no near vision deep anterior chamber, tremulous iris, jet black pupil, absent iridectomy, hypermetropia without accommodation fundus normally unless there is pre-existing pathology. The vision may improve with high hypermetropic correction.

Aphakia

Aphakia is the total or partial absence of a lens in the pupillary area. The commonest cause is surgical removal; if the lens is removed completely, it is called intracapsular lens extraction; if part of the lens is left behind without the nucleus, it is called extracapsular lens extraction. Examples of extracapsular lens extraction are needling, aspiration, classical extracapsular lens extraction, and phacoemulsification. If an IOL is put in the eye, the condition is called pseudophakia. The IOL may be put in the anterior chamber or in the posterior chamber.

Symptoms

Symptoms of surgical aphakia consist of greatly diminished distant vision and absent near vision. Both of which are correctable optically when there is no other cause that can be related to non-improvement.

Signs

Signs of aphakia are the presence of a surgical scar, a deep anterior chamber, tremulousness of the iris, a jet black pupil exceptfollowingextracapsular lens extraction where the posterior capsule with some cortex is left behind the condition is called after cataracts. Surgical aphakia is invariably associated with iridectomy, and a high error of refraction, which is generally associated with astigmatism. The glasses required generally are +10 DSph with +1 DCyl to +2 DCyl at 180°, with the addition of +3 DSph for near.

Pseudophakia

Pseudophakia is a condition where the lens has been removed and an artificial lens has replaced it. The replaced lens is often referred to as the IOL. The IOL may be placed either in the anterior chamber or in the posterior chamber. This can follow either manual extracapsular lens extraction or phacoemulsification. The anterior chamber lenses can be placed both following intracapsular and extracapsular lens extraction.

The features of IOL are:
- There is a history of surgery.
- The scar from the surgery is very small.
- The anterior chamber is deeper than normal but not as deep as the aphakia.
- The iris is not tremulous.
- Generally, there is no iridectomy.
- The lens can be either in front of the iris or behind the iris.
- The pupil is centrally circular.
- The papillary area has a glassy look.
- The Purkinje images are brighter than normal transparent lenses.
- The distant vision may be normal or less than normal, which requires glasses.
- The accommodation is absent and requires correction.

EXAMINATION OF THE SQUINT (STRABISMUS)

Squint is a condition where both eyes do not point in the same direction. It also means misaligned eyes. The eye loses parallelism; it can be congenital or acquired. The children are more affected by squints. The child may be brought with an obvious squint of various degrees in one eye or alternately in two eyes. Bilateral squint is rare and, when present, is congenital in origin.

There are two types of squint, i.e., latent heterophorias and manifest heterotropias. Neither the patient nor the onlookers are aware of the latent squint. It is diagnosed only by an expert. The manifest squint or tropias can either be non-paralytic or paralytic. The non-paralytic squint is called the concomitant squint. The following chart shows various types of manifest squints **(Flowchart 5.4)**.

Some Terms Used in Concomitant Squint

- It is an obvious squint; the onlooker may make out its presence, but rarely are the patients aware of it, especially in paralytic squints.
- The deviating eye is called the squinting eye, and the non-squinting eye is called the fixing eye.

Flowchart 5.4: Various types of squint.

```
                          Squint
                            │
              ┌─────────────┴─────────────┐
         Pseudo-squint                True squint
                                          │
                              ┌───────────┴───────────┐
                         Manifest                   Latent
                         (Tropia)                   (Phoria)
                             │                         │
              ┌──────────────┼──────────┐       ┌──┬──┬─────┬─────┐
         Unilateral   Alternate comitant  Bilateral  Eso Exo Hyper Cyclo
              │              │                │         │
        ┌─────┴─────┐        │           Con-comitant  Non-comitant
   Con-comitant Non-comitant │                           (Rare)
        │           │        │
   ┌──┬─┴─┬─────┐   │    Paralytic   Restrictive
   Eso Exo Hyper Cyclo
```

Note: *Pseudo-squint is a state of false squints where the eyes appear to be squinting without it really being so; the eyes are straight in primary position with normal parallelism not moving under cover. It is a congenital bilateral-symmetrical condition. The commonest cause is bilateral epicanthus. It can be convergent or divergent; the former is more common. Most of the pseudo-squints due to the epicanthic fold disappear with age, even without treatment.*

- When one eye habitually squints, the condition is called uniocular squint. That may be right or left.
- In some cases, the squint changes sides. The patient may have a right squint sometimes, and the left eye is straight and fixed. Sometimes the left eye squints and the right eye deviates by the same degree in the same direction. This is called an alternate squint. The squint may be present at some hours of the day and straight at others; this is called intermittent squint.
- If the eye deviates inward, manifest squint is called esotropia **(Fig. 5.30)**, and external manifest squint is called exotropia **(Fig. 5.31)**. Similarly, upward deviation is called hypertropia **(Fig. 5.32)**, and downward deviation is called hypotropia.

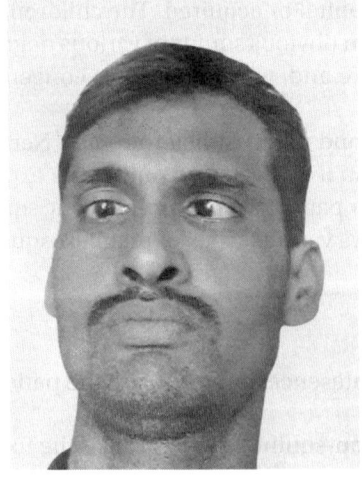

Fig. 5.30: Esotropia.

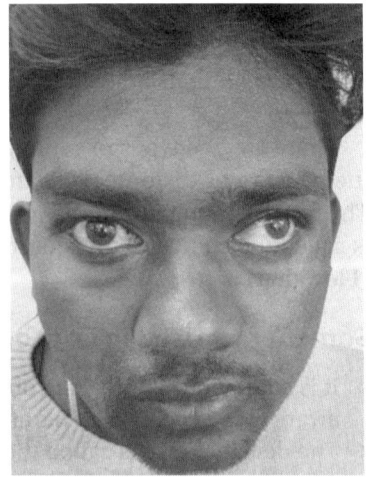

Fig. 5.31: Exotropia.

- The deviation of the squint is measured by the following methods:
    i. Corneal reflex test (Hirschberg test*).
    ii. Prism Bar
    iii. Synoptophore

Hirschberg test*
The test is a simple outdoor procedure that should be performed on each patient with or without ocular deviation. It does not require any special instrument; all that is required is a bright torch light focused on a pinpoint. The patient sits at a distance of 1 meter from the examiner; his head is kept straight, and his eyes are immobile. Both eyes are kept open. The examiner throws the pinpoint light into the cornea or the patient; in a patient without a squint, the light gives a white, shining image in the center of the pupil. The image formed away from the center denotes a concomitant squint. If the image is formed on the lateral side, the eye is deviated inward (esotropia), and vice versa, in cases of upward deviation, the image is formed below. The deviation is measured by the amount of shift in the reflex. If the image is formed in the center of the pupil, there is no deviation. If it is at the pupillary margin, the deviation is 20°, the image at the limbus shows a deviation of 40°, and beyond the limbus, the deviation is more than 45° (**Fig. 5.33**).

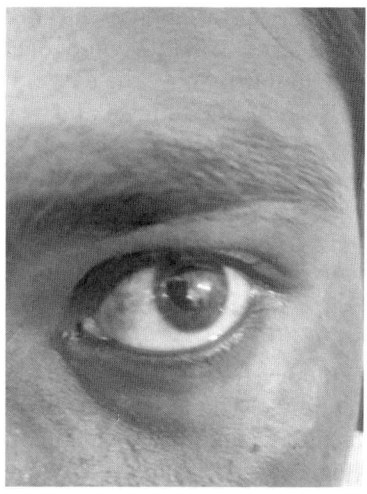

Fig. 5.32: Hypertropia.

Symptoms of Heterotropia

- Obvious squint
- Diminished vision
    - Generally, uniocular tropia has diminished vision that can either be corrected or not corrected by glasses. The correction with glasses may partially or completely eliminate squints. The commonest cause of non-improved vision is untreated amblyopia.
    - In an alternate squint, either there is no visual loss or the loss of vision is minimal and equal in both eyes.
    - Diplopia: diplopia is one of the commonest symptoms of paralytic squint.

Characteristics of the Paralytic Squint

1. Sudden onset
2. Diplopia

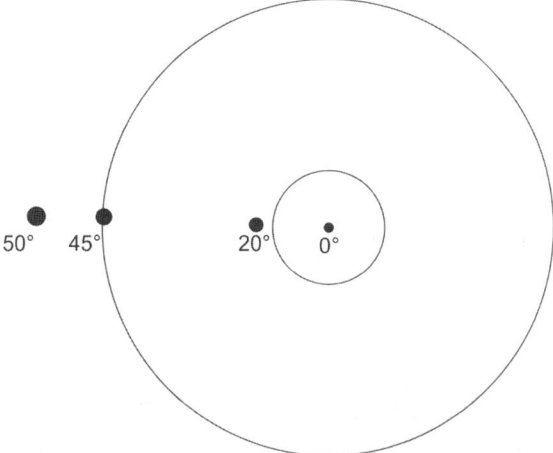

Fig. 5.33: Angle of deviation as measured by corneal reflexes (Hirschberg test).

- Obvious deviation of the affected eye
- Restriction of movement of the involved muscle
- Inability to move the eye equally in all directions
- Turning and tilting of the head
- Elevation or depression of the chin
- Head ache, vomiting, and giddiness

The primary deviation is the deviation of the squinting eye when the non-squinting eye fixes an object; the secondary deviation is the deviation of the sound eye when the squinting eye is forced to fix an object. The secondary deviation is greater than the primary deviation.

Charting of Diplopia

Diplopia charting is required to pin point the muscle involved to record progress and for future reference. The Hess chart is most suitable for the process **(Fig. 5.8)**. The other method of recording diplopia is on a diplopia chart that divides the field into nine quadrants, as shown in **(Fig. 5.34)**.

To chart diplopia, the patient puts on a diplopia glass consisting of one red and one green glass. As shown in image **(Fig. 5.35)**.

The patient puts the red glass in front of the right eye and the green glass in front of the left eye and looks at a lighted candle held by the examiner standing 3–4 feet away. To the right eye, the flame looks red, and to the left eye, it looks green. The image that disappears by closing one eye is called the false image.

The patient is asked to look straight without turning or tilting the head; he is instructed to follow the movement of the lighted candle; and he is asked to say if the two images are superimposed on each other or separated. The procedure is repeated in all nine quadrants. If there is separation

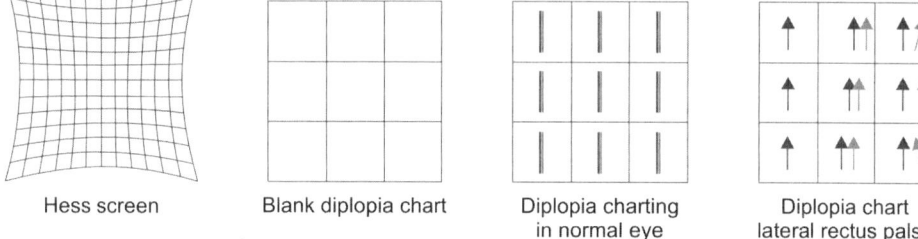

Fig. 5.34: Diplopia chart. (*For color version, see Plate 1*)

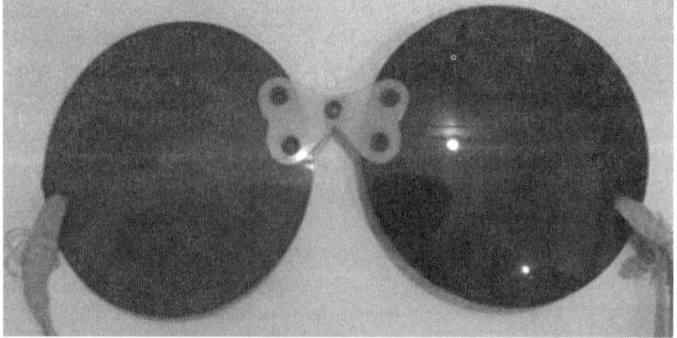

Fig. 5.35: Diplopia glasses. (*For color version, see Plate 2*)

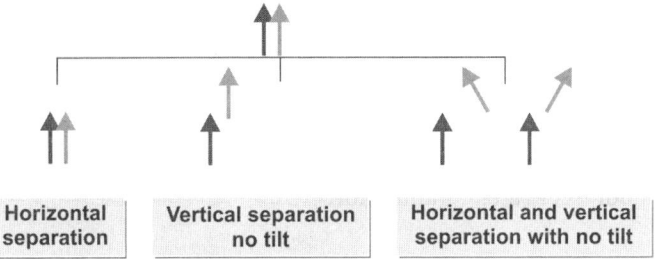

Fig. 5.36: Position of false image in paralytic squint.

between the two images, the patient has diplopia. Diplopia may be present in one or more quadrants. The separation may be horizontal, vertical, or tilted. Horizontal separation indicates paralysis of horizontally acting muscles. While vertical separation and tilting show the involvement of cyclovertical muscles **(Fig. 5.36)**.

EXAMINATION OF A CASE OF GLAUCOMA

Glaucoma is a condition where the intraocular pressure is more than 21.00 mmHg with field loss, a change in the optic nerve, and diminished vision. The condition can be congenital or acquired. Acquired glaucoma is more common than congenital glaucoma. If the cause of the raised intraocular pressure is known, it is called secondary glaucoma; otherwise, it is primary. 2% of the population suffers from some type of glaucoma or another. The tension in the eye is recorded by an instrument called a tonometer. There are two types of tonometers: indentation and applanation. The applanation tonometer may be one where the instrument touches the cornea. The other is where it does not touch the cornea. Out of these, the indentation tonometer of the schiotz tonometer is the most widely used **(Fig. 5.37)**.

The raised intraocular tension may be gradual or sudden. The gradual increase may be so slow that the patient is not aware of it unless it has produced a visual defect. This is called wide-angle glaucoma. The sudden raised intraocular tension is always associated with symptoms of color halo, redness of the eye, watering, diminished vision, and pain. This is called narrow-angle glaucoma. The angle is measured by an instrument called a gonioscope.

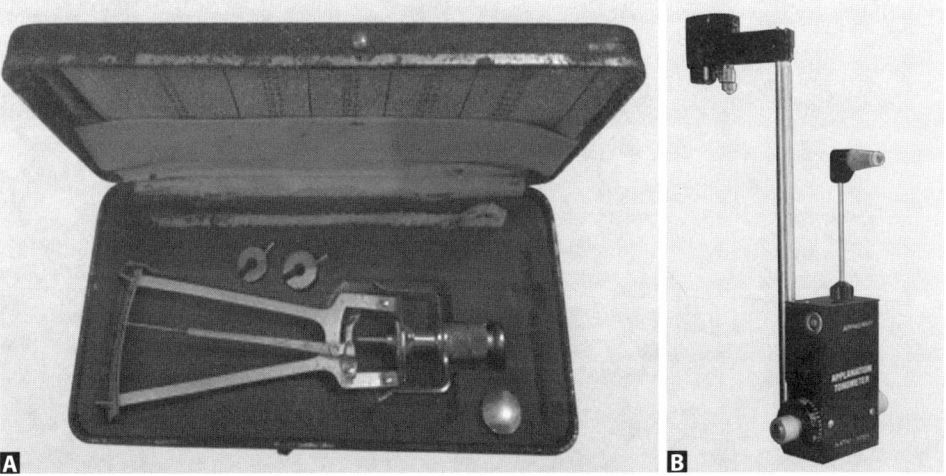

Figs. 5.37A and B: Types of tonometers. (A) Schiotz indentation tonometer; (B) Applanation tonometer to be used with slit lamp.

Internal Examination of the Eye

This consists of an examination of the posterior segment of the eye that is not visible with oblique illumination. It consists of an examination of the ciliary body, choroid, retinal optic nerve, and vitreous. The areas are examined by various instruments. They are direct and indirect ophthalmoscopes, gonioscopes, slit lamps with special attachments for operating microscopes, ultrasonography, fluorescein angiography, and OCT.

6 CHAPTER

Disorders of the Lids

Disorders of the lids are very common in clinical practice, seen from birth to ripe age. They are very obvious and mild. Some are so common that persons do not think it serious enough to be shown to a medical person. They may be painful and sudden enough to prompt medical intervention. They could be unilateral or bilateral; when bilateral, they need not be symmetrical and simultaneous. The disorders are broadly divided into two parts, i.e., congenital and acquired.

The congenital conditions are:
- Ptosis
- Epicanthus
- Blepharophimosis
- Ankyloblepharon
- Coloboma
- Distichiasis

The acquired conditions are: trauma, infection, allergy, and neoplasm (tumor).

PTOSIS

Ptosis is a condition where the upper lid covers more than 2.00 mm of the upper part of the cornea in an adult eye. It is the most common congenital anomaly of the lid. It is unilateral more often than bilateral and may be symmetrical or asymmetrical. It is broadly divided into two groups depending on the action of the levator palpebral superior. The causes of the underaction of LPS may be in the muscles or in its nerve supply. This is called true ptosis, in contrast to pseudoptosis, where the action of the levator is present. The main causes of pseudoptosis are increased bulk of the upper lid (edema, tumor **Fig. 6.1**) or loss of support to the lid (enophthalmos).

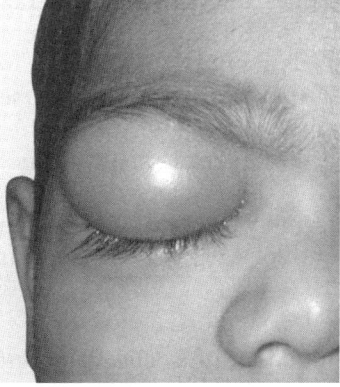

Fig. 6.1: Pseudoptosis.

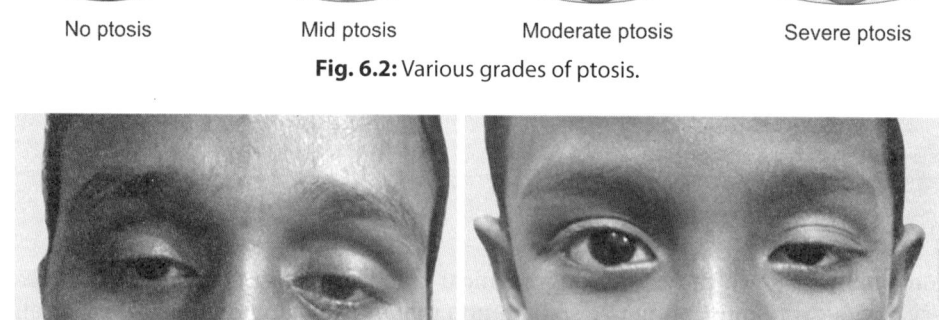

Fig. 6.2: Various grades of ptosis.

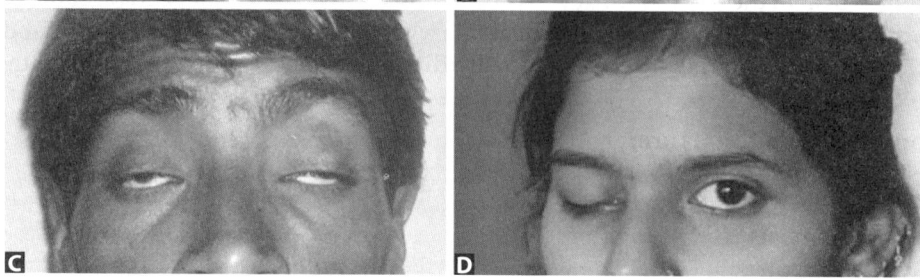

Figs. 6.3A to D: Clinical pictures of various grades of ptosis. (A) Bilateral mild ptosis; (B) Left moderate ptosis; (C) Bilateral severe ptosis; (D) Right total ptosis.
(*Courtesy*: Professor Dr Anand Deshpande)

Clinically, the ptosis has been divided into mild, moderate, and severe, depending on the available function of the LPS **(Figs. 6.2 and 6.3)**. When there is no action of LPS, it is called total ptosis.

Congenital Ptosis

Congenital ptosis is called simple ptosis when only the levator muscle is involved. The involvement of other structures along with simple ptosis is called complicated ptosis.

Simple Congenital Ptosis

It is present at birth but may be missed unless it is bilateral and severe. The other cause of missing it is the sleep habit of the child. The child sleeps almost 18 hours a day. The parents become aware of it when the child is about 2–3 months old. Mild bilateral ptosis are observed still late. The condition is generally unilateral. In moderate to severe cases, the toddler may keep his chin up and his brows raised; on examination, the lid crease is absent, the interpalpebral fissure is narrow, and the furrow of the forehead is marked. The action of the levator is fairly good in mild to moderate ptosis. The vision is not affected unless the pupil is covered. The common error of refraction is astigmatism; amblyopia is common. There is no medical treatment for the condition; the condition does not resolve with age. The only treatment is surgical.

Complicated Congenital Ptosis

Association of the following conditions are put collectively under the term complicated ptosis:
- Poor action of the superior rectus

- ❖ **Blepharophimosis syndrome**: This is less common than the above; it is bilateral, consisting of epicanthus, blepharophimosis, and telecanthus (the distance between the two eyes is more than normal). The only treatment available is surgical.
- ❖ **Ptosis with jaw winking**: This is unilateral, moderate, congenital ptosis that disappears with opening and closing of the mouth; in some cases, it may disappear as the child grows.

Acquired Ptosis

This can develop any time after birth. Most of the time it is unilateral, the common causes are:
- ❖ Trauma to the LPS, third nerve
- ❖ Neurogenic
  - Third nerve palsy
  - Horner's syndrome
- ❖ Myogenic
  - Myasthenia gravis
  - Ocular myopathy
- ❖ Mechanical: This is a pseudoptosis due to the increased bulk of the upper lid (**Fig. 6.1**).

Ptosis in third nerve palsy is more common in adults; it is generally unilateral. It is complete when there is no action of levator. It is generally associated with paralysis of other extraocular muscles and paralysis of the pupil, except in diabetic neuropathy, where the pupil is normal. Ptosis secondary to third nerve involvement may be seen in the following situations: diabetics, aneurism, intracranial space-occupying lesions, and infection.

Horner's Syndrome

Horner syndrome is a rare unilateral condition with features of mild ptosis, miosis, enophthalmos, and the absence of sweating on the side of ptosis. The condition is caused by a lesion in the sympathetic chain.

Myogenic Ptosis

Commonest myogenic ptosis is myasthenia gravis, a bilateral, slow-progressing systemic disease with ocular manifestation, out of which periodic ptosis and paralysis of extraocular muscles are most frequent. The main complaint of the disorder is diplopia after exertion. Diplopia may follow ptosis or precede; both are due to the involvement of muscles supplied by oculomotor cranial nerves; symptoms initially disappear with rest. Only to recur after exertion. The pupils are normal, and the treatment is medical.

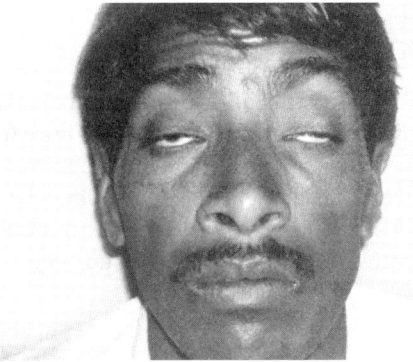

Fig. 6.4: Ocular myopathy.

Other myogenic ptosis seen in ocular myopathy is progressive external ophthalmoplegia (**Fig. 6.4**). Which is rarer than myasthenia. It is bilateral, progressive, and symmetrical. The main signs are gradually developing ptosis with progressive extraocular muscle palsy involving all the extraocular muscles; in the late stages, there is severe ptosis with immobile eyeballs. Other muscles of the body may be involved. There is no treatment.

EPICANTHUS

Epicanthus is a congenital fold of the skin over the medial canthus **(Fig. 6.5)**. The fold covers the medial part of the sclera more than normal. Giving an impression of pseudo-esotropia. Which disappears following pinching of the skin fold in most cases. The condition passes off with age; by the third or fourth year, it is fully abolished. Except in blepharophimosis syndrome.

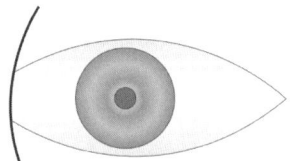

Fig. 6.5: Epicanthus.

BLEPHAROPHIMOSIS

Blepharophimosis is a bilateral congenital, nonprogressive disorder where the length and width of the IPA are greatly reduced. If it is associated with epicanthus, it is called blepharophimosis syndrome. The treatment is surgical.

ANKYLOBLEPHARON

The condition is congenital, where few strands of skin are found between the upper and lower lids. The adhesion can be anywhere on the IPA but is more frequent on the lateral side. The tags may be single or multiple; the treatment is cutting the tags to free the lids **(Fig. 6.6)**.

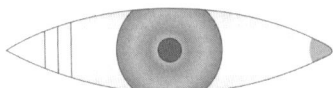

Fig. 6.6: Congenital ankyloblepharon.

COLOBOMA OF LIDS

The colobomas of the lids are full-thickness defects in the lid margin that may just be a notch or may involve a large part of the lid. It is more frequent in the upper lid, generally unilateral. The colobomas of the upper lids are more common in the medial one-third of the lid. The coloboma of the lower lid is less visible, shallower, and longer than the upper lid coloboma, situated on the lateral side of the lower lid. Large upper lid colobomas may cause exposure to the cornea. The definitive treatment is surgical correction **(Fig. 6.7)**.

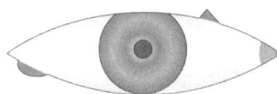

Fig. 6.7: Congenital coloboma—upper and lower lid.

DISTICHIASIS

Distichiasis is a rare congenital anomaly of the lashes of any lid. The lashes are turned in; generally, only a few lashes may be involved. The misdirected lashes arise in place of the tarsal gland opening **(Fig. 6.8)**. The treatment is epilation.

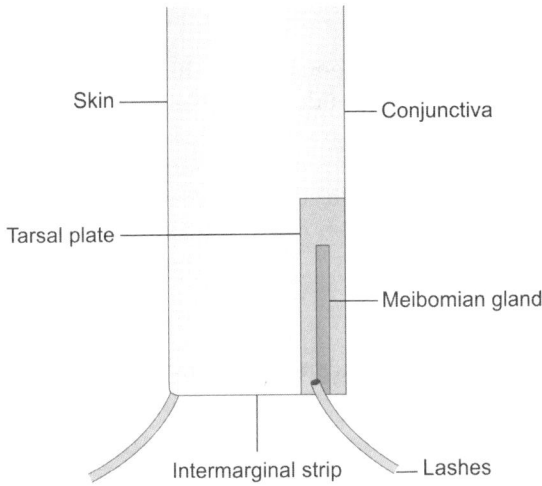

Fig. 6.8: Distichiasis.

ACQUIRED DISORDERS OF THE LIDS

The acquired disorders may include infection, inflammation, allergy, trauma, and new growths.

The infections of the lid may be divided into the following parts:
Infection of the skin and subcutaneous tissue, infection of the lid margin that can involve the skin of the lid margin, and glands of the lid margin. The glands involved are the glands of Zeis and Moll and the meibomian glands.

Infection of the skin may be acute, chronic, or recurrent and may be unilateral or bilateral. They may be seen in one or more than one at a time.

The infection is associated with redness, pain, tenderness, and edema. The pain and tenderness may be localized or generalized. The acute infection is often associated with edema of the lid. The common causes of edema of the lids are: Boils, cellulitis, and abscesses.

The edema of the lid margin is common in stye and infected chalazion. The infection of the lid may be associated with eruptions on the lids, i.e., chickenpox and herpes zoster. It could be seen in acute allergies as well; the allergy could be seen in angioneurotic edema. The lid may be swollen in an acute infection of the conjunctiva. They are ophthalmia, neonatorum, purulent conjunctivitis, membranous conjunctivitis, and acute viral conjunctivitis. The lids are often swollen in cases of orbital cellulitis, acute dacryoadenitis, acute iridocyclitis, endophthalmitis, and panophthalmitis. The most common injuries that cause edema of the lids are craniofacial injuries.

The acute infections of the skin and subcutaneous tissue are boils, vesicles, cellulitis, and abscesses:

Boils

Boils are acute infections of the hair follicle caused by pus-forming organisms. It may be single, there may be many. They are common in children in summer but can develop at any age. Adults with recurring boils should be investigated for diabetes. The boils are more common on the upper lid; they are painful, tender, raised red areas with a white center (pus). The surrounding skin is swollen. They may subside without any treatment or pass into cellulitis of the lid, or even the lid abscess.

Cellulitis, Lid, and Lid Abscess

Cellulitis is an infection of the subcutaneous tissue. The lid is swollen without fluctuation; the cellulitis is generally associated with pseudoptosis **(Fig. 6.1)**.

Once the cellulitis starts fluctuating, the condition is called a lid abscess, which invariably develops a weak spot from where the pus may come out; with subsidence of swelling and pain. If it does not happen, the best option is to surgically drain the abscess by standard procedure. The treatment of cellulitis consists of dry-hot fomentation, systemic antibiotics, and analgesics. The local drops and ointments do not have any therapeutic value.

Vesicles

The common causes of vesicles on the lid are herpes zoster ophthalmicus, herpes simplex, and chickenpox, molluscum and warts.

Herpes Zoster Ophthalmicus

Herpes zoster is caused by a virus called the varicella zoster. This virus causes chickenpox in children and a herpes zoster infection in adults. Infection of the eyes and their adnexa is called herpes zoster ophthalmicus (HZO) **(Fig. 6.9)**.

It is unilateral; the lesions do not cross the midline of the face. It mostly follows the first division of the fifth nerve. It starts with unwellness, fever, and pain on the involved side of the face. The pain is followed by redness of the skin, swelling, and the development of vesicles. The fluid in the vesicle gradually turns white, like pus. After a few days, it bursts and starts healing with the formation of a crust. That ultimately falls, leaving a punched-out, shallow scar. Pain persists even after a complete cure. This is called postherpetic neuralgia, which may linger for years. Besides the skin of the lid, the infection involves the conjunctiva, iris, and cornea. The involvement of the cornea is always associated with a lesion at the tip of the nose.

The conjunctiva may present with acute conjunctivitis and vesicles. The cornea develops both superficial and deep keratitis, a loss of sensation, and the anterior uvea is involved in the form of acute iridocyclitis. Scleritis is less common, and the neurological involvements are: optic neuritis, ophthalmoplegia, facial palsy, and paralysis of the opposite limb.

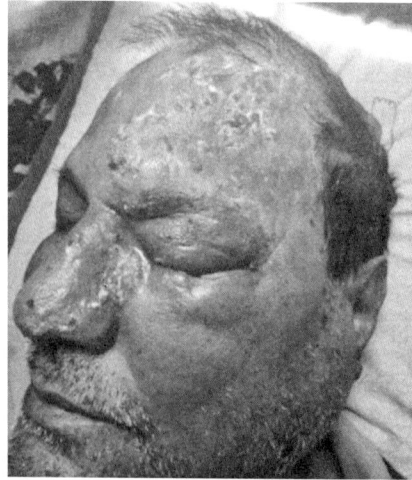

Fig. 6.9: Herpes zoster ophthalmicus. *(For color version, see Plate 2)*

Management

Management is divided into two parts: ocular and systemic.

The treatment for ocular involvement is acyclovir ointment applied three times a day to the skin lesion along with broad-spectrum antibiotic ointment. The corneal lesion requires appropriate atropinization and the installation of acyclovir eye ointment. Administration of systemic acyclovir tablets reduces postherpetic neuralgia and shortens the duration of the disease. Systemic involvement is better left to physicians to manage.

Herpes Simplex

The lid involvement in herpes simplex is caused by herpes simplex virus (HSV) type 1; presenting as multiple vesicles on the lid without any predilection for side or distribution of nerves, it is often missed. It can be seen in neonates as well. The lid infection does not require any specific treatment, unless there is systemic involvement. The child may develop corneal lesions years after the lid involvement; it is a self-limiting disease.

Chickenpox (Varicella)

Varicella is caused by the same virus that causes herpes zoster but presents clinically in a different way. The lesions of chickenpox are vesicles all over the body on both sides of the midline. Generally, it develops in children, but most of the time it heals by itself. However, sometimes it may be serious enough to cause systemic involvement. That may be fatal, but the disease is preventable by a vaccine given after one year of age. The ocular involvement is the same as in herpes zoster ophthalmicus, but milder in nature, not resulting in postherpetic neuralgia. The cornea is rarely involved, and corneal sensation is retained. The conjunctiva may develop a vesicle that looks like phlycten. The disease is preventable by vaccines.

Molluscum Contagiosum

It is a chronic disease of the skin anywhere on the body. It is caused by the pox virus, which spreads through intimate body contact. In the lid, it starts as a painless, translucent nodule with a depression in the center. The number of nodules varies from one to many. A thick, milky material loaded with infective viruses comes out on rupture of the vesicle. Nodules on the lid margin cause keratoconjunctivitis. The disease is self-limiting, not requiring any specific treatment unless the conjunctiva and cornea are involved. The infection is severe and seen all over the body in AIDS. Antiviral treatment should be started under the supervision of a person specifically trained in the management of AIDS.

Warts (Verruca)

Verruca is a common viral infection of the skin caused by papovavirus. They are seen in adults; in the lid, they may develop anywhere from the lid margin to the eyebrow. The number varies from one to many. The size varies from millimeters to centimeters. They are nonpedunculated and raised, with an irregular border and rough surface. The growths on the lid margin cause toxic keratoconjunctivitis. Some of them are self-limited; they do not show a tendency for malignancy. They do not respond to antiviral drugs.

Treatment consists of the application of cryo, lasser, or bipolar diathermy. The next alternative is to remove it surgically.

Acquired Disorders of the Lid Margin

The acquired disorders of the lid margin can be infective, inflammatory, allergic, new growths, or trauma. The infective/inflammatory disorders are called blepharitis.

Blepharitis

Blepharitis is a chronic inflammatory condition of the lid. They extend from the base of the lashes to the posterior edge of the lid margin. Infection from the skin of the lid margin may pass to the tarsal gland opening. Blepharitis is generally bilateral, involving all lid margins. They are more common in children and young adults, have a long course, are difficult to treat, and recur. They have been divided into two groups. Nonulcerative, commonly called squamous blepharitis and ulcerative blepharitis. The following table gives a comparison between the two.

The exact cause is not well known, but the following have been held responsible: Seborrheic dermatitis, allergy, and chronic staphylococcus infection of the conjunctiva **(Table 6.1)**.

Treatment

There is no specific treatment for blepharitis. The common practice is to correct refractive error, practice personal hygiene, rub the lid margin with a warm swab, and apply antistaphylococcal antibiotics.

Parasitic Infestation of the Lid Margin

The disorder is caused by a common parasite, lice. This can be one of the following: head lice or body lice. The former does not cause inflammation of the lids. The body lice is known by various names; the lice that infects the lid margin is called crab lice (Phthiriasis palpebrarum). It involves the base of the lashes. It can be seen at any age; the child gets it from carers, including infected parents. In adults, it is a sexually transmitted disease. The parasites cling to the base of

Table 6.1: Shows comparison between ulcerative and squamous blepharitis.

Features	Squamous blepharitis	Ulcerative blepharitis
Age	Children and young adult	Children and young adults
Side	Both	Both
Lids	All	All
Complaints	Powder like, dry white scales in the lasher	Matted lashes, yellow coarse wet flakes
	Can be removed with ease	Difficult to remove
	No ulceration on removal of scales	Small ulcers on removal of scales
	Mild	Progressive
	Loss of lashes less frequent	Loss of lashes more frequent
	Lashes grow back after loss	Lashes may not grow after loss
Complication	None	Tylosis, madarosis, and trichiasis
	Dandruff of scalp	Chronic conjunctivitis, staphylococcal infection

the lashes and reproduce. The presence of parasites results in irritation, itching, and redness of the lid margin. The parasite and their nits are visible under oblique illumination even without magnification; at magnification, the parasite may be seen wiggling on the lid margin. The best treatment consists of the personal hygiene of the career and sexual partners. The parasites are best treated by a weak solution of anti lice lotion.

Inflammation of the Glands of the Lid Margin

The two types of glands found on the lid margin are sebaceous (sweat glands) and meibomian (tarsal glands).

The former are found at the base of the lashes; they are called the glands of Zeis and Moll. The tarsal glands open between the base of the lashes and the posterior edge of the lid margin. The **(Fig. 6.10)** is composite drawing of various infective conditions of the lid.

The two inflammatory conditions of the glands of the lids are stye and chalazion.

Stye

Stye is an acute suppurative infection of the glands of Zeis and Moll, the other name of which is Hordeolum externum. Styes are more common among children under ten. They are so common and recurring that some parents consider them to be natural, as they are self-limiting in most cases. Recurrence is common; the styes are known to develop on all lids. More common in the upper lid, it presents as a red, tender, painful swelling round the glands of Zeis and Moll. Only to be converted into pus-bearing boils. The lid round the stye is swollen; in severe cases, the

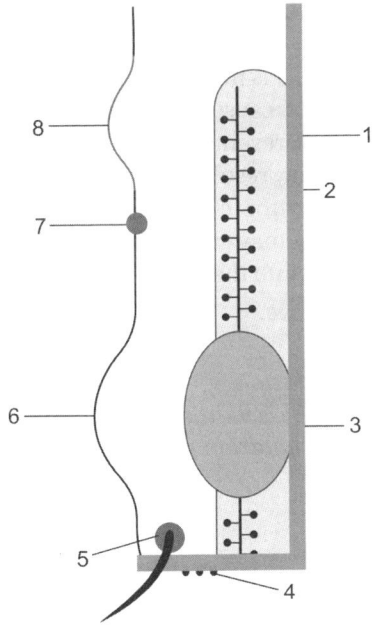

Inflammatory Lesion of Lid

1. Tarsal conjunctiva
2. Tarsal gland
3. Calazion
4. Blapharitis
5. Stye
6. Bulge in the skin over calazion
7. Boil
8. Lid abses

Fig. 6.10: Various infective conditions of the lid.

whole of the lid may be swollen, and the preauricular lymph nodes are enlarged. Photograph A stye at the canthus is more painful and may involve the adjacent lid.

The treatment consists of dry hot fomentation three times a day, and analgesic systemic antibiotics are not needed. Local antistaphylococcus broad-spectrum ointments are applied to prevent adjoining glands from getting infected. If the pus points, the swelling may be pressed between the thumb and index finger to express the pus. That immediately brings relief to the patient. If pus forms at the base of a lash, epilation of the offending lash will have the same results. However, if there is cellulitis of the lid, systemic antibiotics are needed. The ancillary treatment comprises correction of errors of refraction, facial hygiene, and cutting down sugar.

Complication: Most important is cellulitis of the lid. Other complications are tylosis and madarosis. The child should be put on a broad-spectrum antibiotic drop in both eyes once a day for the next 3 months. This is supposed to prevent a recurrence.

Chalazion

Chalazion is as common as Stye in the same age group. It is a chronic inflammation of the tarsal glands. It may involve only one lid or more than one lid. The disorders may be single or multiple in the same lid. It is painless and slow-growing, starting as a pin-sized nodule away from the lid margin.

The swelling is better felt at this stage than seen. As time passes, the swelling increases in size and becomes visible on the skin on the lid. The skin can be moved over the growth, but the chalazion cannot be moved in the tarsal plate. On eversion of the lid, the conjunctiva over the inner surface of the chalazion looks translucent with a bluish pink tinge. The preauricular glands are not involved.

The exact cause of chalazion is not known; it is most probably due to a low-grade infection in the lid margin that travels in the tarsal duct, causing edema of the epithelium of the duct. Resulting in the obliteration of the duct. That prevents the drainage of meibomian secretions. The accumulated secretion acts as an irritant, resulting in a granuloma. The predisposing factors are family history, error of refraction, chronic blepharitis, and diabetes (adults). Some of the chalazia resolve without treatment. Rest may get infected, causing hordeolum interna*; burst on the conjunctival surface and convert into the tarsal cyst.

*Hordeolum Interna**

This is an acute bacterial infection of the chalazion, a very painful and tender condition that prevents eversion of the lid and may cause severe cellulitis of the lid. Noninfected chalazion does not require systemic antibiotics, but infected chalazion requires broad-spectrum antibiotics. It should be differentiated from stye.

Treatment

There is no specific treatment for noninfected chalazia. Repeated, hot, dry fomentation is said to help its resolution. The definitive treatment is surgical, by incision, drainage, and curettage. Recurrence at the same place does not occur. Adults with recurrence have a chance of developing adenocarcinoma of the tarsal gland. This makes it mandatory for histological examination of the curated material to exclude possible malignancy. Children do not develop malignancy in chalazion. The surgery is effective only in a particular chalazion that has undergone surgery. It does not prevent the development of chalazion in other tarsal glands.

ACQUIRED STRUCTURAL ANOMALIES OF THE LIDS

They are mostly post-inflammatory:
1. Trichiasis
2. Entropion
3. Ectropion
4. Tylosis
5. Madarosis

Consisting of the following: They are shown in the **Figure 6.11.**

Trichiasis

Trichiasis is a condition where eyelashes or lashes turn in; it may be a single lash or multiple lashes. It may happen without entropion or with entropion. The main symptoms are watering from the eyes due to rubbing of the lashes on the cornea, or conjunctiva. The causes are idiopathic, trauma, infections like trachoma, leprosy, and chronic blepharitis.

The **treatment** is epilation if the number of lashes is few. This gives temporary respite to the patients, because this is not a permanent solution. The lashes grow again within a few weeks of epilation. The best treatment is to destroy the offending lash follicle by diathermy. If the number of lashes is numerous, the best treatment is plastic repair of the lid margin, as done in cicatricial entropion.

Entropion

Entropion is a condition where the lid margin along with lashes are turned in. It may involve a single or more than one lid. There are two types of entropion, i.e., senile (spastic) entropion and cicatricial entropion:

- ❖ **Senile entropion** is seen in the lower lid only, initially involving one eye; the other eye follows soon. It is generally seen in elderly, thin, and malnourished persons of both sexes. The main cause of entropion is the laxity of the orbicularis and skin. Loss of orbital fat is an important factor. The symptoms are watering from the eye and recurrent redness of the eyes. The treatment is an improvement in nutrition and surgical correction of the deformity.

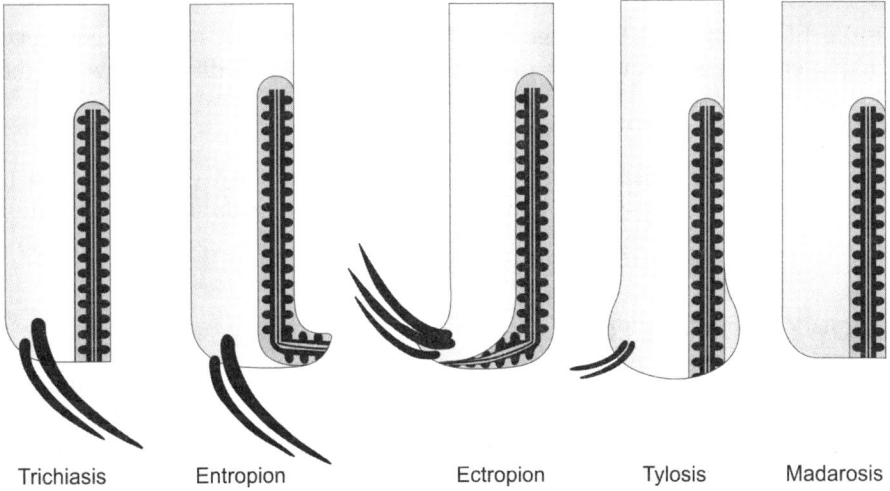

Fig. 6.11: Acquired structural anomalies of the lids.

❖ **Cicatricial entropion** is caused by the deformity of the tarsal plate and the shortening of the tarsal conjunctiva. It is seen mostly in the upper lid and may be unilateral or bilateral. Generally, one eye is involved early. The commonest cause is stage four trachoma. The other causes are leprosy and chemical burns. The symptoms are similar to spastic entropion, i.e., watering, redness, and photophobia. The cicatricial entropion is responsible for superficial vascularization of the cornea and diffuse corneal opacity, which is the main cause of blindness in trachoma. The treatment consists of treatment of trachoma in the initial two stages by chemotherapy, which becomes ineffective in stages three and four. Once entropion develops, the only remedy is surgical correction of the entropion from the conjunctival surface.

Ectropion

Ectropion is the outward turning of the full length of the lid. Ectropion can be seen in the following conditions: (1) Senile; (2) Paralytic; (3) Cicatricial:

❖ **Senile** ectropion is generally bilateral and mild, with the symptom of persistent watering from the eyes. It is generally bilateral.
❖ **Paralytic** ectropion is seen in lagophthalmos the common causes of which are leprosy, Bells palsy, and injury to the facial nerve. Leprosy is the commonest cause of bilateral lagophthalmos, hence a prominent cause of ectropion of the lower lid. Bell's palsy and trauma are unilateral. On examination, the lid margins are everted and may be mild to moderate. The tarsal conjunctiva, when exposed, causes chronic conjunctivitis and exposure of the cornea in the lower part. The main symptom is watering. Treatment: Most of the cases do not require any treatment, especially in Bell's palsy. In leprosy, the best treatment is tarsorrhaphy.
❖ **Cicatricial** ectropion is secondary to a scar formation over the lid. The most common are trauma, acid, alkali, and thermal burns. Both lids may be involved; in severe cases, the conjunctiva is everted, thickened, and red. The patient may not be able to close the lids. The symptoms are watering, redness, and pain. The treatment consists of the removal of the offending scar, followed by a skin graft.

Tylosis

Tylosis is the thickening of the lid margin. The lid margin is rounded and loses contact with the globe. This is generally associated with madarosis. The treatment is directed towards the cause.

Madarosis

Madarosis is the loss of eyelashes. It may be in patches on the single eye or on all the lids. It is generally associated with tylosis. The common causes of madarosis are ulcerative blepharitis, trachoma, leprosy, and thermal and chemical burns. There are hardly any symptoms. The treatment is directed towards the cause.

NEW GROWTHS ON THE LIDS

New growths on the lids can arise from any tissue of the lid. They can be congenital, inflammatory, degenerative, or malignant. On the lid skin arise warts, molluscum, xanthelasma, basal cell carcinoma, squamous cell carcinoma, malignant melanoma, and xeroderma pigmentosum. Hemangiomas arise from the blood vessels and neurofibromas from peripheral nerves. The growth can be malignant (cancerous) or benign noncancerous. The benign growths are warts and molluscum (discussed above), xanthelasma, hemangioma, neurofibroma, and nevus.

The malignant growths are basal cell carcinoma, squamous cell carcinoma, adenocarcinoma, xeroderma pigmentosa, malignant melanoma, and Kaposi sarcoma.

Xanthelasma

Xanthelasmas are common bilateral, slowly developing superficial, nonmalignant growth of the lids, mostly in women past 40 years, frequently in the upper lid, on the medial side. There is a strong family history. The growths are dirty white with a rough surface and an irregular border; they are curved sausage-shaped. They may be single or more than one; they are painless, non-tender, and move with the lid. The patients have generally raised lipid levels in their blood and may be diabetic or hypertensive. They do not develop malignancies. No treatment is required unless the patients want them removed for cosmetic reasons. Recurrence following removal is common; they can be removed by excision or destroyed by laser.

Hemangioma

Hemangiomas are present at birth; they are unilateral and may cross the midline. They are generally pink to red in color, irregular in shape, not raised above the surface of the lid, called port wine stain, or may be seen as growth on the surface called strawberry nevus and become prominent when the child cries. The third variety is cavernous hemangioma. The capillary hemangiomas are either stationary or disappear after 6–7 years of age. The cavernous hemangiomas do not regress. Large hemangiomas cause pseudoptosis, anisometropia, astigmatism, and amblyopia. The Sturge-Weber syndrome consists of unilateral hemangioma involving the upper part of the face, along with hemangioma of the uvea and associated secondary glaucoma. Convulsions are common and indicate intracranial involvement. Most capillary hemangiomas do not require any treatment; intralesional injections of steroids have been advocated without equally satisfactory results.

Neurofibromatosis

This, too, is present at birth and involves peripheral nerves. They may be localized in the lid and orbit or may be seen in other parts of the body, including the brain and spinal cord. In the lid, they cause diffuse swelling of the lid with an S-shaped curve. The hole of the lid is thickened, causing pseudoptosis with its usual complications. The skin may have a coffee-colored stain. There may be small nodules on the iris; involvement of the uvea predisposes to glaucoma. The treatment is a plastic reconstruction of the lid.

Nevi

Nevi are common benign tumors of the lid. May involve all the lids and skin anywhere in the body. They generally develop in young adults of both sexes. The incidence increases with age; they may be flush with the skin or raised over the surface. Sometimes there may be more than one on each lid. The nevi do not cause any ocular problems; hence, they are not required until the patient wishes them to be removed.

MALIGNANT GROWTH OF THE LIDS

Basal Cell Carcinoma

This is the most common malignancy of the lids. It is seen after 50 years of age, mostly in the lower lid. It is a slow-progressing tumor that does not spread to distant parts. The growth starts as a raised black spot on the lid that slowly spreads all round with a depression in the center. The edges are raised and pigmented.

The treatment consists of confirmation of the condition by histopathology. If the diagnosis is confirmed, the standard treatment is surgical removal of the growth followed by plastic repair. The next treatment is radiotherapy, which is less effective than surgical removal; chemotherapy is in effective.

Squamous Cell (Epidermoid) Carcinoma

This is less common than basal cell carcinoma but more malignant. It may develop anywhere on any lid. It developed after 50 years of age. The tumor starts as a nodule, which, over months, develops either as a nodule without ulceration or with ulceration. The metastasis is common. The treatment is surgical removal using standard methods. The tumor is not radiosensitive and is not amenable to chemotherapy.

Adenocarcinoma of the Lid

This is rarer than both basal and squamous cell carcinomas. It develops in the tarsal glands; hence, it is called meibomian gland carcinoma. It may rarely develop in the caruncle. Involvement of the upper lid is more common and seen more frequently in females over 50 years of age.

It is the most common adenocarcinoma of the lid. The typical mode of presentation is a growth in the tarsal plate that looks like a chalazion and is treated as such, i.e., surgical drainage and curettage. In simple chalazion the growth does not recur in the same site following surgery. The adenocarcinoma develops at the same place and is usually retreated by surgery. Only to recur with vengeance, a biopsy at this stage reveals its being an adenocarcinoma. This makes it mandatory to subject each tissue removed from the so-called chalazion for histopathology in all cases of recurrence after 50 years of age.

The treatment is surgical removal with plastic repair of the lid.

Xeroderma Pigmentosa

This is a rare, wide-spread malignancy of the skin. The condition is seen in children between 5 and 25 years old. It involves the face and all the lids. It has a strong genetic preponderance; more than one person in the preceding generation may have the malady. It is common to find many siblings affected. The growth starts as little spots on the parts of the body that are exposed to sunlight. The lids are involved in the early stages. The spots develop fine vessels on the surface; the spot is converted into a nodule and becomes malignant. The diagnosis is confirmed by histopathology. The results may turn out to be any of the following malignancies: basal cell carcinoma, epidermoid/squamous cell carcinoma, and malignant melanoma. The condition proves fatal as it is widely spread without any treatment. The children generally die before 25 years; the management consists of protecting the skin from sun rays by wearing a full-sleeve shirt and trousers. The condition also involves the conjunctiva and cornea.

Malignant Melanoma

This is a rare malignant tumor of the lid that may occur in any part of the body. It is highly malignant and fatal. The tumors are black in color in the early stages; they look like moles. The moles do not grow in size, but the melanoma grows. Making it mandatory to do a histopathology of the biopsy from all fast-growing growths of the skin. There is no known treatment for malignant melanoma.

Kaposi Sarcoma

The tumor was thought to be rare before systemic HIV became rampant. It is a fatal vascular tumor that may start either in the skin of the lid or the conjunctiva. There is no specific treatment; the main attention is directed to the treatment of AIDS under the supervision of a person specially trained. The conjunctival and small lid lesions are treated by excision; the small lesions are treated by cryotherapy and external beam radiation.

Trauma to the Lids

The lids can be involved either mechanically or chemically directly, or they can be associated with craniofacial injuries that involve both sides. The primary injury to the lid may be as small as an abrasion, or there may be total tissue loss. The most common mechanical injuries are abrasion lacerations and punctured wounds with or without a retained foreign body. Simple lid injuries do not cause any visual loss; however, a small injury to the outer third of the eye brow may prove to be a precursor to a more serious indirect injury to the optic nerve that may cause permanent loss of vision.

Abrasions are caused by the rubbing of the superficial surface of the skin against a rough, hard object. They are mild in nature, with an irregular border and slight bleeding. They cause burning and pain in the lid; they are treated by cleaning the wound with antiseptic lotion (Betadine) and dusting with broad-spectrum antibiotics. They heal within a few days without a scar.

Laceration (Tearing) of the Lid

Laceration is the tearing of the lid margin; it may also be without involvement of the margin. Those involving the lid margin cut through all the layers of the lid margin. May be a small notch or may extend up to the orbital margin. They are generally irregular and triangular in shape, with a base at the lid margin. All lacerated wounds may involve the globe as well. The treatment is the plastic repair of the wound in layers.

Punctured wounds are caused by short, hard-pointed objects like needles, thorns, knives, and darts. The punctured wounds involve the full thickness of the lid. This makes the globe vulnerable to puncture wounds, which should get priority in management.

Blunt Injuries to the Lid

The blunt injuries to the lids are caused by hard, stationary, or moving objects. The common moving objects are fists, sticks, cricket balls, shuttlecocks, etc. The objects are generally larger than their orbital diameter. They may abrade the skin. The more common is ecchymosis of the lid, commonly called black eye. The black color is due to changes in the blood accumulated under the skin. The ecchymosis may be edematous or flat. The color is initially pink but changes to black over the next few days. The ecchymosis may develop within a few hours to a few days after the injury. The lid is swollen with pseudoptosis, commonly associated with subconjunctival hemorrhage. The globe should always be examined for associated injuries. The treatment of simple ecchymosis is the immediate application of a cold compress. The patient should be told that it will take 7–8 days for the ecchymosis and subconjunctival hemorrhage.

CHAPTER 7

Disorder of the Lacrimal System

The lacrimal system consists of two parts, i.e., the secretory and drainage systems.

The former consists of the lacrimal gland and accessory glands. The later comprises of lids, puncta, canaliculi, lacrimal sac, and nasolacrimal duct. The secretory system is responsible for the production of tears; its function of the later is to drain the tears. Tear is an important fluid that forms a thin layer on the conjunctiva and cornea. It is constantly produced and drained with equal efficacy. Derangement of the drainage system results in epiphora. The tear film has three layers, i.e., lipid, aqueous, and mucus.

DRAINAGE OF TEARS

The aqueous part of the tear is produced by the lacrimal glands; to this, lipid is added from the meibomian gland of the lids and mucus from the goblet cells, or conjunctiva. The tear flows from superotemporal to inferomedial part of conjunctiva crossing the conjunctiva and cornea, it drains through puncta and canaliculi to the lacrimal sac. The lower puncta drains about 80% of the tear. The tear is squeezed down the nasolacrimal tube into the nasal cavity. Non-functioning of any part of the drainage system will cause an overflow of tears, causing epiphora. The decreased production and increased evaporation of tears are called ocular surface disorder or dry eye syndrome. The functions of the tear are that it keeps the cornea and conjunctiva wet, flushes out external particles in the eye, and forms optical layers on the cornea. It prevents microbial infection; the virulence of the microbia is reduced to some extent due to the presence of an enzyme, lysozyme, present in the tear. The disease of the lacrimal system can be an abnormal tear, an abnormality of drainage, or diseases of the lacrimal glands and drainage system. The abnormality of the drainage system causes epiphora, which is different from the more common type of watering, i.e., lacrimation. The former is an overflow of normally produces tears; due to derangement anywhere between the lid margin and the opening of the nasolacrimal duct in the nose. The latter is caused by overproduction of tears in the presence of normal drainage. It can be superimposed over epiphora, worsening it. The lacrimation is generally acute and may last until the causative factor has been removed. The causes of lacrimation and the location of the causative factor are given in **Table 7.1**.

Table 7.1: Causes of lacrimation.

Sl. No.	Structures involved	Causes
1.	Lid	Trichiasis, entropion, ectropion, lagophthalmos, foreign body in the tarsal conjunctiva
2.	Conjunctiva	Acute conjunctivitis, allergic conjunctivitis, phlycten
3.	Cornea	Corneal foreign body, corneal abrasion, phlyctenular keratoconjunctivitis, corneal ulcer, keratitis, buphthalmos, acute keratoconus
4.	Uvea	Acute iridocyclitis, endophthalmitis

The causes of epiphora and the location of the causative factor are given in **Table 7.2**.

Table 7.2: Causes of epiphora.

Sl. No.	Structures involved	Causes
1.	Lid	Ectropion of lower lid, lagophthalmos, coloboma of lower lid
2.	Puncta	Absence of puncta, pin-point puncta, obstruction of puncta by foreign body, eversion of puncta
3.	Canaliculus	Absence of canaliculus, obstruction of canaliculus due to infection, laceration of canaliculus
4.	Lacrimal sac	Chronic dacryocystitis, absence of sac (surgical removal of sac), granuloma of sac
5.	Nasolacrimal duct	Congenital obstruction, acquired obstruction due to fracture of nasal bone

DRYNESS OF THE EYES

A normal eye should have a moist conjunctiva and cornea. Any condition that reduces the wetness of the ocular surface is called dry eye syndrome or an ocular surface defect. That can be brought about by either a deficiency in layers of tear film or a defect in the ocular surface by way of a defect in the lid, conjunctiva, and cornea. The common causes of deficiency in components are less production of tears in the glands in old age, menopause, thyroid disease, and drugs. The lipid deficiency is caused by chronic blepharitis and meibomianitis. The mucous defect is brought about by reduced goblet cells in the conjunctiva.

The defect in the ocular surface is seen in anatomical defects in the lid, vitamin A deficiency, trachoma, keratoconjunctivitis, and chemical burns.

The symptoms of dry eyes are never severe. A person with mild to moderate dry eye may not be aware of the condition. All that the person complains about is an unexplained foreign body sensation. The other symptoms are recurrent, unexplained redness of both the eyes, mucus secretion, fluctuation of vision, and intolerance to light. On examination, the eyes do not show any pathology. The signs are elicited when examined specifically. The tests are Schirmer's test showing <20 mm of wetting, tear break-up time <15 seconds, and scattered corneal stain by fluorescence without staining of conjunctiva. Positive stain of both conjunctiva and cornea by Rose bengal. The lissamine green only stains the cornea.

Treatment

Treatment of the condition is difficult and prolonged. The principle of treatment is to increase the tear artificially by using a group of drops collectively called artificial tears or lubricants. Some patients may be comfortable with the instillation of the lubricant just twice a day. Patients with severe dry eye may require as frequent instillation as hourly. The second line of treatment is the correction of associated blepharitis. Along with lubricants, associated tarsitis is treated with a low dose of an appropriate long-acting antibiotic for 4–6 weeks. Systemic conditions, such as thyroid disease and arthritis should also be treated. The condition per se does not cause blindness.

DISEASES OF THE LACRIMAL DRAINAGE SYSTEM

Diseases of the lacrimal drainage system are more common than diseases of the lacrimal glands. The diseases of the drainage system could be congenital or acquired. The former is seen in neonates and children **(Fig. 7.1)**.

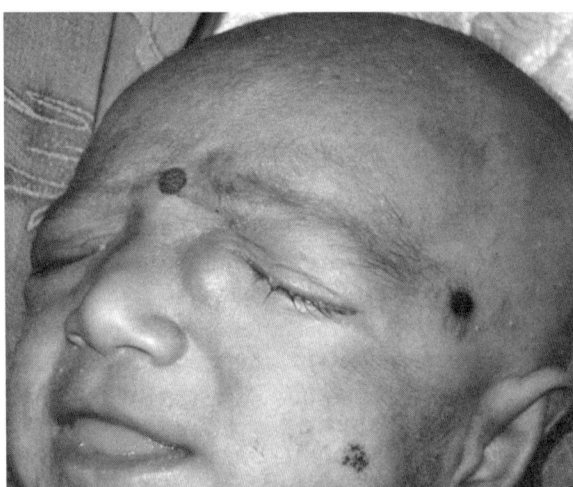

Fig. 7.1: Congenital cyst of lacrimal sac.

The latter is seen in adults; and the main symptoms of defective lacrimal drainage are epiphora. The other symptom is positive regurgitation of mucus or pus on application of pressure over the sac. These symptoms are seen in chronic obstruction without infection. Infection of the drainage system causes pain, tenderness, and swelling over the sac and surrounding tissue. The epiphora is caused by obstructions in drainage anywhere from the puncta to its opening in the nose. Out of all the components of the drainage system, the sac is the most important structure involved.

The causes of epiphora that can be related to sacs are:
1. **Absence of sac:** Due to surgical removal of the sac, which is called dacryocystectomy (DCT) in short.
2. **Failure of dacryocystorhinostomy (DCR):** This means the surgical creation of a passage between the sac and the nasal mucosa.
3. **Infection:**
    i. Chronic dacryocystitis
    ii. Acute dacryocystitis
    iii. Granuloma of the sac—rhinosporidiosis
4. **Obstruction of the nasolacrimal duct:** This can be present at birth or acquired in adults.

Congenital Nasolacrimal Duct Obstruction

This is commonly known as congenital dacryocystitis, which is a misnomer. The pathogenesis of the condition is non-canalization of the nasolacrimal duct. The nasolacrimal duct should be open throughout its length at birth. This may not happen if some epithelial debris is left in the duct at the time of birth. This happens in one-third of neonates and takes about 2–3 weeks to be patent. In a small percentage of these children, it may fail to canalise even after three weeks. These are the children who will develop congenital dacryocystitis. In the majority of cases, it is unilateral; there is a positive history of such incidents in 20% of parents that may be told by the grandparents.

The lacrimal glands do not start functioning before three weeks after birth; hence, watering starts only after three weeks. Thus, any watering from the eyes before two weeks is not due to

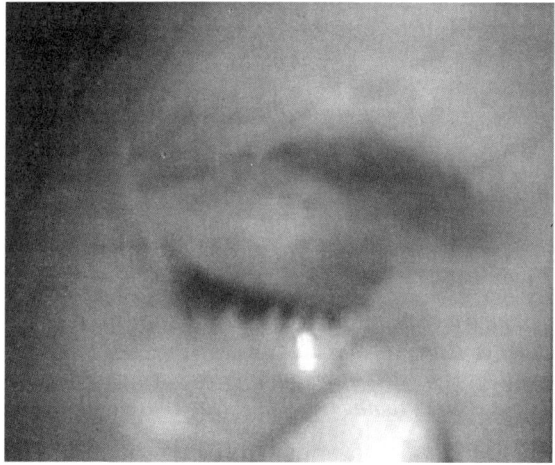

Fig. 7.2: Untreated case of congenital dacryocystitis. *(For color version, see Plate 2)*

congenital nasolacrimal duct obstruction. Other causes of watering before 3 weeks are birth trauma and ophthalmia neonatorum. Hence, children with congenital nasolacrimal ducts are brought for consultation after 3 weeks. On examination, there is a diffuse, painless swelling over the sac, which, on pressure, produces regurgitation of mucoid discharge **(Fig. 7.2)**. That comes from the walls of the sac, and after three weeks, a tear reaches the sack, carrying microbes and initiating infection of the pent-up secretion of the discharge. This is actual neonatal dacryocystitis. If the organism invading the sac is virulent, a state of pericystitis will set in, the signs of which are diffuse tender swelling over the sac and adjacent skin and subcutaneous tissue.

The **management** of neonatal dacryocystitis is simple and effective if the caregiver can carry it out properly. It consists of gentle pressure over the sac 3–4 times a day. The pressure will force the contents into the nasolacrimal duct and make them patent. At the same time, some fluid will regurgitate from both the puncta. The first pressure will produce maximum regurgitation, which will be reduced with subsequent pressure. The regurgitate material is swabbed, followed by the instillation of a broad-spectrum eye drop in the conjunctiva. The procedure should be explained to the caregiver and asked to be demonstrated to the clinician. They should be told that the results solely depend on their ability to follow the instructions. In 3–4 days, there will be no regurgitation from the puncta, yet the procedure should be carried out for at least for one month **(Figs. 7.3A to C)**. This will cure the condition in 90% of cases. Those who do not improve with this simple, non-invasive procedure will have to undergo probing and syringing under general anesthesia in experienced hands. A single procedure is sufficient; otherwise, the

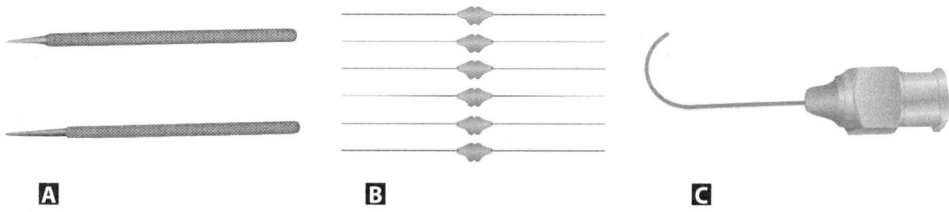

Figs. 7.3A to C: Appliance used for lacrimal syringing: (A) Punctum dilator; (B) Lacrimal probe; (C) Lacrimal cannula.

child will require repeated probing* and syringing**. Children not responding to probing and syringing are predisposed to chronic dacryocystitis in later life.

Probing

Probing consists of dilatation of the upper puncta and passing a probe of suitable diameter through the upper canaliculus; once it has reached the sac, the probe is moved upwards to align it with the nasolacrimal duct. The probe is then gently pushed through the nasolacrimal duct. Once it has passed the nasolacrimal duct, it is kept in the same position for a while and gently withdrawn, followed by passing the lacrimal cannula attached to a two-mL syringe filled with saline. The saline is pushed gently down the cannula; a free flow ensures the opening of the duct.

Syringing

Lacrimal syringing is a method to detect any defect or occlusion and to check the structural integrity of the lacrimal drainage system following probing.

Acute pericystitis in neonates is treated by an appropriate systemic antibiotic in consultation with a neonatologist. Regurgitation tests and probing should be delayed until the acute infection has subsided.

Complication of congenital dacryocystitis consists of persistent epiphora conversion of mucocele to pyocele → pericystitis → lacrimal abscess → lacrimal sinus → lacrimal fistula. **Figure 7.4** shows a child with lacrimal sinus.

Chronic Dacryocystitis

Chronic dacryocystitis is a slowly progressing disease of the lacrimal sac.
It has been divided into two broad groups:
1. Chronic dacryocystitis under 20 years
2. Chronic dacryocystitis above 20 years

Chronic Dacryocystitis in Children

Chronic dacryocystitis in children are less common than adult chronic dacryocystitis. It is seen equally in boys and girls. It is more often bilateral (**Figs. 7.4 and 7.5**). The features are similar to those found in adults; the difference lies in the cause. The causes are—untreated or partially treated congenital dacryocystitis, following measles and chickenpox, facial injury, and rhinosporidiosis. The treatment is the same as in adult chronic dacryocystitis.

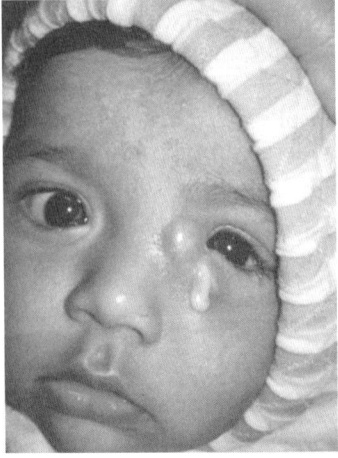

Fig. 7.4: Lacrimal sinus in untreated neonatal nasolacrimal duct block.
(*Courtesy:* Dr Preeti Gupta)

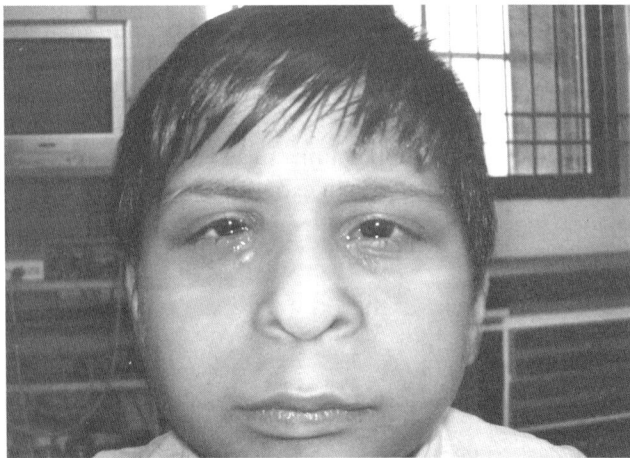

Fig. 7.5: Chronic bilateral dacryocystitis in a child.
(*Courtesy:* Dr Preeti Gupta)

Chronic Dacryocystitis in Adults

This is the most common cause of epiphora in adults, mostly unilateral. It is more common in females because they have a narrower nasolacrimal duct that predisposes to obstruction. The other causes in both sexes are swollen inferior nasal turbinates, deviated nasal septums, nasal polyps, and growths in the nose.

The infection from the nose spreads to the nasolacrimal duct, causing swelling and congestion of the mucosa. This initially causes a partial block that terminates in a complete block if not treated early. Thus, secretions from the sac wall and tears from the canaliculi start accumulating in the sac, distending the sac. To this is added infection from the conjunctiva. The most common organism isolated from the contents of the sac is *Pneumococcus*. The effect of the above factors is cause of epiphora and conjunctival congestion and a visible round subcutaneous, compressible swelling over the sac. The skin can be moved over the swelling. Pressure over the swelling causes regurgitation of the contents. The procedure is called a positive regurgitation test. The swelling of the sac is called the mucocele of the sac **(Fig. 7.6)**; if it gets infected, it is called the pyocele of the sac, where the regurgitated material is pus **(Fig. 7.7)**. If there is block in both the canaliculi along with nasolacrimal duct block, the condition is called encysted mucocele of the sac **(Fig. 7.8)**, which produces a non-compressible, firm swelling without regurgitation.

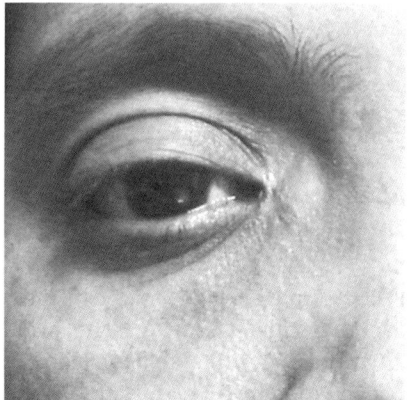

Fig. 7.6: Mucocele of the sac.

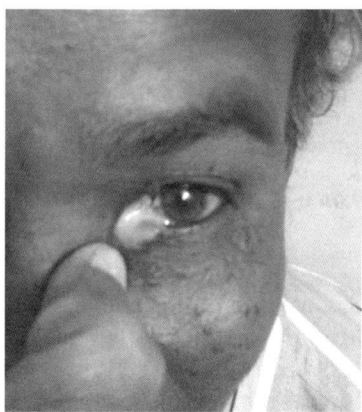

Fig. 7.7: Pyocele of the sac.

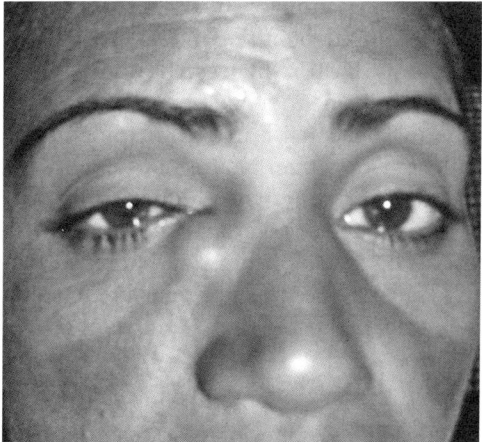

Fig. 7.8: Encysted mucocele of the sac.

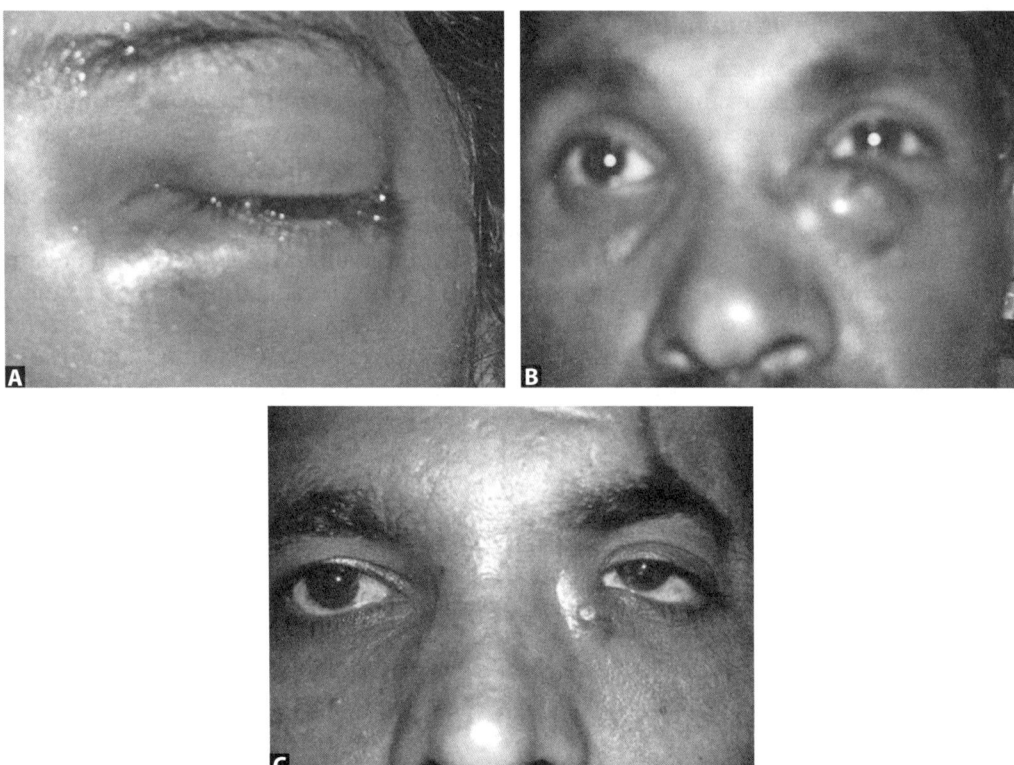

Figs. 7.9A to C: Various stages of chronic dacryocystitis: (A) Pericystitis; (B) Lacrimal abscess; (C) Lacrimal fistula.
(*Courtesy*: Dr Preeti Gupta)

If the infection passes through the sac wall, it infects the tissues round the sac, causing cellulitis. This is a state of pericystitis, wrongly called acute dacryocystitis **(Fig. 7.9A)**. The swelling may spread to the lids as well. Pericystitis, if not treated, forms a lacrimal abscess **(Fig. 7.9B)**. An untreated lacrimal sac ruptures on the skin surface, evacuating the pus and establishing a tract between the atmosphere and the sac, resulting in a lacrimal fistula **(Fig. 7.9C)** through which the contents of the sac pour out. This abolishes epiphora with subsiding pain and swelling. The sac, when infected, remains a source of infection for the cornea.

The management of the conditions depends on the stage of the disorder. The gold standard of treatment is dacryocystorhinostomy (DCR), which can be done either through the skin or through the nasolacrimal duct by endoscope. The management of acute dacryocystitis is similar to that of cellulitis anywhere in the body. That consists of dry-hot fomentation, administration of broad-spectrum antibiotics for a sufficient long time, local application of antibiotics have no role to play. Once the cellulitis has subsided, the patient may undergo surgery. In the absence of facilities to do DCR, the sac is removed through the skin surface; the procedure is called dacryocystectomy (DCT). A properly done DCR results in establishing tear drainage, which makes the patients free of epiphora. DCT removes the sac but does not give relief to the epiphora. Intraocular surgery is contraindicated in the presence of an infected sac.

DISEASES OF THE LACRIMAL GLAND

Disorders of the lacrimal glands are less common than disorders of the lacrimal sac. The three common disorders of the lacrimal glands are inflammation, tumor and hyposecretion (rare).

The inflammation of the lacrimal gland is called dacryoadenitis, which can be acute or chronic. Acute dacryoadenitis is more common than chronic. The organisms that cause dacryoadenitis are viruses, such as mumps, measles, and influenza. The bacterial infections are less common; the list is headed by *Gonococcus*, followed by *Streptococcus* and *Staphylococcus*.

The most common cause of acute viral dacryoadenitis is mumps, which is a systemic condition seen mostly in children and less commonly in adolescents who have not been immunized against mumps. The signs associated with mumps are swelling of the parotid glands, a bilateral condition seen in both unimmunized sexes. It starts with fever, shivering, pain, and upper respiratory symptoms; when bilateral, both sides are not equally involved. The gland is swollen, tender, and painful. The ocular signs are swelling of the lacrimal gland, causing mild proptosis; the direction of the proptosis is forward, down, and medial. The swelling spreads into the upper lid, causing pseudoptosis. The conjunctiva in the superior temporal quadrant is congested. The condition is self-limiting but is known to cause serious systemic viral infections. In boys, it is often associated with orchitis, and in girls, it is associated with oophoritis.

Management

Mumps is fully preventable by immunization with MMR as per the National Programme of Immunization. There is no specific treatment for acute dacryoadenitis. The antiviral and antibacterial drugs are infective, and the pain is managed by oral analgesics.

Chronic dacryoadenitis is less common than acute and is seen in adults. It is commonly bilateral, slow-progressing, non-tender, and painless, and may be associated with mild ptosis and proptosis. The condition is caused by tuberculosis, leprosy, and syphilis. The treatment is the treatment of a primary systemic infection.

Tumors of the lacrimal glands can be benign or malignant. Out of the two, benign tumors are more frequent. The most common benign tumor is called a mixed tumor of the gland. Which develops after 50 years of age, is unilateral and slow to progress. The features are the ptosis S-shaped curve of the lid margin, visible and palpable growth in the superior and outer quadrants of the orbit, and mild proptosis. The lymph nodes are not enlarged. The treatment is the surgical removal of the gland. The malignant tumor is adenoid cystic carcinoma, which has the same features as a mixed tumor. The only difference is that it progresses fast with enlarged preauricular lymph nodes. The treatment consists of the removal of all the contents of the orbit, including the eye.

8

CHAPTER

Disorders of the Orbits

The disorders of the orbits are—displacement, infection, inflammation, growths, and trauma. Out of these displacements, the most common cause may be primary or secondary. The displacement may be forward or backward. The forward displacement is known by proptosis and exophthalmos. While posterior displacement is called enophthalmos, the term anophthalmos should be strictly used to denote the congenital absence of an eyeball. The condition; more common than anophthalmos is microphthalmos, which means an overall congenital reduction of the eyeball. A soft eye is called phthisis bulbi, and the removal of the structures is called an emptysocket. Removal of all the orbital structures, including the periorbita, is called exenteration; removal of intraocular tissues leaving the sclera intact is called evisceration; and removal of eyeballs with intraocular structures is called enucleation.

PROPTOSIS AND EXOPHTHALMOS

In the past, the two terms were used to denote separate conditions. The term proptosis was used to denote a passive bulge of the globe due to retrobulbar or peribulbar mass. The term **exophthalmos** was exclusively used to denote thyroid oculopathy **(Fig. 8.1)**. Nowadays, the two are used to denote the forward displacement of the globe due to any cause.

Proptosis

Proptosis can be congenital or acquired; the second is more common than the first.

Congenital Proptosis

Congenital proptosis is due to underdevelopment of the orbit, generally associated with maldevelopment of the skull and face. The eyes, which are normal in all dimensions, are too large for the shallow orbits hence are pushed forwards. The eyes have poor vision due to associated

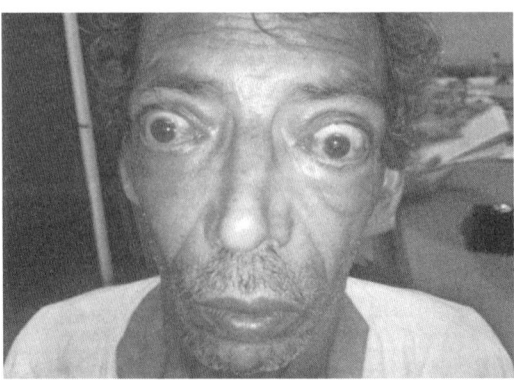

Fig. 8.1: Exophthalmos.

optic atrophy; squints and mental retardations are common. Rarely there may be an abnormal congenital mass in a normal orbit, causing proptosis. The causes of deformed skulls are seen in Crouzon and Apert syndromes. The proptosis is generally bilateral and symmetrical.

Acquired Proptosis

Acquired proptosis is generally unilateral. The main causes of proptosis are tumor, benign or malignant. The malignancy can be primary, secondary, or an extension from the surrounding structures. The mass can be inflammatory and called pseudotumors of the orbit. The other causes are hematoma (blood), abscess (pus) parasites cysts, dermoid, mucocele of paranasal sinuses, meningoencephalocele, and meningocele **(Fig. 8.2)**.

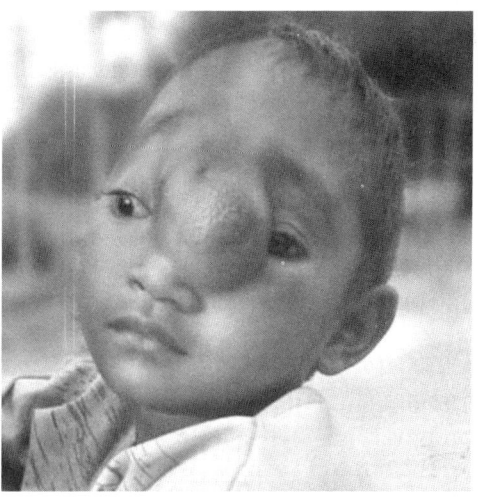

Fig. 8.2: Meningocele.
(For color version, see Plate 2)

The common tumors causing proptosis in children are orbital retinoblastoma, leukemia, rhabdomyosarcoma (RMS), and optic nerve glioma.

The common tumors in adults that cause proptosis could be primary or secondary.

The **primary** tumor causing proptosis are—optic nerve meningioma, neurofibroma, orbital varices, dermoid, cavernous hemangioma, and orbital lymphomas.

The **secondary** tumors deposited in the orbit are from the bronchus, breast, prostate, kidney, and lymphomas. The malignancies that arise from the intraorbital and paraorbital structures are growths from the globe, lacrimal glands, paranasal sinuses, and brain. The malignancies from the globe that invade orbit are retinoblastoma and malignant melanoma. From the lacrimal gland arise the mixed lacrimal gland tumors. The mucocele invading the orbit are mucocele from the paranasal sinuses. The meningocele and meningoencephalocele arise from the brain. The other cause consists of parasitic cysts and retained foreign bodies.

Table 8.1 shows the causes of unilateral and bilateral proptosis.

Table 8.1: Causes of unilateral and bilateral proptosis.		
	Proptosis	
Sl. No.	Unilateral	Bilateral
1.	**Congenital**: Meningocele, encephalocele, and dermoid	Oxycephaly
2.	**Tumors** • Primary tumors—retinoblastoma, rhabdomyosarcoma (RMS), hemangioma, optic nerve glioma, meningioma leukemia, lymphoma neuroblastoma. • Extension from surrounding structures • Secondaries from distant organs	Retinoblastoma, lymphoma, lymphosarcoma, and leukemia
3.	• **Infective lesion:** Orbital cellulitis, cavernous sinus thrombosis	Cavernous sinus thrombosis, Wegener granuloma, tuberculosis, and fungal granuloma
4.	• **Inflammatory:** Pseudotumors of the orbits	Pseudotumors
5.	• **Others:** Orbital thyroid disease, parasitic cyst, foreign body, orbital varix	Orbital thyroid disease

Note: Some of the unilateral conditions become bilateral.

Proptosis can be Acute or Chronic

The acute proptosises are generally associated with pain and are unilateral. Proptosis as per onset can be acute or chronic, as shown in the **Table 8.2.**

Pseudoproptosis

These are the conditions where the globe seems to bulge out of its orbit without actually being so. **The causes are:** Unilateral high myopia, unilateral buphthalmos, unilateral large ciliary staphyloma, retraction of the upper lid, unilateral lagophthalmos, contralateral microphthalmos and phthisis, contralateral mild ptosis, and familial.

Direction of Proptosis

The direction of proptosis and its extent point many a time towards the possible cause of proptosis.

The direction of proptosis can be any of the following or in combination. **They are:**
1. **Axial:** straight forward due to any growth inside the muscle cone **(Fig. 8.3)**. Common causes are glioma of the optic nerve and meningioma of the optic nerve sheath.
2. Downwards due to growth from the roof of the orbit.
3. Upwards due to growth from the floor of the orbit.
4. Down towards and medial lacrimal gland tumors
5. Down towards the ear, growth from the frontal sinus

Extent of proptosis can be measured by simple inspection or by employing various types of instruments called exophthalmometers. The fully developed proptosis is too obvious to miss;

Table 8.2: Acute or chronic proptosis.	
Acute onset	**Gradual onset**
Retrobulbar hemorrhage, surgical emphysema of the orbit, acute orbital cellulitis, cavernous sinus thrombosis, panophthalmitis, acute dacryoadenitis, and fast-growing rhabdomyosarcoma (RMS)	Craniofacial dysostosis, pseudotumor of the orbit, dysthyroid orbitopathy, orbital tumor, orbital parasites, leukemia, periorbital tumor, optic nerve glioma, optic nerve meningioma, aneurysm of the ophthalmic artery, orbital varices

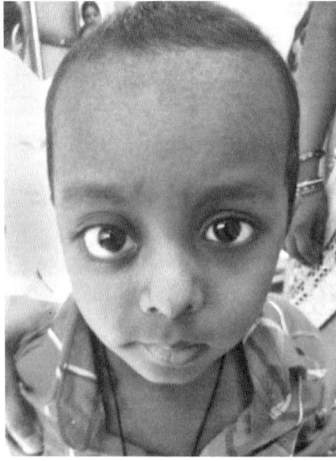

Fig. 8.3: Unilateral axial proptosis.

difficulty arises when the proptosis is mild or minimum. To inspect, the patient is made to sit in a chair with the observer standing behind, and the patient's head is bent backwards. The observer looks down and notices the position of the cornea in relation to the upper orbital rim. In a normal orbit, the apex of the cornea is not visible in this position; if the cornea is visible beyond the upper lid margin, the patient suffers from proptosis **(Fig. 8.4)**. Proptosis can be accurately measured by exophthalmometers.

INFECTIOUS DISEASES OF THE ORBIT

The infectious diseases of the orbit could be intraorbital or from the walls and periosteum of the orbit. The common sources of infection with the orbital contents are any of the following, i.e., paranasal sinuses, blood, or penetrating injury. The infections of the contents are called orbital cellulitis, which could be acute, chronic, or recurrent.

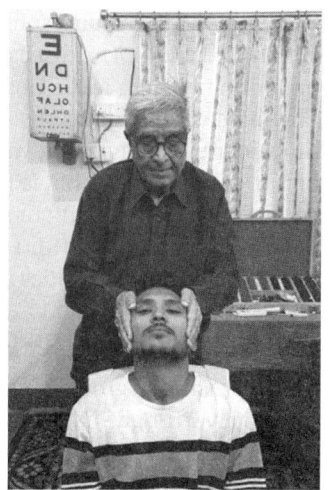

Fig. 8.4: Inspection of proptosis.

Acute Orbital Cellulitis

This is an ocular emergency, specially in children requiring urgent attention; it is the most common cause of acute, painful unilateral proptosis. More common in children, it is associated with fever, chills, headaches, and pain in the orbit and periorbital structures. The most common source of infection is from acute or chronic paranasal sinuses. The signs consist of swelling of the lids, pseudoptosis congestion, and chemosis of the conjunctiva. Proptosis is mild to moderate. The movement of the globe is restricted. Diminished vision and sluggish pupillary reaction due to involvement of the optic nerve. The condition should be differentiated from preseptal Cellulitis, cavernous sinus thrombosis, panophthalmitis, retained foreign body, X-ray, shows presence of foreign body and evidence of sinusitis. CT is better than X-rays as it delineates specific sinuses involved, especially the ethmoid. It also reveals subperiosteal abscesses and intracranial involvement. Ultrasonography is also helpful in the diagnosis of orbital cellulitis. It shows the involvement of individual muscles. The management consists of the administration of an appropriate intravenous, broad-spectrum antibiotic in an age-related dose. Orbital cellulitis, if not treated well, will result in the formation of an orbital sinus opening on the skin. Partially treated orbital cellulitis passes into a stage of recurrence or chronic orbital cellulitis, which rarely may be converted into an orbital abscess.

Orbital Abscess

An orbital abscess is a collection of pus behind the orbital septum; its most common sign is mild to moderate proptosis, generally axial. The amount of proptosis depends on the size of the abscess. The other signs are restricted movement of the globe and diminished vision. The diagnosis is confirmed by ultrasonography and CT. A CT will reveal the exact position and size of the abscess. The treatment is a broad-spectrum systemic antibiotic. No attempt should be made to drain the abscess blindly.

Cavernous Sinus Thrombosis

This is yet another ophthalmic emergency that requires consultation with neuro physicians. The condition is an acute infection of the cavernous sinus situated just behind the orbit, receiving venous blood from many sources. Infections of the nose and face are most likely to cause cavernous sinus thrombosis. The disease starts on one side; the other side gets involved a few days later. The patient has a high fever, headache, and vomiting with diplopia and mild to severe proptosis. The effected side develops edema of the lids, and the conjunctiva is chemosed and red. The movements are restricted with diminished vision. The other eye commonly develops paralysis of the lateral rectus. That is followed by a clinical picture similar to the other eye involved. The condition should be differentiated between orbital cellulitis and ophthalmitis. The diagnosis is confirmed by CT and MRI. The treatment is multidisciplinary and requires the administration of broad-spectrum antibiotics and a life-support system.

Chronic Inflammation of the Orbit

This consists of a group of chronic inflammatory conditions of uncertain origin. The conditions are mostly wrongly diagnosed as malignancies of the orbit. They are called pseudotumors of the orbit. That may involve any structure in the orbit or even the lacrimal gland. The condition is supposed to be an autoimmune disease. The other causes are tuberculosis, syphilis, ruptured dermoid, leaking orbital abscess, and ruptured parasitic cyst. The condition is generally unilateral. Seen in the fourth to fifth decade, equally in both sexes. The symptoms are variable; they are mild to moderate proptosis. Swelling of the lids, puffiness of the conjunctiva, restricted muscle movement, and diminished vision. The diagnosis is by exclusion. X-rays has hardly any used in diagnosis; better results are found by USG, CT, and MRI. When the superior orbital fissure through which pass. All the cranial nerves serving the eye are involved; the condition is called superior orbital fissure syndrome. If the apex of the orbit is involved, it is called orbital apex syndrome. The superior orbital fissure syndrome presents with the underaction of single or many extraocular muscles. In the orbital apex syndrome, the optic nerve is also involved, along with the extraocular muscles.

Tumors of the Orbit

The orbit contains tissues of varied origin; it is surrounded by many extraorbital structures, such as paranasal sinuses; and it communicates with the brain as well. The orbital tumors may arise from its structures, invasion from neighboring structures, and secondaries from distant organs. The tumors of the orbit can be congenital or acquired. **Flowchart 8.1** shows the classification of orbital tumors.

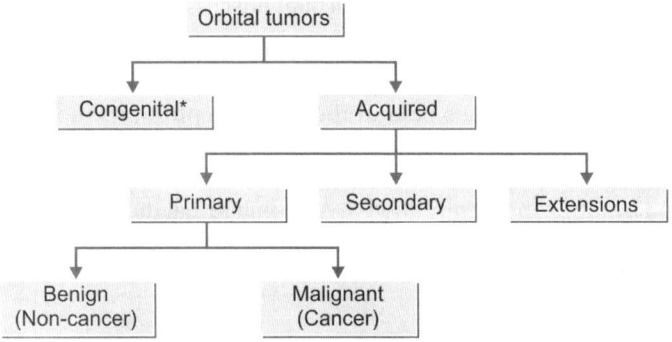

Flowchart 8.1: Classification of orbital tumor.

Congenital*
The congenital growths are dermoid, hemangioma, encephalocele, meningocele, and meningoencephalocele. The congenital growths are non-cancerous. They may be obvious at birth or diagnosed in the next few months or years.

Dermoids

Dermoids are very common tumors encountered in orbital and paraorbital structures. They are cystic growths; they contain skin, hair, and fatty tissue. They may arise anywhere in the orbit; the growths behind the orbital septum cause proptosis, the amount of which depends on the position and size of the growths. The preseptal growths do not cause proptosis; the common sites of the tumors are the superomedial and superiotemporal ends or orbital margin **(Fig. 8.5)**. The dermoids present in front of the septum are visible and palpebral. They are spherical, firm growths over which the skin can be moved, non-tender, and fixed to the bone underneath. The growths are slow to develop, showing an increase in size at puberty; otherwise, they are symptoms-free. The diagnosis is confirmed by X-rays and CT, and the definite treatment of all dermoids is surgical removal without rupturing the wall. There is no recurrence following surgical removal; retroseptal dermoids are difficult to remove. They are removed by various orbitotomies.

Hemangioma of the Orbit

They are benign tumors of vascular origin, generally congenital, that remain asymptomatic and were discovered on routine imaging with a well-defined capsule. They are seen mostly in the fourth and fifth decades, causing the gradual onset of proptosis. The type and degree of proptosis depend on the position and size of the tumor. The standard management is surgical removal through an appropriate orbitotomy.

Meningocele (Fig. 8.2)

A normal orbit does not contain meninges that stop beyond the apex of the orbit. If the meninges find access to the orbit, they may lie dormant throughout their lives or may convert into a round cystic swelling. They may be pre- or retroseptal; the retroseptal growths are responsible for proptosis. They are best seen on CT and MRI. The treatment is surgical removal. If brain tissue finds its way into the meningocele, it is called a meningoencephalocele; still rare is the encephalocele, where brain tissue finds its way into the orbit. The treatment for all the above conditions is surgical removal.

Acquired Orbital Tumors

Acquired orbital tumors can be benign or malignant; the malignant tumor can be primary, secondary, extension from neighboring structures.

The common benign orbital tumors are hemangioma, glioma of the optic nerve, meningioma of the optic nerve, neurofibroma, and mixed tumor of the lacrimal gland.

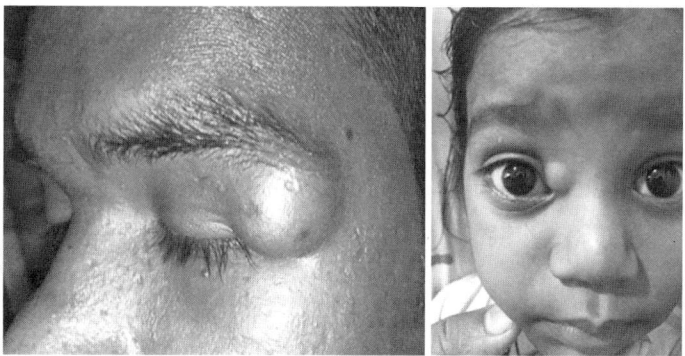

Fig. 8.5: Preseptal dermoids in different ages not causing proptosis.

The common primary malignant tumor of the orbit are rhabdomyosarcoma*, orbital lymphoma**, and carcinoma of the lacrimal gland.

Rhabdomyosarcoma (RMS)*
Rhabdomyosarcoma is a rare malignant tumor of soft tissue anywhere in the body, at all ages. It is a sarcoma that spreads rapidly. Orbital Rhabdomyosarcoma is the most common primary malignancy of orbit in children; 90% of them are seen before 15 years of age, with the average age being 5–7 years. The boy-to-girl ratio is 5:3 without any racial predisposition without any genetic background. Ophthalmologists are first to see them. The child is brought in with fast-growing puffiness of the lid with mild to moderate proptosis. That has not responded to the usual broad-spectrum antibiotics because it is often missed and diagnosed as slow-growing orbital cellulitis. The treatment consists of a combination of chemotherapy and radiation following an excisional biopsy by an oncologist.

Orbital lymphoma**
Primary orbital lymphoma is a rare malignant disorder of the orbit. It presents as gradual, progressive swelling of the lid and conjunctiva lacrimal gland with mild to moderate proptosis. The treatment consists of **surgery, radiotherapy, and chemotherapy by an oncologist.**

Common malignant tumors that invade the orbit are from eyeballs and neighbouring structures. The two intraocular malignancies that extend into the orbit are retinoblastoma in children and malignant melanoma. The second group consists of malignancies in the paranasal sinuses, nasopharynx, and brain. The metastatic tumors of the orbit in children are neuroblastoma, nephroblastoma, and Ewing's sarcoma. In adults, they are from the breast, lung, stomach, and prostate.

Clinical Presentation of an Orbital Tumor

They can be seen in any age in all races in both the sexes can be unilateral, bilateral, malignant, or non-malignant **(Figs. 8.6 and 8.7)**. Some of which respond well with treatment, occurrence following treatment is common. The symptoms depend on the location and size of the lesion and its nature, i.e., malignant or non-malignant. The most common symptoms are—proptosis, reduced movement diplopia—diminished vision pain in and around the orbit associated with symptoms of the primary tumor.

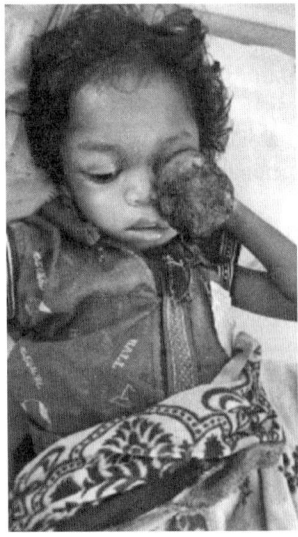

Fig. 8.6: Late presentation of unilateral retinoblastoma.

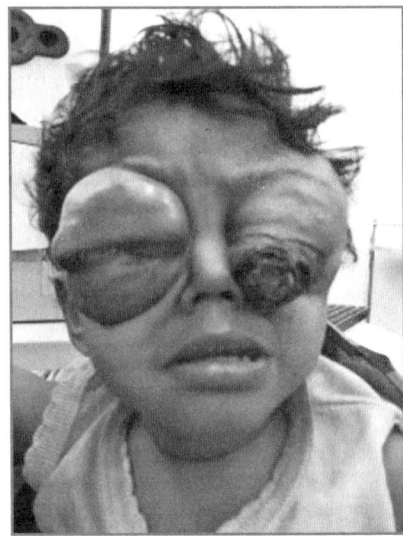

Fig. 8.7: Late presentation of bilateral retinoblastoma.

Signs of Orbital Tumors

- **Proptosis:** Tumors in the muscle cone cause axial proptosis **(Fig. 8.3)**, tumors outside the cone cause eccentric proptosis away from the growth. Tumor from superiotemporal aspect cause proptosis down and in **(Fig. 8.8)**, growth from superomedial cause proptosis down and out **(Fig. 8.9)**.
- Restricted movement
- Variable diplopia
- Lagophthalmos
- Diminished vision
- Corneal and conjunctival exposure
- The eyeball may/may not be pushed back by pressure

The diagnosis is confirmed by:
- X-ray, USG, CT and MRI
- Biopsy
  - Fine needle biopsy
  - Excisional biopsy

Treatment

Treatment depends on the nature of the tumor, the benign tumors are best removed surgically, while primary malignant tumors are treated by surgery, chemotherapy, and radiation. May be alone by one method or combination. The tumors extending from the neighboring structures and the metastatic tumor require treatment of the primary tumor along with ophthalmic treatment, both under the supervision of an oncologist.

Exophthalmos

The term exophthalmos is used to denote the forward placement of the eyes in thyroid orbital diseases. It generally happens in hyperthyroidism, can be seen in hypothyroidism, or even without

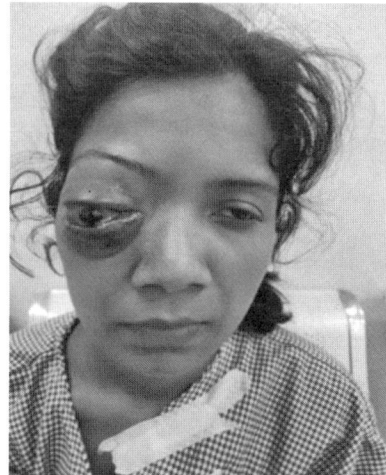

Fig. 8.8: Eccentric proptosis due to growth from superomedial orbit.
(*Courtesy:* Professor Somen Misra)

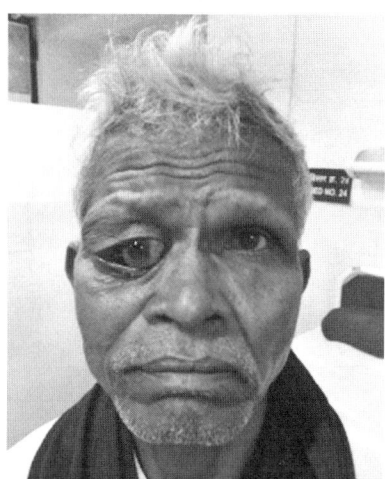

Fig. 8.9: Eccentric proptosis due to growth from superiotemporal orbit.
(*Courtesy:* Professor Somen Misra)

involvement of the thyroid. It is more commonly seen in women; it may start in one eye. When bilateral, the amount of exophthalmos need not be the same in the two eyes. The patients may not be aware of developing exophthalmos because it is slow and progressive. The first clinical feature is lid retraction, followed by lid lag and diplopia. The exophthalmos is clinically divided into mild, moderate, and severe grades; in the late stages, there may be exposure to the cornea, causing irritation and lacrimation. The corneal exposure may lead to corneal ulceration. Hyperthyroidism and hypothyroidism are treated by endocrinologists. The ocular features are managed by the ophthalmologist.

Enophthalmos

Enophthalmos is the backward placement of a normal or small eyeball in relation to the normal position. The causes of these are microphthalmos **(Fig. 8.10)**, phthisis bulbi, and fibrosis of the muscle, fracture of the flow of the orbit following squint surgery, retraction syndrome, and Horner's syndromes. The signs of enophthalmos are a narrow interpalpebral aperture and the appearance of pseudoptosis; the curvature is less; the vision is low and cannot be corrected; the only treatment is either to increase the orbital volume or to place an artificial eye **(Fig. 8.11)**.

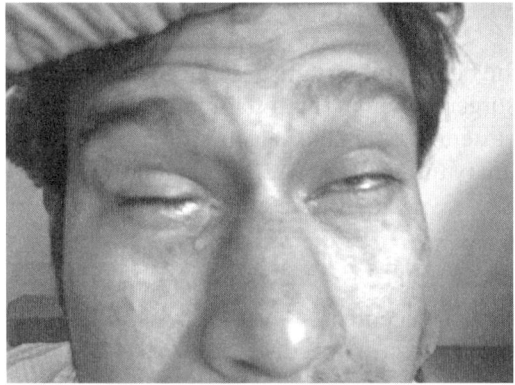

Fig. 8.10: Bilateral enophthalmos.

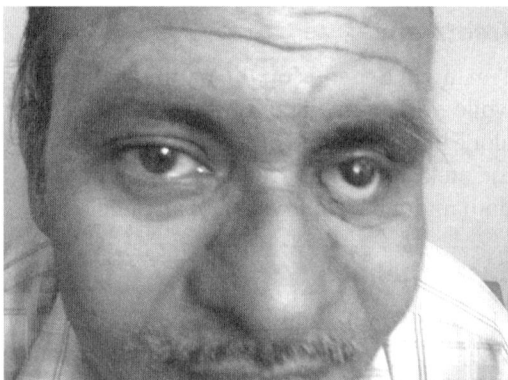

Fig. 8.11: Left artificial eye due to microphthalmos.

CHAPTER 9

Disorders of Conjunctiva

Disorders of conjunctiva are very common in all ages from birth onwards. Congenital anomalies of the conjunctiva are rare, but when present, they are associated with anomalies of the lids. The conjunctiva extends from the intermarginal strip of the lid to the limbus, covering the back of the lid and the front of the sclera. The junction of the two is the fornix **(Fig. 9.1)**.

The conjunctiva is well supplied by blood vessels and nerves with sufficient lymphatic drainage.

The diseases of the conjunctiva are:
- Congenital
  - Rare
- Acquired
  - Infection
  - Allergy
  - Nutritional
  - Degenerative
  - Neoplasm
    - Benign
    - Malignant

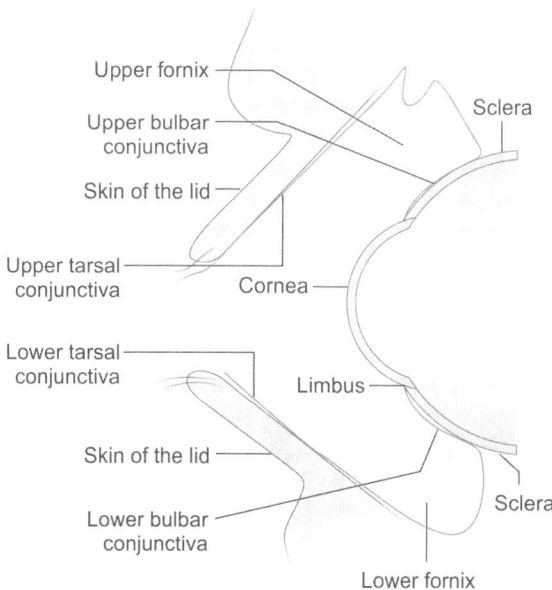

Fig. 9.1: Parts of conjunctiva.

COMMON CLINICAL FEATURES OF CONJUNCTIVAL DISORDERS

- Lacrimation
- Hyperemia
- Subconjunctival hemorrhage
- Chemosis (puffiness)
- Discharge
- Itching
- Xerosis
- Phlycten
- Episcleritis
- Pinguecula
- Pterygium
- Symblepharon
- Growth

Lacrimation

Lacrimation is a common symptom of conjunctival disease, both inflammatory and allergic. It is more prominent in acute conjunctivitis, which is invariably associated with discharge. Besides conjunctival disorders, it can also be seen due to disorders of the cornea, uvea, and reflex. To find out the cause of lacrimation, the following examination should be done: exclude epiphora, examine the cornea for injury, minute foreign body keratitis, examine the tarsal plate for hidden foreign bodies, and look for evidence of iritis.

Hyperemia

Inspite of the rich blood supply, the conjunctiva does not look red or pink, except for a few blood vessels travelling from the periphery not reaching the limbus. This property is responsible for its transparency. In hyperemia, the number of blood vessels, both arteries and veins, increases. The redness is directly proportionate to the number of blood vessels. As the conjunctiva vessels spread from the fornix to the center, conjunctiva hyperemia is at its maximum in the fornix. There are three types of redness in the conjunctiva. They are conjunctival congestion, circumciliary congestion, and episcleral congestion. The three are differentiated by their distribution.

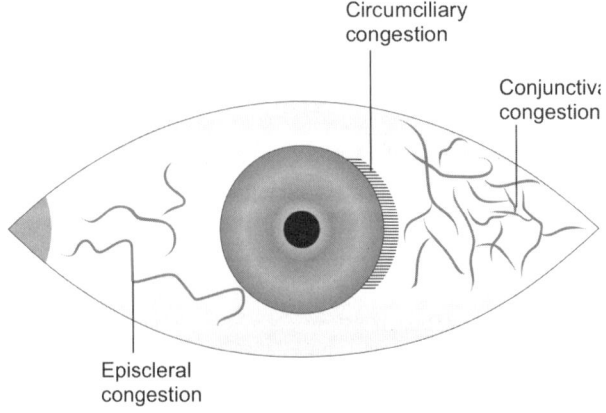

Fig. 9.2: Three types of conjunctival congestion.

Conjunctival Congestion

Conjunctival congestion starts in the fornix **(Fig. 9.3)** and spreads towards the cornea, not reaching the limbus. They are bright red in color, move with the movement of conjunctiva, the blood flow is from the periphery to the center, and the congestion disappears with the instillation of vasoconstrictor, generally associated with discharge **(Fig. 9.4)**.

Conjunctival congestion **(Fig. 9.5)** is generally bilateral. Unilateral conjunctival congestion is rarely infective, which is the commonest cause of conjunctival congestion. The other cause is allergic conjunctivitis; the conjunctival congestion disappears with treatment. There is no pain in pressing over the globe, which is common with circumciliary congestion.

Circumciliary Congestion

Circumciliary congestion **(Fig. 9.6)** is maximum at the limbus and fades towards the fornix. It does not extend more than 2–3 mm all-round the limbus. Rarely may it be localized to begin with; the color is lighter than seen in conjunctival congestion, in the early stages; it is called a circumciliary flush. It is invariably associated with ciliary tenderness. The common causes are keratitis, iridocyclitis, and acute congestive glaucoma. Posterior uveal inflammation and chronic simple glaucoma do not cause circumciliary congestion. It is the first to disappear

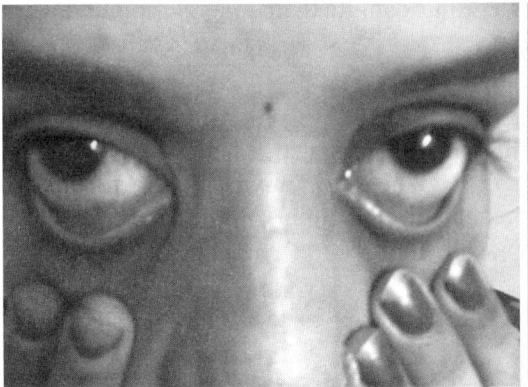

Fig. 9.3: Early conjunctival congestion. *(For color version, see Plate 3)*

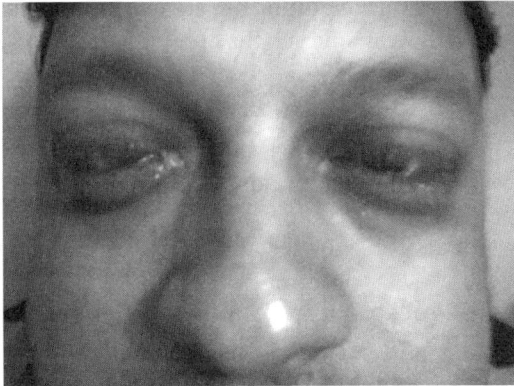

Fig. 9.4: Bilateral conjunctivitis congestion with discharge.

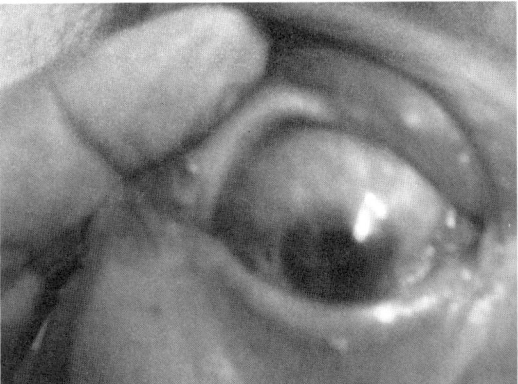

Fig. 9.5: Fully developed conjunctival congestion with subconjunctival hemorrhage. *(For color version, see Plate 3)*

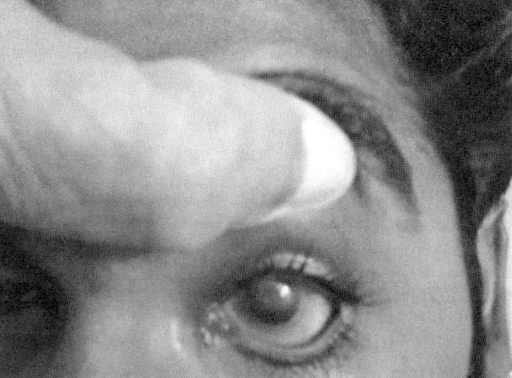

Fig. 9.6: Circumciliary congestion. *(For color version, see Plate 3)*

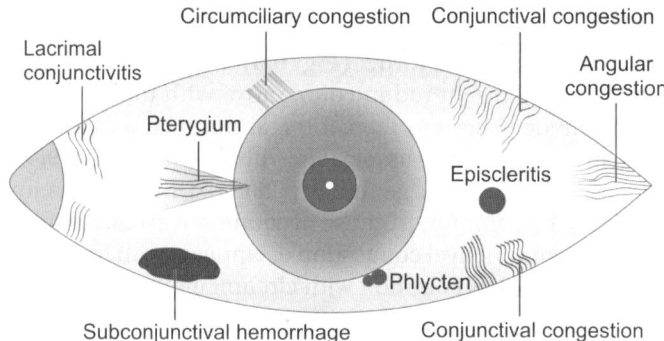

Fig. 9.7: Various types of conjunctival congestion.

with treatment; its disappearance does not indicate a cure of iridocyclitis or acute congestive glaucoma. It may sometimes be associated with conjunctival congestion, and the condition is then referred to as mixed congestion.

The conjunctival congestion can be generalized or localized **(Fig. 9.7)**. The causes of conjunctival congestion are acute conjunctivitis, chronic conjunctivitis, allergic conjunctivitis, and chemical injury to the conjunctiva.

Episcleral Congestion

Episcleral congestion is less frequent than the above two. It is due to the dilatation of episcleral vessels. The commonest cause is benign absolute glaucoma. The vessels start from the periphery, proceeding towards the limbus. Before reaching the limbus, they bifurcate and take a lateral course to meet the adjoining vessels **(Fig. 9.2)**.

Causes of Localized Conjunctiva Congestion
- Infection
- Allergy
- Trauma

Causes of localized conjunctiva congestion are:
- Trauma
- Pterygium
- Phlycten
- Episcleritis
- Circumciliary congestion
- Angular conjunctivitis
- Growth of the conjunctiva

Subconjunctival Hemorrhage (Blood Under Conjunctiva)

Logically, the term subconjunctival hemorrhage should be used to denote blood under the transparent conjunctiva; however, clinically, the term is used for intraconjunctival hemorrhage. Subconjunctival hemorrhage can develop anywhere in the conjunctiva. It only attracts attention when it is in the bulbar conjunctiva. Generally, it is unilateral. It can be localized or generalized **(Figs. 9.8A and B)**.

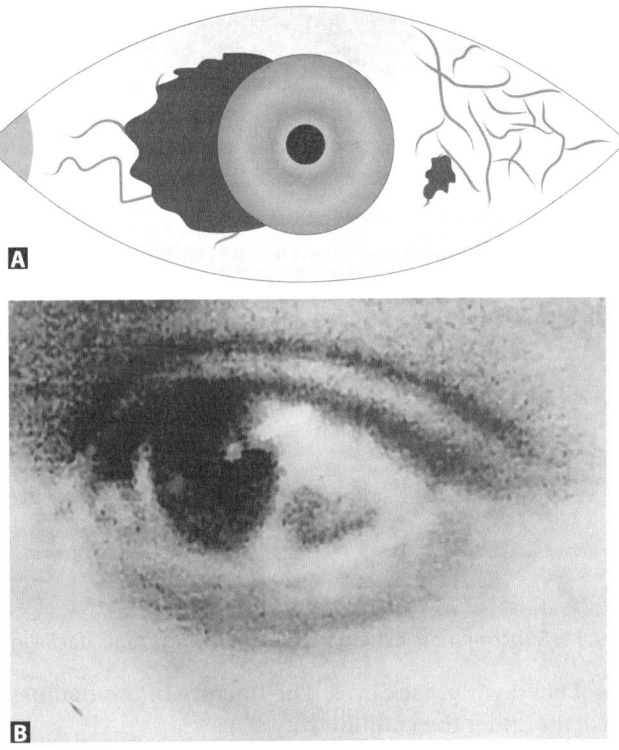

Figs. 9.8A and B: Localized subconjunctival hemorrhage, periphery visible.

Causes of Localized Subconjunctival Hemorrhages

- Trauma
- Whooping cough (commonest cause in children)
- Idiopathic (when no cause can be found)
- Blood dyscrasia (abnormal blood)

Causes of Generalized Subconjunctival Hemorrhage

- **Severe microbial infection:** They may be uniform, covering the whole conjunctiva or petechial **(Fig. 9.9)**, caused by *Pneumococcus*, acute hemorrhagic conjunctivitis, and epidemic keratoconjunctivitis.
- **Injury:** (i) Head injury; (ii) Orbital injury
  These hemorrhages occur after few hours to few days of injury. They spread from the periphery to the center; their peripheral borders are not seen **(Figs. 9.10 and 9.11)**.

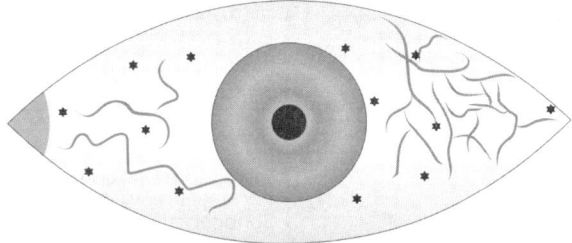

Fig. 9.9: Petechial hemorrhages.

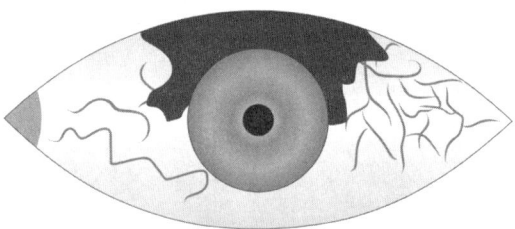

Fig. 9.10: Subconjunctival hemorrhage, periphery not visible, may be due to head injury.

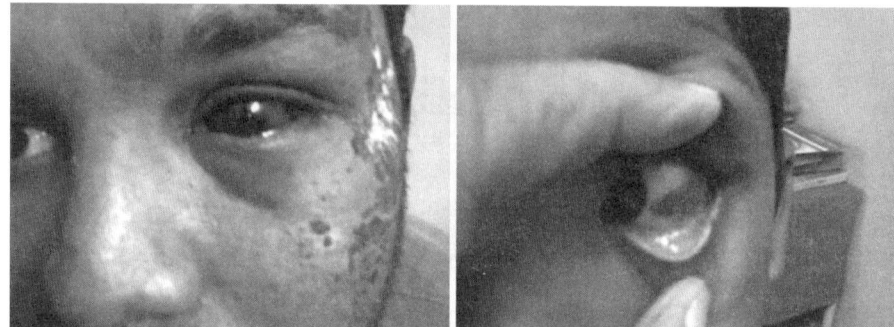

Fig. 9.11: Subconjunctival hemorrhage following cranial facial injury.

They are often associated with black eyes. The fracture of the paranasal sinuses results in the accumulation of air under the conjunctiva

Chemosis (Puffiness)

Chemosis is the accumulation of fluid under the conjunctiva; the conjunctiva is lifted away from the sclera, causing a diffuse, translucent edema of the conjunctiva. The edema can be reduced by pressure, only to reappear when the conjunctiva is congested. It is not painful; the commonest cause is acute allergic conjunctivitis. That can be unilateral or bilateral; most of the time, it disappears within an hour without treatment. If it persists, a local drop of steroids can be used. Chemosis of conjunctivitis is also seen in severe infections of conjunctiva by gonococcus and leptospirosis. It is common in severe endophthalmitis and panophthalmitis.

Discharge

Presence of discharge from the eyes denotes conjunctival disease. The quality of discharge differs in its character; it could be watery, mucoid, mucopurulent, and purulent.

The causes of these types of discharge are given in **Table 9.1.**

Table 9.1: Types and causes of discharge.	
Type	*Cause*
Watery	Allergic and viral conjunctivitis
Mucoid	Simple conjunctivitis
Mucopurulent	Severe bacterial conjunctivitis
Purulent (pus)	Gonococcal conjunctivitis

The discharge contains tears, mucus, epithelial cells, pus, and organisms.

Itching

Itching may be mild, moderate, or severe; persons with mild itching generally do not seek medical help. The most troublesome itching is due to allergies: spring catarrh, seasonal allergic conjunctivitis, perennial allergic conjunctivitis, and giant papillary conjunctivitis. The itching in acute allergic conjunctivitis is short-lived. The discharge in spring catarrh is ropy.

Xerosis (Xero = Dry)

In xerosis of the conjunctiva, the conjunctiva loses its shine, brightness, and wetness. It is generally bilateral and does not need to be symmetrical. On the temporal side of the conjunctiva, it may involve the whole bulbar conjunctiva and spread over the cornea. Involvement of the conjunctiva and cornea is called xerophthalmia. The commonest cause of xerosis of conjunctiva is vitamin A deficiency seen in children. The conditions may be associated with night blindness. The xerotic area looks dirty, white, wrinkled, slightly raised, and dry. As xerosis is a precursor to xerophthalmia, it should not be taken lightly. Xerosis of the conjunctiva at this stage, if treated, prevents xerophthalmia, which is an important cause of blindness in children.

The other causes of xerosis, independent of vitamin A deficiency, can be seen in all ages and may be unilateral or bilateral; they are coloboma of the upper lid, lagophthalmos proptosis, trachoma, severe dry eye syndrome, and chemical injury to the conjunctiva.

Bitot's Spot

Bitot's spot is a triangular raised whiter than underline sclera with a rough surface. The base of the Bitot's spot is towards the limbus. It is mostly seen on the temporal side. It can be rubbed off with a swab, only to reappear. It does not stain with fluorescein or Rose Bengal but stain with kohl (kajal) which is the best sign for the parents to bring the child for consultation. It is a common sign of vitamin A deficiency and disappears following complete treatment with vitamin A as per the national program.

Prevention and Treatment of Xerophthalmia

- **Administration of vitamin A**: All pregnant mothers should get 100,000 IU of vitamin A between 6 and 9 months of pregnancy.
- All children should be immunized as per national program.
- All children should get 100,000 IU (55 mg retinyl palmitate) orally every 6 months up to 6 years of age. Oral vitamin A syrup is available in all primary health centers and Anganwadi free of cost.
- All children suffering from measles should get 100,000 IU of injectable vitamin A.
- Children suffering from chronic diarrhea should be treated by qualified persons.
- All newborn should be fed with the colostrums (The first thick yellow breast milk).
- All children should be breastfed for the first six months. Thereafter, solid food should be added to the diet without stopping breast feeding. Breast feeding should continue till 3 years of age of the child. If mother milk is not sufficient, the child should drink animal milk, i.e., cow or buffalo milk, undiluted.

Phlycten

Phlycten is a common localized delayed allergic conjunctivitis due to delayed allergic to endogenous allergens. In the past, the allergen was thought to be tubercular in nature, which remains an important cause in underdeveloped countries. Nowaday other nontubercular causes too have been thought to cause phlycten. They could be bacterial, viral, fungal, or intestinal parasites; occasionally, no cause can be found.

It is a disorder of childhood. The patients have single or multiple lesions, consisting of small yellow-gray nodules called phlyctenules that commonly appear on the limbus, lasting for few days to few weeks, and either disappear without treatment, not leaving any conjunctival scar, or may ulcerate. The girls are affected more than the boys.

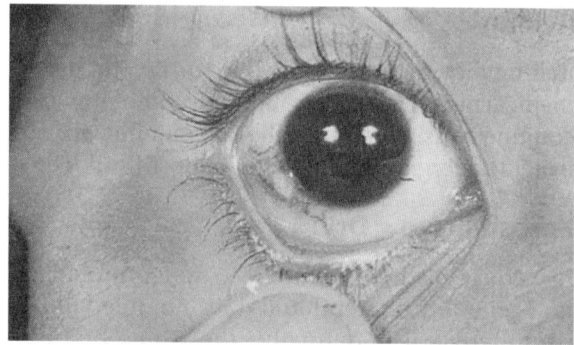

Fig. 9.12: Limbal phlycten.
(For color version, see Plate 4)

The condition is bilateral; both eyes may be involved simultaneously or separately; the number of phlyctens varies from single to multiple; when multiple, they may be seen at different places on the limbus or in a group of 3–5 arranged adjacent to each. They do not recur in the same place after healing. The phlyctens, when sitting astride the limbus, are called phlyctenular keratoconjunctivitis (for corneal involvement, see chapter on cornea). Though the commonest site of phlycten is the limbus in children (**Fig. 9.12**), it has been reported in the tarsal plate intermarginal lid, even at the bulbar conjunctiva, away from the limbus. In children, it is generally associated with conjunctivitis, which has no role as a cause of phlycten. The management of conjunctival phlycten is a weak solution of corticosteroid 3–4 times a day. Only a few drops will resolve a phlycten but will not prevent its recurrence. All children with phlycten should be dewormed regularly.

Episcleritis

Episcleritis is not a disease of the conjunctiva; it is a disorder of the tissue that binds the conjunctiva to the sclera. It is a localized diffuse area of conjunctival congestion (**Fig. 9.13**). The lesion is nontender in contrast to scleritis, which is a disease of the sclera and is painful and tender. It is seen in adults; it is generally unilateral and often confused with phlycten and pinguecula. It does not encroach on the cornea. It is an autoimmune disease commonly associated with pain in the joints. Treatment is a weak solution of local steroids.

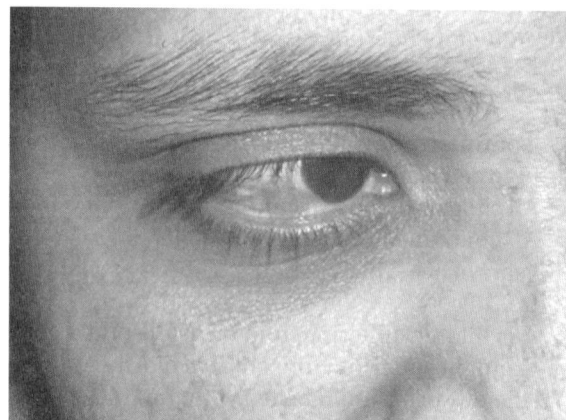

Fig. 9.13: Episcleritis.
(For color version, see Plate 4)

Pinguecula

Pingueculae are frequent noninfective or inflammatory nodules seen on the bulbar conjunctiva, generally on the medial side away from the cornea. They are 1–2 millimeters in size and can be moved, with the conjunctiva being white in color without any vessels on it. It is seen in adults and, once developed, lasts for life. Does not require any treatment.

Pterygium

Pterygium is a noninfectious, non-inflammatory benign growth of the conjunctival seen in the third decade, more common in males who lead outdoor lives. The exact cause of the condition is not well understood. It is thought to be a degenerative condition. Pterygium is a noninfectious, noninflammatory benign growth of the conjunctiva seen in the third decade, more common in males who lead outdoor lives. The exact cause of the condition is not well understood. It is thought to be a degenerative condition. Ultraviolet rays are supposed to increase the chance of the development of pterygium.

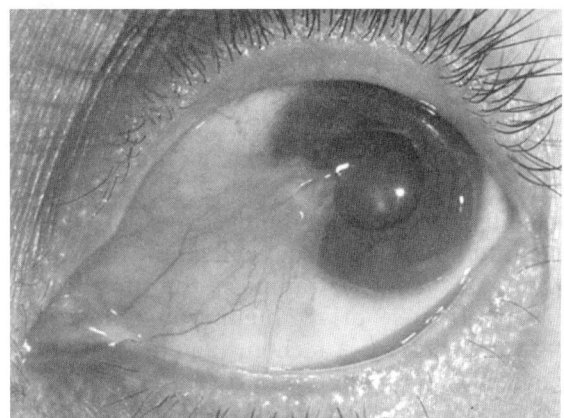

Fig. 9.14: Pterygium.

It is a triangular, fleshy, hyperemic area of conjunctival tissue with an apex on the cornea. The apex is called the head of the pterygium; the rest is the body of the pterygium. It is a vascular, fleshy mass. The hyperemia is more than the adjoining conjunctiva, standing out prominently.

It fans out towards the canthus; it cannot be lifted from the conjunctiva. There is no space between the growth and the sclera. Hence, probes cannot be passed under. It is generally seen on the medial side of the cornea **(Fig. 9.14)**. Less commonly on the lateral side, rarely on both sides. It has been put into various stages and grades.

The first among them is as follows:
Stage 1: The lesion is a flat pink structure at or a little away from the limbus.
Stage 2: The lesion reaches the limbus, and the vascularization is minimal with a slightly raised triangular area.
Stage 3: The lesion spreads like a fan, reaching the medial canthus. The limbal area spreads over the cornea, ending in between the limbus and the pupil.
Stage 4: The pterygium covers the pupil.
Stage 5: The pterygium crosses the pupil.

The grades are progressive, stationary, and atrophic. In the progressive stage, the pterygium grows fast. It takes 2–3 years to reach the cornea. Once on the cornea, it may stop growing and become stationary; otherwise, it may grow to cover the pupil or may cross the pupil. It can develop at any stage and atrophy. The first symptom is the presence of a red, triangular area on the medial side of the cornea for many months without responding to any treatment. The next symptom is the presence of pterygium. The third symptom is diminished, uncorrectable vision. The pterygiums do not cause diplopia.

Treatment

There is no medical treatment. The only treatment is the removal of the growth and the prevention of its recurrence. Recurrence is common following improper surgery.

Symblepharon

Symblepharon is an abnormal adhesion between the tarsal conjunctiva and the bulbar conjunctiva. Rarely, the tarsal conjunctiva may be adherent to the cornea. It is a unilateral condition. There are two types of symblepharon: common anterior symblepharon, where the tarsal conjunctiva gets attached to the bulbar conjunctiva, or cornea **(Fig. 9.15)**. The second is the posterior symblepharon, where there is no visible adhesion. It is seen in Fornices that the fornix is shallow. The causes of symblepharon can be trauma, infection, or autoimmune disease. Out of all the traumas, chemical trauma is the most frequent cause of symblepharon. The infective causes are trachoma and herpes zoster. The autoimmune diseases are Stevens-Johnson syndrome (SJS) and ocular cicatricial pemphigoid (OCP). If both lids are adherent to the globe all over the bulbar conjunctiva, it is called total symblepharon. Treatment of symblepharon is surgical.

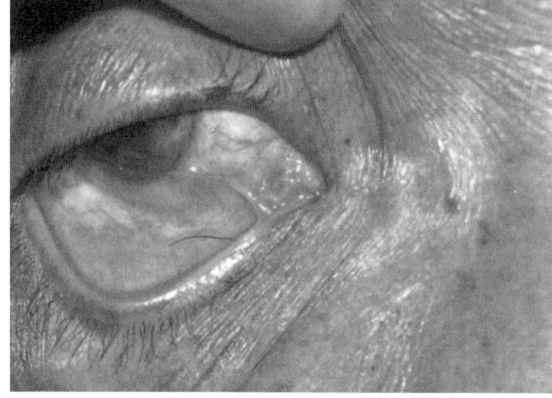

Fig. 9.15: Symblepharon.

Growth

The growth of the conjunctiva can be congenital or acquired. The first example is the conjunctival dermoid **(Fig. 9.16)**. The acquired causes can be infective or noninfective. The causes of infective growths are burst chalazion **(Fig. 9.17)**, foreign body granuloma, and rhinosporidiosis **(Fig. 9.18)**.

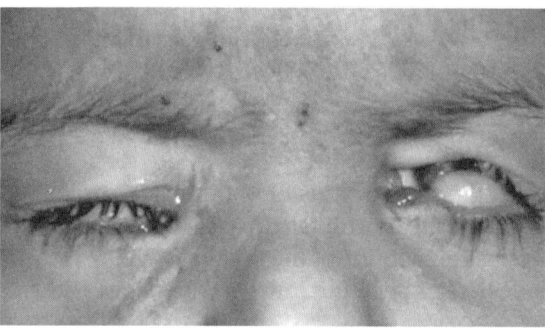

Fig. 9.16: Limbal dermoid.

The causes of noninfective growths are benign and malignant. The benign growths are: nevus, limbal dermoids, dermolipoma, papilloma, hemangioma, and neurofibroma. The malignant growths are epidermoid carcinoma, basal cell carcinoma, and malignant melanoma.

CONJUNCTIVITIS

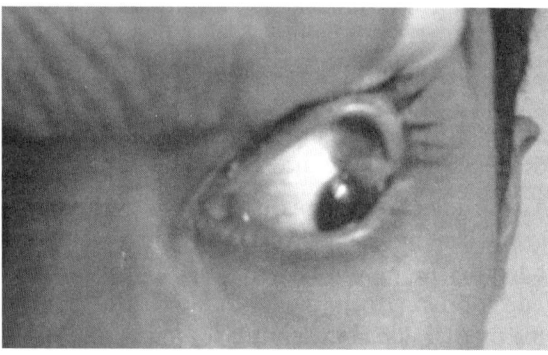

Fig. 9.17: Burst chalazion.

The term conjunctivitis is used to denote an infection or allergy of the conjunctiva.
The infective conjunctivitis can be bacterial, viral, or chlamydia.

Bacterial Conjunctivitis

Bacterial conjunctivitis can be hyperacute (Ophthalmia neonatorum), acute, and chronic; it is seen in all ages in both sexes and is more common in children. Acute conjunctivitis begins in one eye and spreads to the other eye. The commonest symptoms are hyperemia,

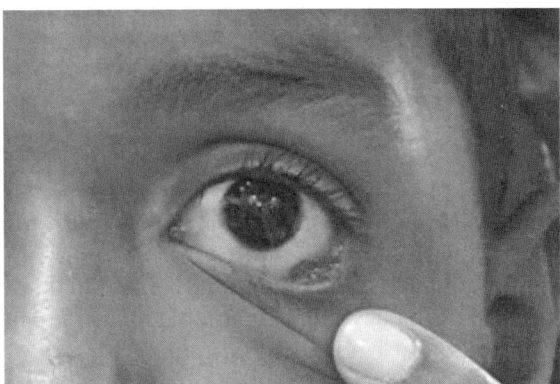

Fig. 9.18: Rhinosporidiosis.

mucopurulent discharge, matting of the lids at night, a foreign body sensation without pain, or diminished vision. The signs consist of mild to moderate swelling of the lids, discharge matted on the lid margin, and a bright red color of the conjunctiva. There may be petechial hemorrhages (pneumococcal conjunctivitis). The blood vessels are dilated, the discharge is mucoid or mucopurulent, the cornea is bright AC, and the pupils are normal. The regurgitation test is negative. The milder form is self-limiting, healing within a few days without leaving any scars. Moderate to severe cases require treatment with frequent local drops of broad-spectrum antibiotics.

The outline of the management consists of:
- Clean the lid margins
- Remove the discharge
- There is no need to wash the conjunctival sac
- No need of hot compress
- Instill broad-spectrum antibiotic drops atleast four times a day, one drop at a time, same antibiotics eye ointment at bedtime.

SOME SPECIFIC TYPES OF CONJUNCTIVITIS

They are: gonococcal, diphtheritic, pneumococcal, and moraxella conjunctivitis.
The first two represent hyperacute conjunctivitis, which is likely to invade the cornea and may be life-threatening, specially in children.

Gonococcal Conjunctivitis

The condition is caused by N-gonococci. The most dangerous part of the infection is that it can pass through intact corneal epithelial cells. Conjunctivitis is found in two forms, i.e., in newborns and adults. In newborns, it is called ophthalmia neonatorum.

Ophthalmia Neonatorum

This is a hyperacute, bilateral conjunctivitis that develops in infants in the first month after birth. It may start within a few hours of birth but may be delayed up to 3–4 weeks. The list of organisms that result in ophthalmia neonatorum is headed by *Gonococcus*. The other causes are pneumococci, staphylococci, hemophilus, herpes simplex, inclusion conjunctivitis, and chemicals.

The clinical presentation of ophthalmia neonatorum is as follows: it develops within 3 days of birth, and the child gets an infection from the mother or from the appliances used to deliver the child. Both the lids are swollen so much that a lid retractor may be used to separate the lids, specially to examine the cornea. The discharge is as thick as pus, and the conjunctiva is bright red.

Management

It is a preventable and treatable condition, and management begins with preventive methods employed by the mother and the child:
- Prophylaxis in mothers should consist of an antenatal examination to exclude evidence of gonococcal infection in the birth passage. If the mother is found to be infected, she is given full antigonococcal chemotherapy before the due date.
- Prophylaxis in newborns consists of cleaning the lidmargins, separating the lidmargins, and instilling one drop of one percent betadine eye drop in each eye. In the absence of betadine, any broad-spectrum antibiotic can be administered one drop in each eye.

Treatment

Treatment of conjunctivitis consists of cleaning the lid margins and instilling one drop of any of the following antibiotic drops: gentamycin, ciprofloxacin, and tobramycin. Every 5 minutes for six times, one drop every 10 minutes for the next one hour, followed by one drop every 4 hours for the next 24 hours. This usually controls the infections. Otherwise, the child should get injectable antigonococcal chemotherapy in consultation with a pediatrician. If the cornea is involved, half a percent atropine sulphate eye ointment is put only once.

The most dreaded complication of ophthalmia neonatorum is a central ulcer that soon perforates, leading to endophthalmitis. If the perforation is sealed by the iris, an adherent leucoma will develop. This prevents the eye from going into stage of endophthalmitis. Such perforations are followed by the development of an anterior polar cataract. That leads to diminished vision and nystagmus.

Gonococcal Conjunctivitis in Adults

The condition is generally unilateral; the infection spreads from the genitals to the eye through contaminated fingers. The ocular infection takes 2–3 days to develop conjunctivitis to develop after genital exposure. The clinical picture is similar to gonococcal conjunctivitis in children, but in a lesser form, which consists of swelling of the lid, conjunctival congestion with chemosis, and purulent discharge. The cornea should be examined at the first visit, and if found to be involved, the condition should be treated as any fast-developing corneal ulcer. The other eye may get involved via infected fingers and clothing. The conjunctivitis is managed by antigonococcal antibiotic eye drops every hour for the first 24 hours. Following that, every four hours for the next 5 days. The patients should get sufficient antigonococcal chemotherapy to prevent and treat systemic involvement.

Diphtheritic Conjunctivitis

This is a hyperacute bilateral conjunctivitis mostly seen in children who have not been immunized as per the national program of immunization. It can occur in adults attending the sick child. The diphtheritic conjunctivitis in adults is milder. Conjunctivitis develops following an infection in the throat. The infection is caused by diphtheria bacilli that can pass through intact corneal epithelium. The clinical picture consists of swollen lids and congested conjunctiva with membrane on the tarsal conjunctiva in both lids or in patches. Sometimes the membrane develops on the bulbar conjunctiva. It is difficult to remove the membrane, which is white in color without vessels on it. Attempts to remove the membrane cause bleeding from the conjunctiva. Cornea may develop an ulcer that requires early attention and management. Besides diphtheria, the other organisms that also cause membrane formation are N. gonorrhoeae, Streptococcus pyogenes, adenovirus, and chlamydia.

Note: All membranes on conjunctiva should be considered to be diphtheritic unless proved otherwise.

Management

The condition is fully preventable and treatable. Immunization in infancy against diphtheria prevents the child from the disease.

Treatment

All cases of diphtheritic conjunctivitis should be treated under the supervision of a pediatrician. Local treatment consists of the instillation of broad-spectrum antibiotics frequently along with age-matched atropine sulphate eye ointment only once. No attempt should be made to remove the membrane. It dissolves with local treatment.

Moraxella Conjunctivitis

This is a chronic bilateral conjunctivitis seen mostly in malnourished adults persons caused by an organism called Morax-Axenfeld bacilli. The condition is also known as angular conjunctivitis, as it develops in the temporal conjunctiva near the outer canthus. The skin of the lid at the outer canthus is eczematous. The other complication is the development of hypopyon. The cornea may show peripheral infiltration.

Treatment

It consists of the instillation of erythromycin or bacitracin along with a drop of Zinc sulphate three times a day. If there is hypopyon, it should be treated by the standard method. Intramuscular injections of vitamin A help with early recovery. The overall nutrition should be corrected.

Viral Conjunctivitis

The viral conjunctivitis is very common and can be divided into two groups. The first consists of pharyngoconjunctival fever (PCF), epidemic keratoconjunctivitis (EKC), and acute hemorrhagic conjunctivitis (AHC). That occurs regularly in epidemic form every year worldwide. Infecting persons of all ages. They are nonblinding. The other group does not occur in epidemic form; they are caused by herpes zoster, herpes simplex, and conjunctivitis associated with measles and chickenpox.

Pharyngoconjunctival Fever (PCF)

As the name suggests, it is associated with fever and pain in the throat. It is generally seen in children and young adults, is bilateral, lasts for a short period, and is self-limiting. Antibiotics and antiviral drugs have very little effect on conjunctivitis. Mild transient corneal involvement is seen in some cases.

Epidemic Keratoconjunctivitis (EKC)

It mostly inflicts children and young adults; there may be many in the community. It is bilateral, with severe conjunctivitis that may develop pseudomembrane, watering, and thin discharge. Corneal involvement is common; that is the cause of lacrimation, photophobia, and blepharospasm. Corneal involvement is the cause of diminished vision. The lesions do not stain as they are subepithelial. The subepithelial lesions may start in the second week or may be weeks after the conjunctival redness has subsided and linger for weeks to months. There are no antibiotics or antiviral drugs available for the condition. Oral painkillers are given to reduce ocular pain.

Acute Hemorrhagic Conjunctivitis (AHC)

This also happens in epidemics, mostly in late summer and early rains, seen in all ages. It is bilateral, beginning with watering and redness without discharge. As the days pass, the conjunctival congestion increases, ending in large areas of subconjunctival hemorrhage. Cornea complications are rare; subconjunctival hemorrhage takes longer time to disappear than conjunctival congestion. There are no antibiotics or antiviral drugs available against the virus.

Herpes Simplex Conjunctivitis

Herpes simplex conjunctivitis is less common than the above; it is unilateral; the involvement of the other eye is independent of the first eye; and it may develop for weeks to months. It is known to cause nongonococcal ophthalmia neonatorum. In children, it is passed through asymptomatic carriers. The conditions may involve the cornea; involvement of the cornea in children is less common; and adults develop microdendrites (MDs) that may be converted to dendritic corneal ulcers, which require antiviral drugs.

Herpes Zoster Varicella Conjunctivitis

They are seen in two forms, i.e., in chickenpox and in herpes zoster ophthalmicus. The first is bilateral acute mucopurulent conjunctivitis that develops in children. The conjunctiva is congested; there may be a vesicle of chickenpox on the lid margin and conjunctiva; the cornea is not involved; however, a vesicle near the limbus that looks like phlycten may cause photophobia. Conjunctivitis in chickenpox subsides with the subsidence of systemic chickenpox. The second is seen in adults and is unilateral, always associated with eruptions on the forehead and lids. It may involve the cornea; episcleritis is less frequent. Treatment is the treatment of herpes zoster ophthalmicus.

Conjunctivitis in Measles

Measles is a contagious systemic viral infection of childhood not seen in adults. It is a fully preventable disease. The disorder presents with rashes all over the body, including the lids. Small vesicles may develop on the conjunctiva and caruncle. The conjunctivitis does not require additional treatment. There are no antiviral drugs effective against the virus; the condition is seen as a depletion of vitamin A; hence, it is mandatory to administer 100,000 IU of soluble vitamin A to every child suffering from measles, irrespective of Immunization status of the child.

Note:
- Besides the viruses mentioned above, many viruses may involve the conjunctiva.
- Most of the viruses do not impart immunity to the person.

CHLAMYDIAL CONJUNCTIVITIS

Chlamydia are a group of microorganisms larger than viruses and smaller than bacteria. They are difficult to culture; there are many types of chlamydia, not all involving human beings.

The chlamydia of ophthalmic interest are: Trachoma, inclusion conjunctivitis in adults, and ophthalmia neonatorum in newborns.

Trachoma

Trachoma is the most common cause of blinding ocular disease produced by any chlamydia. Trachoma used to be a major cause of bilateral blindness in India; presently, it has been eradicated from most of the states in India. However, it still remains a formidable cause of blindness in underdeveloped countries.

The trachoma is not known to involve intraocular structures. It mostly involves the conjunctiva and cornea. Involvements of the lids are secondary to involvement of the tarsal conjunctiva. The cornea is involved either due to conjunctival vessels growing on its surface or secondary to entropion of the lids. The condition is chronic keratoconjunctivitis, with an acute onset in childhood and a chronic course in adults. It is seen in a dry, hot climate in a crowded locality with unhygienic surroundings. It is a disease of the community; many members of the same family may display various stages of the disease.

The acute attack is missed in childhood and treated as mild conjunctivitis; in children with good immunity, the disease may automatically get cured. Reinfection is common, which brings another subacute attack. Lasting for many months to years and involving the cornea and tarsal conjunctiva. This is the most infective stage. Presenting with symptoms of redness, foreign body sensations, and watering. On examination, follicles are seen in the tarsal conjunctiva and lower fornix. The cornea gets involved every few months or years. The corneal changes are superficial keratitis and superficial vascularization. The vascularization is called pannus; there are follicles at the limbus that are converted into shallow pits called Herbert's pits, which are diagnostic of well-developed trachoma. At the same time, changes in the tarsal conjunctiva progress to a stage of fibrosis. Deforming the lid margin, developing trichiasis, and entropion. The above two start with superficial vascularization, ulceration, and opacity formation. The above factors are responsible for constant watering, persistent redness, and diminished vision that may ultimately end in bilateral blindness. Trachoma spreads from one percent to another through infected fingers and flies. It is common for a trachomatous eye to be invaded by flies that help spread the disease in the community. The secondary bacterial infection predisposes to corneal ulcers and deep opacities. This stage is called the blinding trachoma stage.

The WHO classification of trachoma is as follows:
TF-Follicles in the upper tarsal conjunctiva
TI-Papillary hypertrophy in the upper tarsal conjunctiva
TS-Trachomatous scarring
TT-Trichiasis and entropion
TCO-Corneal opacity
Trachoma is infectious in the TF stage only, after which it becomes noninfectious.

Management of Trachoma

The management is divided into:
- Prophylaxis
- Management of the acute stages
- Management of established trachoma
- Management of blinding trachoma
- Management of complications

Prophylaxis

The disease can neither be prevented by immunization nor by chemotherapy. The prophylaxis is directed to the persons at risks, and is in suffering from TF stage. This is divided into two groups: The first group comprises those who are trachomatous. The second group comprises those who are free of trachoma but are likely to get infected; those who are already in the first group are given antibiotic eye ointment two times a day for 5 days a week for one month, with a gap of two months. Only two repeat the previous regime. The common antibiotic ointments used are tetracycline 1%, erythromycin 0.5%, and chloromycetin 1%. The members of the community should be explained about personal hygiene, specially that of the face and hands. The methods of cleaning the face and hands should be demonstrated to all the children in the school or at their residence by health workers. The community should be explained dangers of open-air defecation and choked drains because they act as breeding places. The flies play an important role in the spread of trachoma.

Management of the Acute Stage

The acute stage is treated by the instillation of:
- 20–30% sulfacetamide drops three times a day in each eye.
- Tetracycline 1%, erythromycin 0.5%, or chloromycetin 1%, two times a day.
- Broad-spectrum antibiotics are added to the above to prevent secondary infections.

Management of Established Trachoma

The treatment described below is continued for at least three months at a dose of capsule tetracycline 500 mg twice a day for three weeks. Children under 10 years of age are not given tetracycline. The alternatives to tetracycline are: doxycycline 100 mg for 15 days; tablet erythromycin 500 mg two times a day for 15 days; or azithromycin 1 gram in a single dose. The systemic antibiotic therapy should be supplemented with local treatment by sulfacetamide drops (20–30%) three times a day for three months with tetracycline or erythromycin ointment two times a day for three months. The importance of personal cleanliness and face washing should be emphasized to the members of the community.

Management of Blinding Trachoma

Consists of management of acute trachoma, intensive treatment of bacterial conjunctivitis, 1% atropine ointment as per requirement, along with personal cleanliness and face wash. Administration of vitamin A under the national program of immunization.

Management of Complications

The complications, except blinding trachoma, do not take place before 20 years. By the time complications develop, the persons are no more infected.

The main complaints of complications begin with watering of the eyes due to trichiasis; the eyes are red and irritable with mucopurulent discharge; the vision is reduced due to corneal vascularization; and opacity. In the late stages, the patients initially develop entropion of the upper lid, followed by the lower lid. No medical treatment can undo the lid deformation; antibiotic drops are given to reduce the bacterial infection. The WHO model of management of complications of trachoma in general and entropion in particular is designated as SAFE, where S stands for surgery, A for antibiotic, F for face wash, and E for environment.

Adult Inclusion: Conjunctivitis

This is a less common, nonblinding, bilateral conjunctivitis in sexually active adults. It starts in one eye, followed by the other. It begins as acute mucopurulent conjunctivitis, passing into the chronic stage. In the late stages, it causes vascularization of the cornea without going into complications of trachoma. The condition is often missed and treated as chronic conjunctivitis. Once the diagnosis has been established, the first step is to treat the genital infection with an appropriate antibiotic. The conjunctivitis is treated with a broad-spectrum antibiotic locally three times a day for 15 days.

ALLERGIC CONJUNCTIVITIS

Allergy is the most common noninfective, nonblinding, bilateral conjunctivitis in children and young adults. The allergic conjunctivitis falls into two main types: The first is due to an external allergen (exogenous). The other is due to endogenous allergens. **Flowchart 9.1** shows various types of allergic conjunctivitis.

The allergic conjunctivitis in both groups can be acute or chronic:

Acute Allergic Conjunctivitis

This is bilateral acute conjunctivitis, beginning with one eye and being followed by the other eye within a few minutes. The exact allergen in most of the cases cannot be pinpointed. The allergen is always organic; the patient suddenly develops instant watering and itching of the eye, followed by a gritty sensation that the patient thinks is due to a foreign body. The conjunctiva is greatly chemosed, so much so that it protrudes out of the interpalpebral fissure all-round the cornea. The condition is generally associated with the running of the nose. The condition subsides even without treatment; if it does not subside within an hour, it is better to start a weak solution of steroids.

Chronic Allergic Conjunctivitis (Simple Allergic Conjunctivitis)

This occurs many times throughout the year in both eyes, mostly in adults. This is caused by the frequent entry of allergens into the conjunctiva. Which is generally chemical or drug-induced. The patient complains of mild, constant itching, redness, watering, and discharge, often misdiagnosed as chronic bacterial conjunctivitis, trachoma, and ocular surface disorder.

Flowchart 9.1: Types of allergic conjunctivitis.

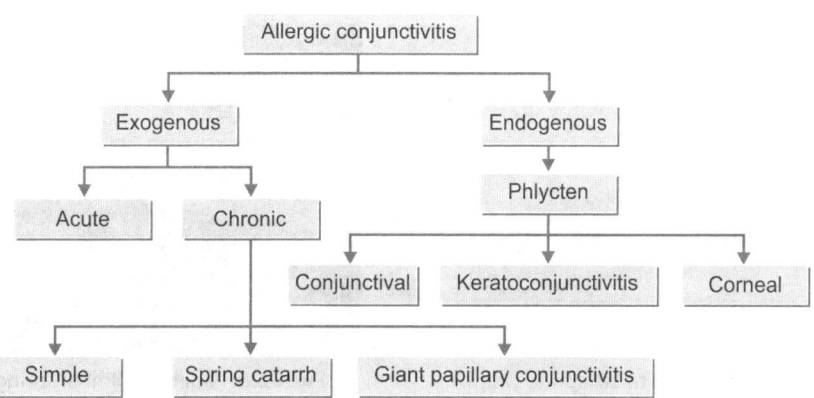

The management is difficult and prolonged. It has been noted that patients may be symptoms-free by changing their drugs, occupation, or place of residence. The patients are put on a weak solution of steroids at the minimum concentration and instillation. Systemic long-acting antihistamine tablets for a few weeks may be required. Instillation of lubricant gives much-needed relief.

Spring Catarrh (Vernal Conjunctivitis)

The name suggests that this type of conjunctivitis develops in spring; hence, it has been called spring catarrh. This is not always true; the condition may be seen throughout the year, specially in hot and dry months. It is a chronic bilateral conjunctivitis seen under 10 years of age, commonly in boys. There may be a family history of spring catarrh among siblings and parents. The disease automatically disappears after puberty; the exact cause is not known. External organic allergens like pollen and flowers have been thought to be common precipitating factors. The chief complaints are intense, itching throughout the waking hours in both eyes with watering and ropy discharge. The disease has been divided into two types: The first is called palpebral, and the second is limbal; in severe cases, both may be present. The palpebral form is more common than the limbal, and the tarsal conjunctiva is more frequently affected than the lower. The tarsal conjunctival develops large, pink, polygonal papillae with a flat top (**Fig. 9.19**). The number of papillae varies from a few to many. The papillae become smaller with treatment and may disappear only to return next year. This can even happen without treatment or a change of habitat. In the long run, there may be slide drooping of the lid, and the skin over the lids develops hyperpigmentation. In the limbal form, papillae similar to those in the upper lid develop. The common sites to be involved are the upper and temporal limbus (**Fig. 9.20**). In long-standing cases, the papillae may encircle the whole of the limbus with mild vascularization of the cornea still later, the cornea may be involved.

Management

The condition is nonblinding in spite of its long duration. The condition requires prolonged treatment with dedication. The aim of the treatment is to use a minimum amount of drugs that give maximum relief. It is essential to counsel the parent regarding the long course of the disease and the possibility of spontaneous regression at puberty. They should also be warned about the use of strong steroid drops that give quick results. The steroids should be of minimal concentration with maximum effect, without side effects that may cause the early development of cataracts and steroid-induced glaucoma. The possibility of secondary infection should not

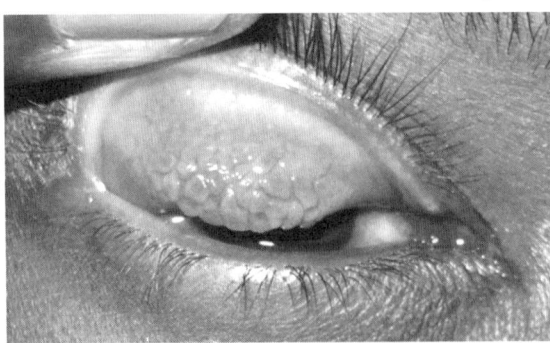

Fig. 9.19: Papillae in tarsal spring catarrh.
(For color version, see Plate 4)

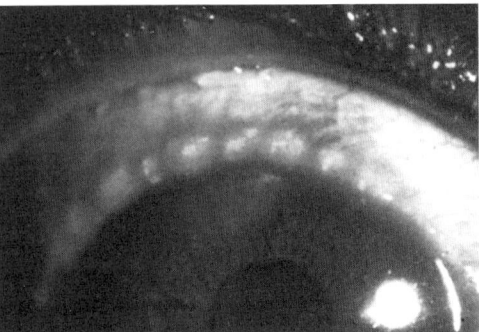

Fig. 9.20: Papillae in limbal spring catarrh.

be overlooked. In its initial stages, the steroid may be used as frequently as four times a day with strong concentration. The steroid drops are tapered as per the practice of the institution. The child may have other systemic manifestations of allergy, like asthma rhinitis and allergic dermatitis; some children may develop secondary keratoconus.

Giant Papillary Conjunctivitis

This is less common than other types of allergic conjunctivitis seen in young adults; this is due to the contact lens itself or its preservative, nylon sutures left after surgery. The condition is mostly unilateral. The symptom consists of mild to severe itching, mucoid discharge, and redness. The papillae of giant papillary conjunctivitis are larger than those in spring catarrh. The essential part of management is to remove the offending factor. Steroids may be tried in extreme cases.

Growths of the Conjunctiva

The growths of the conjunctiva can be infective granulomas or neoplastic, which may be benign or malignant. Malignancies of the conjunctiva are rare:

Infective growths of conjunctiva are:
- Burst chalazion
- Foreign body granuloma
- Rhinosporidiosis

The benign tumors of conjunctiva are:
- Nevus
- Limbal dermoids
- Dermolipoma
- Papilloma
- Hemangioma
- Neurofibroma

The malignant tumors of the conjunctiva are:
- Epidermoid carcinoma
- Basal cell carcinoma
- Malignant melanoma

CHAPTER 10

Disorders of the Cornea

DISORDERS OF THE CORNEA

The disorders of the cornea may be slight enough not to result in loss of vision or serious enough to cause blindness. The main function of the cornea is optical; the other function is protective, along with the sclera. The cornea is the transparent anterior one-sixth of the globe; the curvature of the cornea is more than that of the sclera. Hence, the junction of the two is not smooth; it is stepped. The corneoscleral junction is called the limbus. The diameter of the adult cornea is 11.7 mm. A cornea with a diameter <10.00 mm is called a microcornea; a cornea >13.00 mm is called a megalocornea. The corneal curvature is 7.80 mm; the posterior curvature is more than the anterior. This makes the cornea thinnest at the centre. The corneal curvature is increased in keratoconus and buphthalmos; it is reduced in microcornea and phthisis. The optical power of the cornea is +43D sphere. The anterior surface of the cornea is shining and smooth; it is kept moist by tear film. The anterior surface of the cornea acts as a convex mirror that forms a small, erect virtual image. In the disease of the cornea, these properties are lost, causing diminished vision. The corneal disease can be congenital or acquired.

The congenital diseases of the cornea are—microcornea, buphthalmos, keratoglobus, sclerocornea, and limbal dermoid.

Microcornea

Microcornea is a congenital condition that may be unilateral or bilateral. The diameter of the cornea is <10.00 mm, and the curvature is <7.80 mm. It is generally associated with microphthalmos. This makes the anterior chamber shallow. The pupil is generally central and circular; it becomes keyhole-shaped when the eye is microphthalmic with coloboma. The eyes have poor to very poor vision. The error of refraction is generally hypermetropic; it is difficult to improve the vision. The child may require low-vision aids.

Buphthalmos

The corneal diameter is >13.00–17.00 mm. The corneal curvature is increased, and the overall thickness of the cornea is reduced. This makes the anterior chamber deep, and the iris may be tremulous. The most common cause is congenital glaucoma; any state of raised intraocular tension will result in secondary buphthalmos. The condition can be unilateral or bilateral. The vision depends on the range of intraocular tension. The treatment involves the management of associated glaucoma. The term keratoglobus oblique megalocornea is used to denote a condition similar to buphthalmos with normal tension and good vision. The condition does not require any treatment except correction of the associated error of refraction.

Sclerocornea

Sclerocornea is a congenital condition where the cornea becomes as opaque as the sclera. The opacity is generalized and vascularized. The corneal curvature is reduced. While the thickness is increased. The condition is rare; it may have a genetic predisposition and may be uni or bilateral. Generally with very poor vision.

The treatment is penetrating keratoplasty, provided other ocular structures are normal. The result of penetrating keratoplasty is not very encouraging.

Limbal Dermoid

Limbal dermoids are congenital, non-malignant growths on the limbus. They vary from pinpoint size to as large as the cornea itself. The most common symptom that brings the child for consultation is a visible growth at the limbus. On examination, the child generally has poor vision due to high astigmatism. The treatment consists of the removal of the growth, followed by improvement with glasses.

Common Features of Corneal Disease

1. Change in Shape and Size

   i. Cornea size is reduced in microcornea, microphthalmos, and phthisis.
   ii. Cornea size is increased in buphthalmos and keratoglobus.
   iii. Corneal curvature is increased in keratoconus and keratoglobus.
   iv. Corneal curvature is irregular in corneal staphyloma.

2. Loss of Transparency

Any disease that involves the cornea results in a loss of corneal transparency, which is called corneal opacity. The opacity may be uni- or bilateral.

The causes of bilateral corneal opacities are as follows:
- **Congenital**: Rare
- **Infection**: Ophthalmia neonatorum, trachoma leprosy, interstitial keratitis, and smallpox.
- **Trauma**: Blast and chemical injury
- **Allergy**: Phlyctenular keratitis
- **Nutritional**: Severe vitamin A deficiency
- **Degeneration**: Arcus senilis (old age), arcus juvenilis (young age, rare), and band keratopathy
- Dystrophy
- Depositions on the cornea

The opacities can be temporary or permanent; the opacities cause diminished vision depending on their position in relation to the pupil; an opacity in front of the pupil causes greater loss of vision than peripheral. The opacity may be single or multiple. The opacities do not stain with fluorescein. Staining of the opacity means active infection/inflammation. The opacities are graded according to their density. They are the nebula, macula, and leukoma. The nebulae are faintest and not visible on usual oblique illumination; they are visible only on a slight lamp, and the maculae are denser than the nebulae and visible on ordinary torch illumination. Leukomas are the densest of all other opacities and can be seen in natural light. The opacities may occasionally be vascularized; incarceration of the iris in any corneal opacity is called leukoma adherent.

3. Inflammation of Cornea

The inflammation of the cornea is called keratitis. It can be infectious when caused by microorganisms and non-infectious when inflammatory. A superficial infective keratitis is called a corneal ulcer, where there is loss of corneal epithelial tissue with infection by microorganisms and an ulcer as a border, edge, and floor. The small staining of the epithelium is called punctate keratitis, which is common in viral infections. The corneal ulcers stain with fluorescein. They are active lesions causing pain, watering, and photophobia. Severe forms of infective corneal ulcers are associated with hypopyon. Deep corneal ulcers on healing leave opacities; most of the corneal ulcers are associated with circumcorneal congestion.

4. Loss of Sensation of Cornea

This is seen in herpes simplex and herpes zoster.

5. Vascularization of Cornea

Normal corneas are avascular; the presence of vessels on the cornea means disease of the cornea. The vascularization can be superficial or deep. The superficial vascularizations develop from conjunctiva vessels and are more common than the deep vascularization that develop from deeper vessels. The superficial vascularization is irregular in distribution, may anastomos with each other, and is bright red in color; the deep vessels are straight, arranged in a bottle brush appearance without anastomosing, and are dull pink in color **(Fig. 10.1)**.

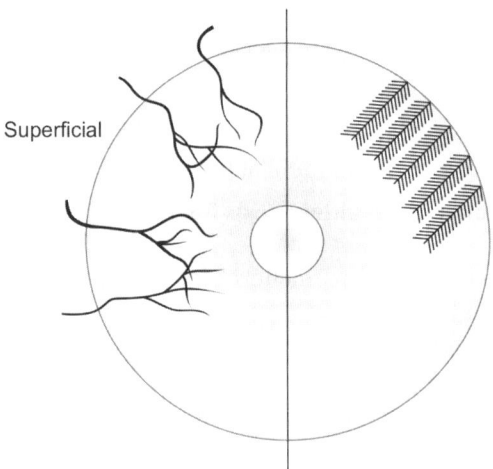

Fig. 10.1: Superficial and deep vascularization of cornea.

Table 10.1 shows the difference between the superficial corneal vascularization and deep corneal vascularization.

Table 10.1: Difference between superficial corneal vascularization and deep corneal vascularization.	
Superficial corneal vascularization	*Deep corneal vascularization*
Start in the conjunctiva and cross the limbus in the epithelium Bright red in color, branching irregularly, join each other. Seen in trachoma, phlycten, and chronic corneal ulcers	Start in the sclera, are not visible at the limbus, and grow in the corneal stroma. Pink in color; do not join see in deep keratitis

Corneal Ulcer

Corneal ulcer is the most common infectious disorder of the cornea, seen in all ages in both sexes, and is more common in underdeveloped countries. The ulcers may be uni or bilateral; when bilateral, they need not be simultaneous or similar. They are caused by microorganisms as the primary cause or develop on previously diseased corneas. The organism can be bacteria, fungi, viruses, or parasites (Acanthamoeba). The viruses are least likely to cause a frank corneal ulcer. The ulcer may be central or peripheral. To develop a corneal ulcer, a breach in the epithelium is mandatory. However, some organisms may invade the corneal substance without a breach. They are: *C. diphtheriae, H. influenza, N. gonorrhoea, N. meningitidis,* and *Listeria*. The bacterial ulcer develops within 24 to 48 hours following the injury. The following conditions predispose to ulcers—chronic dacryocystitis, trichiasis, entropion, ectropion, lagophthalmos, corneal foreign body, loss of sensation, and diabetes.

The bacterial corneal ulcer has an acute onset with foreign body sensations, pain, watering, redness, and diminished vision. On examination, the conjunctiva is congested along with circumciliary congestion. The ulcer looks gray and stains with fluorescein. Hypopyon develops in severe bacterial infections. A small, uncomplicated corneal ulcer should heal by itself, even without treatment. This is rare. A large corneal ulcer not only spreads towards the periphery but also in depth. A deep corneal ulcer gets its first resistance from the Descemet's membrane, which can resist moderate infection; it bulges forward as a translucent bulge from the floor of the ulcer. The bulge is called a descemetocele or keratocele. If the descemetocele ruptures, a small hole develops in the cornea; this is called perforation of the corneal ulcer. As soon as the ulcer perforates, aqueous leaks from the anterior chamber, causing the anterior chamber to collapse. The iris moves forward to plug the perforation. Once the perforation has been sealed, the anterior chamber is reformed, leaving the iris attached to the cornea. This is called leucoma adherence; if the perforation is large, the corneal cells from the periphery start migrating towards the center to bridge the gap. This results in the formation of a pseudocornea. The pseudocornea is a thin, irregular white week spot that does not with stand normal intraocular tensions; this makes it bulge, and the condition is called anterior staphyloma. The staphyloma may be localized or may involve the whole of the cornea, called total anterior staphyloma. When the perforation is large and not healed by the formation of pseudocornea, the lens and vitreous may flow out, and the eye goes into a state of phthisis. If the infection passes into the anterior chamber, the uvea gets infected, causing severe uveitis ending in endophthalmitis. The following figure shows the natural history of a corneal ulcer. **Flowchart 10.1** shows the natural history of corneal ulcers.

Hypopyon Corneal Ulcer

The pus in the anterior chamber is called hypopyon. Hypopyon commonly develops in severe bacterial and fungal keratitis. It can also happen without a corneal ulcer, i.e., severe iridocyclitis. Hypopyon is sterile unless it has been infected by bacteria that can pass through the intact corneal epithelial, and infection can be introduced through a contaminated wound. Hypopyon contains WBC and fibrin; it may be fluid or fibrinous; the former settles at the bottom of the anterior chamber with a horizontal fluid level towards the pupil **(Fig. 10.2)**. The fluid hypopyon changes its position as per the position of the head. The fibrinous hypopyon commonly seen in fungal keratitis does not change its position. A hypopyon corneal ulcer is an ophthalmic emergency that should be attended to promptly. The treatment of hypopyon ulcers involves extensive treatment of corneal ulcers by atropine twice a day and broad-spectrum drops hourly till the hypopyon disappears. Subconjunctival injections of broad-spectrum antibiotics give prompt relief. The other causes of white material in the anterior chamber are: cortical matter **(Fig. 10.3)**, nucleus of the lens **(Fig. 10.4)**, complete lens, and malignant cells (retinoblastoma). Non-inflammatory

Flowchart 10.1: Natural history of corneal ulcers.

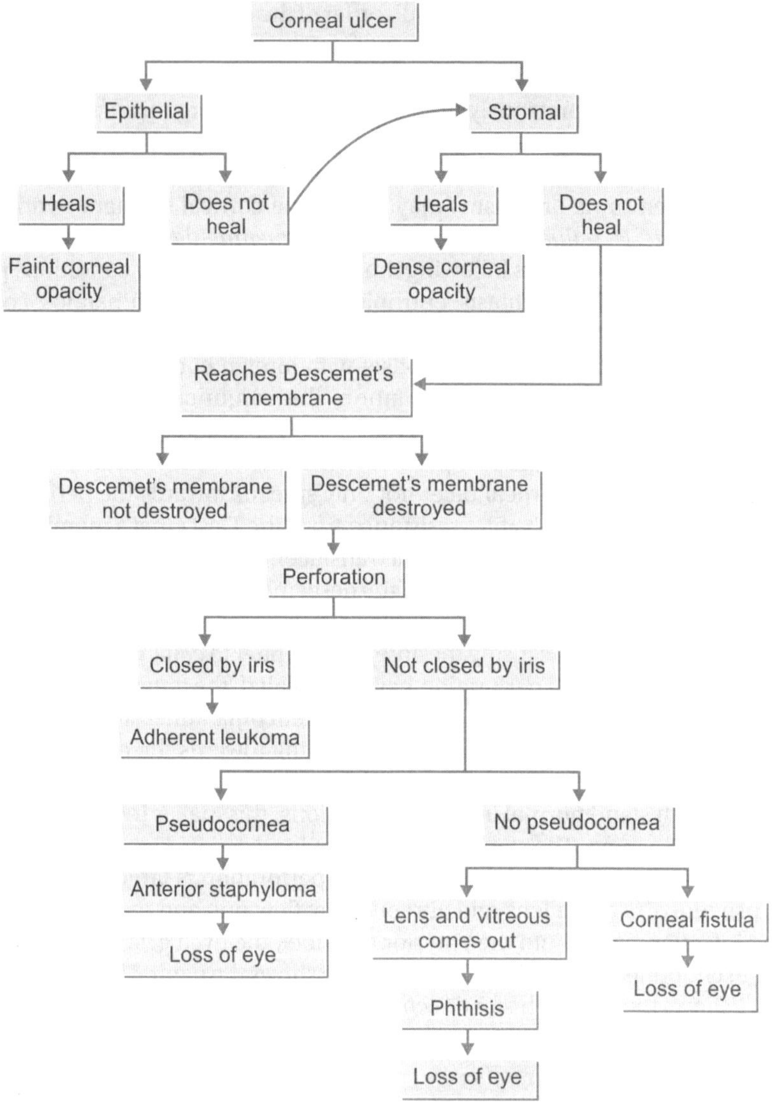

```
                        Corneal ulcer
                       /            \
                 Epithelial         Stromal
                 /     \            /      \
              Heals   Does not   Heals    Does not
                      heal                  heal
                |       |          |          |
            Faint     →→→→→    Dense corneal
            corneal              opacity
            opacity
                        Reaches Descemet's
                           membrane
                         /           \
              Descemet's membrane   Descemet's membrane
              not destroyed         destroyed
                                        |
                                   Perforation
                                   /         \
                          Closed by iris   Not closed by iris
                                |                |
                          Adherent leukoma
                           /         \
                    Pseudocornea   No pseudocornea
                         |            /         \
                   Anterior     Lens and      Corneal
                   staphyloma   vitreous      fistula
                         |      comes out        |
                    Loss of eye     |        Loss of eye
                                Phthisis
                                   |
                               Loss of eye
```

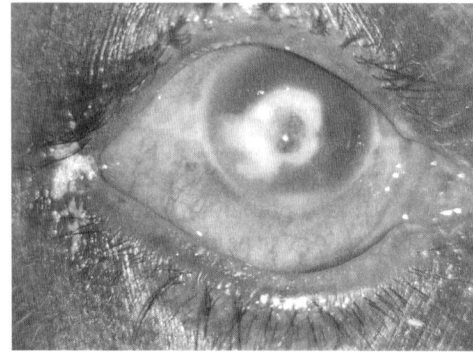

Fig. 10.2: Hypopyon with descemetocele.

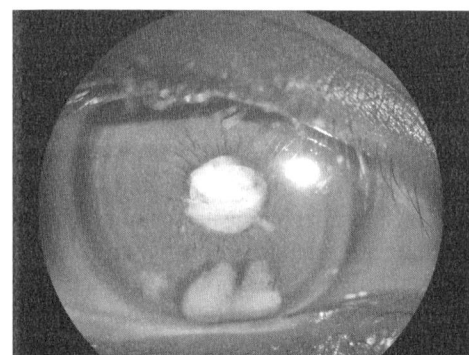

Fig. 10.3: Cortical matter in the anterior chamber.

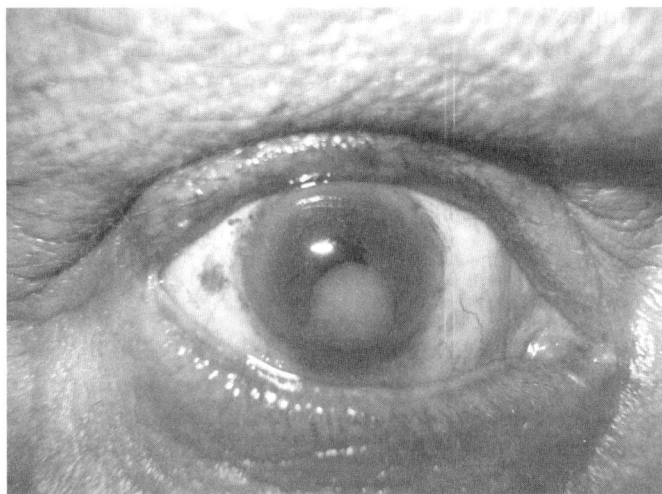

Fig. 10.4: Nucleus in anterior chamber.

hypopyons are called pseudohypopyons. All the white matter in the anterior chamber should be considered infective unless proved otherwise.

The hypopyon is generally seen at the bottom of the anterior chamber. It is called inverse hypopyon, where the white matter is seen in the upper part of the anterior chamber with a flat border towards the pupil. The cause of which is silicone oil injected following a vitrectomy. Silicone oil, being lighter than aqueous, floats upwards, forming an inverse hypopyon. This does not respond to the usual treatment of hypopyon.

Management of Corneal Ulcers

A corneal ulcer, once confirmed, should be treated as an emergency because an apparently small ulcer may turn severe enough to cover the whole of the cornea. A central ulcer requires earlier management than a peripheral ulcer. The treatment consists of—cleaning of the lid margin; removal of discharge; there is no need to wash the conjunctival sac. Instill broad-spectrum antibiotics hourly during the day and ointment with the same antibiotic at night. I applied a pad and bandage at night. Atropine, in appropriate consultation, should be instilled twice a day along with antibiotics; systemic antibiotics are not needed. Mild to moderate corneal ulcers should heal with this regime in about 5–7 days. If the ulcer does not respond, the next step is to search for the cause that is preventing healing. They include lid deformity, missed foreign bodies, loss of corneal sensation, use of ineffective antibiotics, and raised intraocular tension.

Viral Keratitis

All viruses that involve conjunctiva can affect the cornea. They generally produce punctate keratitis scattered all over the cornea without forming an ulcer-like bacterial infection. The two common viruses that require special attention are herpes simplex and herpes zoster keratitis.

Herpes Simplex Keratitis

Herpes simplex keratitis is met with in all ages, from neonates to old age. In neonates, it is mild and self-limiting. In adults, it is recurrent and difficult to eradicate. Herpes simplex keratitis is found in two forms, i.e., primary and recurrent.

Primary herpes simplex keratitis is seen between 6 months and 10 years. It is transferred from a person infected by herpes simplex to a non-immune child. The primary herpes keratitis is unilateral, with herpes blepharitis on the same side that has herpes vesicles on the skin of the lid. The conjunctiva has follicular conjunctivitis. Keratitis develops as punctate staining spots without going to the typical dendritic shape seen in recurrent keratitis among adults. The primary keratitis may heal or may pass into a recurrent stage that may take a few months to years. The treatment of primary herpetic keratitis is the instillation of local antiviral drops for a few days.

Recurrent Herpes Simplex Keratitis

This is more common than the former seen in adults; it may be localized to the epithelium or may involve deep layers and anterior uvea.

The epithelial lesions generally develop in the following way:
Superficial punctate keratitis → Dendritic ulcer → Geographic ulcer → Keratitis meta-herpetica.

Dendritic Ulcer

Dendritic ulcer is a superficial ulcer caused mostly by the herpes simplex virus; the zoster virus can also cause dendritic ulcer. It can develop anywhere on the cornea. The most common site is the central cornea. It is an irregular, linear, branching ulcer that stains brightly with a fluorescein 2% drop kept in contact with the cornea for 5 minutes and seen under cobalt blue light **(Fig. 10.5)**. The ulcer heals on one end and progresses on the opposite end. The corneal sensation is reduced; a dull corneal sensation is diagnostic of herpetic keratitis. The keratitis may heal without treatment; a dendritic ulcer not responding to the usual management of corneal ulcers should be treated with appropriate antiviral drops. Systemic antiviral drugs are not required. The dendritic ulcer may progress to a stage of geographic ulcer, also called ameboid ulcer. They are larger than the dendritic ulcer; if the dendritic ulcer does not heal with usual treatment, it passes into a state of keratitis metaherpetica. This is the most advanced and difficult form of herpetic keratitis that may involve the stroma and endothelium and cause anterior uveitis. A simple dendritic ulcer does not cause hypopyon unless it is infected secondarily by bacteria. Debridement and carbolization are no longer used.

Recurrent herpetic keratitis is common in untreated cases and may develop following treatment as well, after weeks or months. It may be epithelial or involve stroma.

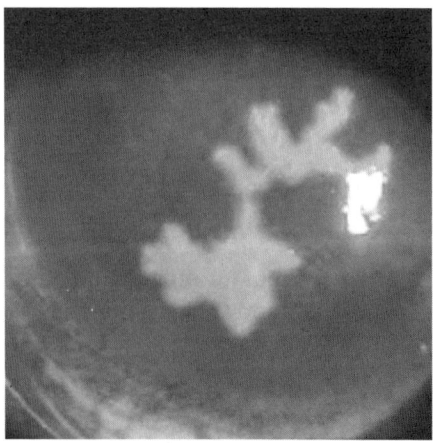

Fig. 10.5: Dendritic ulcer staining seen under cobalt blue light. *(For color version, see Plate 5)*

Chapter 10: Disorders of the Cornea

The following is the natural history of recurrent herpetic keratitis:
Superficial punctate keratitis → Dendritic ulcer → Geographic ulcer → Keratitis Meta herpetica.

Deep keratitis may be in the form of any of the following—stromal keratitis, disciform keratitis, or trophic keratitis. These lesions are seen in adults due to the reactivation of primary lesions from childhood.

Fungal Keratitis (Mycotic Keratitis)

Mycotic keratitis is the most severe and potentially blinding corneal ulcer that is difficult to manage and is caused by filamentous fungi and yeast. Mycotic keratitis is mostly caused by trauma from vegetative matter. They are most common among farmers. Mycotic keratitis develops following an injury by organic matter causing a breach in the corneal epithelium that initially results in simple bacterial keratitis and is treated as such. The suspicion of fungal involvement arises only when the ulcer does not heal with usual treatment. The typical ulcer develops a week or two after the initial injury. As a large yellowish spot with an irregular margin, the edge is surrounded by an area of stromal edema. The eye is unexpectedly congested, and the vision is diminishing. The anterior chamber soon develops a thick, immobile, yellowish hypopyon. It is generally unilateral. The treatment of fungal infections is difficult and prolongs. The success of treatment depends on the efficacy of the antifungal drug. A successful treatment always leaves a dense central opacity. The treatment consists of—Atropine ointment twice a day along with antifungal drops 4–6 times a day. Along with systemic antifungal drugs. If there is suspicion of raised intraocular treatment, oral Diamox should be added.

Prophylactic use of antifungal drops following an organic injury does not prevent fungal corneal ulcers. The old treatment of debridement of the ulcer and carbolization is no more in use. If all the medical treatments fail, the eye may be subjected to penetrating keratoplasty. The advantage of penetrating keratitis is that it removes the infected cornea along with the residual fungal load. The results of penetrating keratoplasties are not encouraging.

Marginal Corneal Ulcers

Most marginal corneal ulcers are non-infective; they are due to hypersensitivity to unknown antigens that may be external or internal. The common marginal ulcers are—phlyctenular ulcer, marginal infiltrates, and Mooren's ulcer. The last is the least common, and the first is the most common. The marginal infiltrates are mildest and non-vision-threatening.

Phlyctenular Corneal Ulcer

They are seen between 3 and 10 years old in malnourished children, more common in girls. They may be unilateral or bilateral. The lesions are generally single but may be multiple at different places on the limbus or in a segment with multiple phlyctens. In severe form, they may invade the cornea, causing keratoconjunctivitis, or they may invade the cornea in the form of a fascicular ulcer. Phlycten on the limbus are very painful; they are the most common cause of blepharospasm in children. The phlycten ulcerates before it heals. A phlycten on the limbus on healing leaves a dome-shaped opacity on the cornea periphery with its apex towards the pupil. A phlycten may heal without treatment, and the other phlyctens may follow in succession at places other than the first. If the limbal phlycten does not heal, it progresses on the cornea towards the pupil, followed by a leash of superficial vessels. The condition is called a fascicular ulcer. Which causes severe loss of vision if it is in the pupillary area. The anterior chamber is not affected by phlyctenular keratitis. The management of keratoconjunctivitis is steroid as per the practice of the institute under the supervision of an ophthalmologist. Recurrences are common (Fig. 10.6).

Marginal Corneal Infiltrates

They are seen in adults and are self-limiting and recurrent, the exact cause of which is not well established; they may be allergic or autoimmune in nature, cause severe pain, and cause photophobia and lacrimation without diminishing vision. In the long run, superficial vascularization may develop on the cornea. They respond well to the local weak solution of steroids; recurrences are frequent.

Mooren's Ulcer

This is an infrequent degeneration of the corneal periphery of unknown cause. It develops in adults on the periphery of the limbus as a small depression that extends on each side and in depth. It is rarely bilateral and does not respond to the usual treatment of corneal ulcers and steroids. They may require immunosuppressive drugs in the form of cyclosporine (1–2%) twice a day for months together.

Corneal involvement of Trachoma

Cornea may be involved in acute or chronic stages. The involvement in the acute stage is not sight-threatening. It can be the primary involvement of the cornea or due to deformity of the lid margin. The corneal changes are divided into early, late, and delayed stages.

In the early stages, the cornea develops punctate keratitis, visible on fluorescein stain under a cobalt blue filter with high magnification of slit lamp. The next stage is the development of micropannus, which are small areas of superficial vascularization not extending more than 1.00 mm on the cornea.

The late stage consists of gross-pannus, Herbert's follicles, and Herbert's pits. Herbert's follicles are seen on the limbus, similar to those seen in the tarsal conjunctiva. They are to be differentiated from the follicles of follicular conjunctivitis. Herbert's follicles rupture to form Herbert's pits at the limbus. They are diagnostic of late-stage trachoma that does not respond to medical treatment.

Vascularization of the Cornea in Trachoma

The vascularization of the cornea in trachoma is a late feature of trachoma. It is generally seen after the third decade; it is superficial in nature and continues with conjunctival congestion. This is called pannus formation. There are two types of trachomatous pannus, i.e., progressive and regressive (Fig. 10.7).

The delayed effects of trachoma on the cornea are—bacterial infection leading to blinding trachoma the other is constant rubbing on the cornea by a deformed lid, worsening the already-present vascularization. The end result of corneal involvement is bilateral corneal blindness.

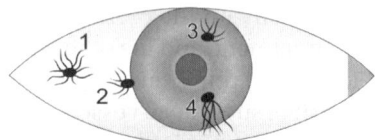

Fig. 10.6: Various types of conjunctival and corneal phlyctens: (1) Conjunctival; (2) Limbal phlycten; (3) Corneal phlycten; (4) Fascicular ulcer.

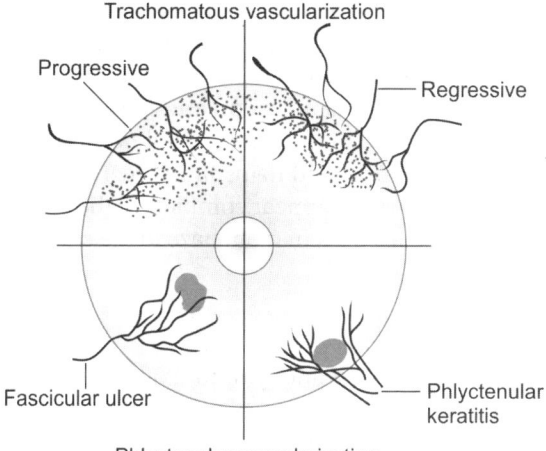

Fig. 10.7: Superficial vascularization of the cornea in trachoma and phlycten.

The management consists of treating the disease in the infective stage with an appropriate antibiotic. This stage does not require surgical intervention. The surgical intervention is directed towards the correction of lid deformities by surgery. Once vascularization has been brought under control, the cornea may undergo keratoplastic surgery.

Deep Keratitis

This is also known as parenchymatous or interstitial keratitis. They basically involve the deeper layer of the cornea; involvement of the anterior uvea is common.

The common causes of interstitial keratitis are:
- Congenital syphilis
- Acquired syphilis
- Tuberculosis
- Herpes simplex (disciform keratitis)
- Herpes zoster (disciform keratitis)

Interstitial keratitis can be divided into two groups, i.e., childhood and adult. Interstitial keratitis in children is more common than in adults. It is seen between first years after birth to fifteen years. Seen equally in boys and girls, it is a bilateral condition. The most common cause of the disease is inherited syphilis; the mother passes the infection to the growing fetus via the placenta. The developing cornea gets sensitized to the organism. The disease most probably starts in the iris, causing iridocyclitis. The condition has an acute onset with a prolonged course. The acute stage starts with intense watering, pain, redness, and photophobia. The eye shows intense circumciliary congestion. The cornea is vascularized, starting from the periphery all-round the pupil in sectors.

They generally develop in front of the pupil. The vessels are straight with a bottle brush appearance, parallel to each other without touching each other. The color of the vascularized are is less red than superficial vascularization. The vascularization gives the cornea a dull pink color. The vascularization stops growing once they have reached the center of the pupil and start regressive. This process takes months to years to complete, and the vessels start disappearing from the periphery. The acute stage lasts for a few weeks to months, while the chronic stage lasts for years. The other features are diminished vision and signs of iridocyclitis; the condition is self-limiting. The other systemic signs are Hutchinson's triad, which comprises interstitial keratitis, malformed teeth, and eighth nerve deafness. Along with a depressed nose bridge.

The child with interstitial keratitis is in agony, requiring prompt attention. The gold standard of treatment is basically treatment of the associated anterior uveitis. That consists of age-matched local instillation of atropine twice a day and hourly administration of a water-soluble corticosteroid drop. The child gets prompt relief after atropinization and steroid instillation. The steroid drops are tapered as per the practice of the institute. The steroid has to be continued for months or years. It promptly controls the symptoms and helps in the regression of the vessels. In spite of prolonged treatment, the vessels do not disappear completely; they remain as empty white lines in the deeper layer of the cornea, giving a permanent haze to the cornea, resulting in diminished vision and amblyopia.

Adult Form of Interstitial Keratitis

The condition is less common, and the signs and symptoms are milder. The condition is unilateral, and the patient develops interstitial keratitis years after exposure to *Treponema pallidum*. It also starts in the anterior uvea. The vascularization starts in the upper limbus, not encircling the cornea. The treatment consists of systemic antisyphilitic chemotherapy under the supervision of a person trained in the treatment of infectious diseases. The local treatment is similar to interstitial keratitis in children. The other cause of adult interstitial keratitis is systemic tuberculosis. It is less common than its syphilitic counterpart; both have similar clinical presentation and management. The patients should get full treatment for tuberculosis.

Disciform Keratitis

This is a localized, mostly unilateral, deep inflammation of the central cornea. The common causes are herpes simplex and zoster. Many a time, no definite cause can be found out. It may be caused by acquired syphilis. It is seen in adults. The lesion looks like a coin, white in color, present in the stroma with/without deep vascularization. The anterior uvea is commonly effected. The treatment is a mild cycloplegic drop once a day with mild steroid drops 2–3 times a day for weeks.

Neurotrophic keratitis and neuroparalytic keratitis are noninfectious keratitis due either to loss of sensation of the cornea or inability to close the lids in the presence of corneal sensation.

Neurotrophic Keratitis

Neurotrophic keratitis develops following a loss of corneal sensation due to involvement of the fifth nerve. The normal corneal sensation is required to protect the cornea by blinking, and Bell's phenomenon.

Bell's phenomenon is an essential protective mechanism to save the cornea from outward injury. It consists of an upward rotation of the globe in an attempt to close the lids. The movement of the globe up is lost in the absence of corneal sensation; in the absence of corneal sensation, the blinking is lost, resulting in exposure keratitis that is soon converted into a frank ulcer that stains with fluorescein. The condition is frequently associated with hypopyon.

The most common cause of absent Bell's phenomenon is leprosy. Where the condition is bilateral and permanent. The other cause is herpes zoster ophthalmicus and surgery on the trigeminal ganglion; in the above two cases, they are unilateral. As there is no corneal sensation, the patient remains unaware of the presence of a corneal ulcer. His attraction is drawn towards redness and watering.

The **treatment** of neurotrophic corneal ulcers consists of early diagnosis and treatment of corneal ulcer by usual method. Protecting the cornea from the onslaught of external factors by way of a soft contact lens and tarsorrhaphy.

Neuroparalytic Keratitis

In this case, corneal sensation and Bell's phenomenon are present. The fault lies in the orbicularis, and the patient is unable to close the lids, exposing the cornea. The inability to close the lid is called lagophthalmos. The neuroparalytic corneal ulcer starts in the lower part of the cornea. The most common cause is leprosy. As the pain is retained, the patient becomes aware of the ulcer with its usual presentation. The ulcer is associated with hypopyon.

The treatment of the condition consists of the usual treatment of corneal ulcers with tarsorrhaphy.

Exposure Keratitis

Exposure keratitis is a superficial corneal ulcer that may be punctate, large, or irregular. This happens when the lids fail to cover the cornea. Commonly seen in proptosis, exophthalmos, lagophthalmos, and coloboma of the lid, ectropion of the lower lid, and patients in coma. The management is the correction of the lid disorders and the reduction of proptosis and exophthalmos with the usual treatment of corneal ulcers.

Bullous Keratitis

This is a painful condition, generally unilateral, with watering. The bullae develop on the epithelial surface secondary to damage to the endothelium. The normal corneal epithelium is loosely attached to the Bowman's membranes and remains bright, flat, and smooth without being detached from the Bowman's membranes with movement of the lid. The cause of bullae is the accumulation of fluid between the epithelium and Bowman's membrane. The accumulation of fluid causes elevation of the epithelium in a small cyst called the bullae. The bullae is painful with a simple movement of the lids. The source of fluid does not lie in the epithelium. Normal endothelium at the back of the cornea prevents aqueous from finding its way into the stroma. If the endothelium is damaged, this protective mechanism is lost and gets into the stroma, causing edema of the stroma followed by bullae formation under the epithelium. The common causes of bullous keratitis are aphakia, pseudophakia, anterior chamber IOL, vitreous in the anterior chamber, retained foreign body in the anterior chamber, long-standing glaucoma, uveitis, disciform keratitis, and some corneal dystrophies. The condition is painful associated with watering and diminished vision. The complication of bullous keratitis is the formation of a corneal ulcer following its rupture.

The usual treatment consists of the instillation of 5% hypertonic saline 3–4 times a day, along with broad-spectrum antibiotic drops frequently, and the use of lubricant in ointment form at bedtime. The other methods are the use of therapeutic contact lenses and penetrating keratoplasty; in the absence of its facility of keratoplasty, a tarsorrhaphy is the best alternative available.

Corneal Degeneration

Degenerations are a group of diseases that develop on the cornea secondary to some primary disorders, such as prolonged iridocyclitis, glaucoma, and injury. They are unilateral and non-hereditary. The two common degenerations are band keratopathy and nodular keratopathy.

Band Keratopathy

This type of degeneration of the cornea is exclusively seen in the exposed part of the cornea, i.e., the interpalpebral fissure. It is more commonly seen in children suffering from chronic anterior uveitis. The typical appearance of band keratopathy is a strip of opacity horizontally from limbus to limbus with a gap between the band and the limbus. The ends of the band are parallel to the limbus; they are denser on the periphery, gradually becoming fainter towards the pupil, and may cover the pupil, causing diminished vision. They rarely cause foreign body sensations or watering. The exact cause of the disorder is not well established. It is thought to be the deposition of calcium under the epithelium. It takes months to years to develop band keratopathy following primary disorders. The treatment is the removal of the opacity by keratoplasty.

Nodular Degeneration of the Cornea

This is less common than band keratopathy, seen in adults with a past history of reaped phlyctenular keratitis in childhood. The lesion is a white nodule in the anterior stroma and Bowman's membrane. The nodule may bulge through the epithelium. The nodule generally does not cover the pupillary area or cause redness or watering of the eyes. The treatment is keratoplasty.

Lipid Keratopathy (Fatty Degeneration of the Cornea)

Lipid keratopathy is a disease seen in adults due to the deposition of fat in the layers of the cornea, leading to the development of opacity that results in subnormal vision. The exact cause of the disease is not known; it may happen without any disorder of the cornea or anterior uvea. It does not cause pain, redness, or watering. The condition is rare. The treatment is keratoplasty.

Corneal Dystrophies

The dystrophies are a group of primary disorders with a bilateral genetic predisposition seen in both sexes. They may be present at birth or become evident at a later age. Generally not associated with systemic disorders, it is progressive in nature. There is no medical treatment.

Corneal dystrophies are rare in the Indian subcontinent. They are bilateral; the patients may not be aware of their presence unless diminished vision is marked. They may involve any layer of the cornea, singly or in combination. All patients with corneal dystrophy do not require any treatment, except keratoplasty when indicated.

Keratoconus (Conical Cornea)

This is a bilateral condition. The age of onset is between 10 and 20 years. It is supposed to be a dystrophy. It involves all the layers of the cornea in the center. The cornea bulges in the center. It progresses slowly up to forty years of age but may stop at any age as well. In some cases, it progresses very fast and ruptures the Descemet's membrane. In such a case, the aqueous enters the cornea. The cornea becomes cloudy and painful, and the vision suddenly falls to hand movement. Otherwise, the only symptom is a fall in distant vision due to irregular myopic astigmatism, which is confirmed by retinoscopy, keratoscopy, keratometer, and videokeratograph.

Retinoscopy Shows

- Myopic refraction with scissor movement. The axes are always oblique.
- The central part shows a black spot.
- A black circle at the base of the cone.

In advanced cases, the corneal bulge is visible when seen from the side.

The treatment of the condition in its initial stages is the prescription of glasses as per retinoscopy or autorefraction. Which turns out to be irregular myopic astigmatism. The patient requires frequent changes in power with ever-increasing curvature. Contact lenses give a better result as they undo the irregularity of the cornea. Keratoplasty also gives good results; the other treatment available is collagen cross-linking.

Arcus Senilis

Arcus senilis is a common, non-vision-threatening condition of unknown cause seen in adults. It is a white ring situated 1.00 mm away from the limbus in a circular manner; a fully developed arcus is visible in natural light. It may have a genetic background. The common theory of its development is the deposition of lipid in the cornea. The condition does not require any treatment; if the arcus develops under 30 years of age, it is called arcus juveniles.

Keratomalacia

Keratomalacia is also known as xerotic keratitis and corneal melting. It causes drying and clouding of the cornea due to vitamin A deficiency. May be associated with night blindness. Night blindness may precede or follow keratomalacia. It is a bilateral vision-threatening condition of childhood in children suffering from vitamin A deficiency along with protein and caloric mall nutrition. On examination, the child is underweight with stunted growth; the conjunctiva is dry, which may show Bitot's spot; and the cornea is hazy and dull. The development of a central corneal ulcer is very common and is often associated with hypopyon. Perforation is also common. The condition is fully preventable under the national program of treatment for xerophthalmia.

CONTACT LENSES

Contact lenses are optical devices that give better results in selected cases of refraction errors; they are used in place of spectacles. Some contact lenses are used to alleviate corneal disease. They are made of specialized plastic materials. They can be corneal or corneoscleral. The corneal contact lenses are smaller than the scleral; they are generally smaller than the cornea. The scleral contact lenses have a larger diameter than the cornea and extend well over the sclera. The contact lenses are curved, transparent discs of variable curvature and thickness. They remain in place in front of the cornea by the surface tension of the tear film; a well-fitting corneal contact lens is not displaced by the movement of the lids. The tear film in between the contact lens and cornea forms an optical unit. That modifies the corneal curvature; common contact lenses correct only the spherical part of the error of refraction. The corneal curvature is measured by a keratometer. The power of contact lenses and spectacle lenses is not the same. The minus power of the contact lens is less than minus power in the spectacle; the plus power of the contact lens is more than plus power in the spectacle. The high degree of astigmatism requires special contact lenses. The contact lenses are given for distant correction unless they are specially modified for near vision. Without this modification, the near vision is corrected by a spectacle worn in addition to the contact lens in presbyopic persons. As per the material used, contact lenses are called hard, soft, or rigid, and gas permeable. Each with its own merits and demerits **(Fig. 10.8)**.

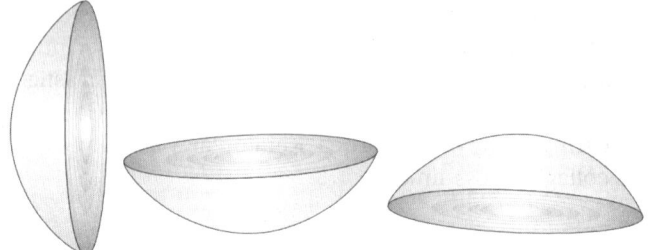

Fig. 10.8: Diagram of corneal contact lens.

Indications of Contact Lens

The most common indication is optical, which includes high errors of refraction, both spherical and astigmatic. They are useful in unilateral aphakia to avoid diplopia. The next indication is anisometropia, where the powers of the two eyes are different. A different of more than three diopters is called clinical anisometropia. Many pupils use contact lenses for cosmetic purposes. Contact lenses can sometimes be used as a low-vision aid; especially manufactured contact lenses are used to deliver uninterrupted delivery of drugs. The contact lenses can be prescribed by trial method or according to the keratometer findings.

Contraindications of Contact Lenses

Contact lenses are not prescribed in the following conditions:
- Diminished corneal sensation
- Dry eye
- Chronic dacryocystitis
- Chronic conjunctivitis
- Deformity of lids
- Lagophthalmos
- Pterygium
- Limbal dermoid
- Vascularization of the cornea
- Exophthalmos and proptosis

Hygiene of Contact Lens

Contact lenses are delicate optical devices that are likely to be scratched and infected. The common source of contamination comes from the conjunctiva and even the contact lens preservation fluid and storage case. The infection may range from as mild as scratching on the cornea to an intractable infection by potent bacteria and parasites (Acanthamoeba). That may cause severe pain, watering, and redness. The contact lenses should be regularly cleaned by a fluid specially made; they should not be cleaned by drinking water or distilled water.

Corneal Surgeries

The corneal surgeries are—repair of wounds, keratoplasty, and refractive keratotomy.

Repair of a Corneal Wound

While repairing the corneal wound, the needle should pass partially through the corneal substance; full-thickness stretching is absolutely prohibited. Care should be taken to free the iris from the corneal wound. The corneal repair should be done under a microscope with proper magnification by a thread not less than 8/0. The use of viscoelastic substances protects the iris and lens from inter-operative trauma; the anterior chamber should be reformed following the surgery.

Keratoplasty

Keratoplasty replaces opaque corneas with transparent corneas acquired from donated corneas (**Figs. 10.9A and B**). There are mainly two types of keratoplasty—penetrating (full thickness) keratoplasty and lamellar (partial thickness) keratoplasty. In full-thickness keratoplasty, a circular button of the cornea containing all the layers from the center of the donated cornea is stitched to the already-made hole in the cornea of the recipient cornea. In lamellar keratoplasty, the disc removed contains up to the stroma of the donor cornea and is stitched to the recipient cornea with corresponding depth and diameter.

The donor cornea is removed from a dead body within 6 hours of death in winter and 2 hours in summer. No eyes are removed from any living person.

The donated eye is transported to the nearest eye bank for future use in a special nutrient fluid. The donated cornea in this situation should be used within 4 days. In eye banks* the unused cornea can be frozen and dehydrated in special refrigerators in nutritional media for 3 weeks. These corneas are suitable for lamellar grafts only.

*Eye bank

Eye bank is different from a commercial bank. In the sense that it is a place to store donated cornea for future use by corneal surgeons and research. It is a non-profit organization that obtains, evaluates, and distributes collected eyes for transplant. The eye bank should have a proper communication and transport system. It can be attached to a hospital or may function from outside the hospital.

Refractive Corneal Surgeries

Refractive corneal surgeries are performed on transparent corneas to improve vision. The most commonly used refractive surgeries are radial keratotomy, photorefractive keratectomy, and lasik. All the refractive surgeries are performed after the error of refraction has stabilised, i.e., after 21 years of age. All refractive surgeries are done under local anaesthesia with an operating microscope.

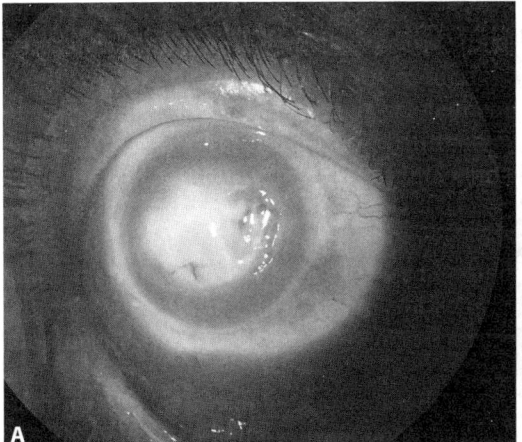 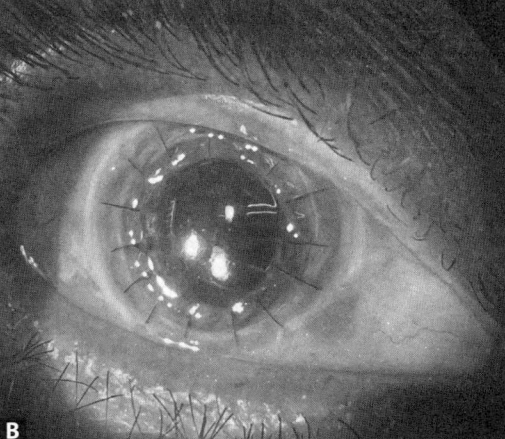

Figs. 10.9A and B: Corneal disease replaced by penetrating keratoplasty.

In the first, multiple partial-thickness incisions are given on the anterior surface of the cornea, leaving the pupillary area; no stitches are required. It is most useful in myopia of moderate degrees. It is not so effective in hypermetropia. High errors may require repeat surgery. The surgery has been mostly given up in favour of photorefractive keratotomy and lasik. That requires a special type of excimer laser.

In lasik surgery, a circular flap is raised that remains hinged to the cornea at one end by a microkeratome. The underlined stroma is treated with a calculated dose of excimer laser. The flap is put back without stitches. The methods give the best result even in high errors of refraction. It also corrects very high astigmatism as well. For the surgery, the patient need not be admitted; improvement in vision is noticed within the next 24 hours.

In photorefractive keratectomy, no flap is raised; only the corneal epithelium is removed, and the cornea is treated by excimer laser. It gives a good result between -6 D to +3 D. It takes a few days to notice an improvement in vision. It is done under local anaesthesia, but the eye remains painful for a few days.

Corneal Trauma

Traumas to the cornea are common causes of diminished vision, ranging from the loss of a few lines to no perception. They are more commonly unilateral but can be bilateral. The causes of bilateral corneal injuries are: Blast injury and chemical burns: the former are generally associated with multiple foreign bodies that may be extraocular or be intraocular in the form of retained intraocular foreign bodies. The injuries may be localised to the cornea with or without iris incarcerated. The injury may extend to the sclera as well **(Fig. 10.10)**.

Mechanical injuries can ranged between simple abrasions to full-thickness injuries. The superficial injuries, if not associated with retained foreign bodies, are treated like corneal ulcers; the embedded foreign bodies should be removed as far as possible. Iron foreign bodies, if not removed within a few hours, form a rust ring all around the foreign body **(Fig. 10.11)**, surrounded by an area of stromal edema. The partial-thickness wounds need not be stitched; they heal by themselves if treated like a corneal ulcer with a pad and bandage. Full-thickness wounds require multiple stitches done under a microscope with 8/0 to 10/0 sutures under a viscoelastic substance. Incarcerated intraocular tissues are removed during primary sutures. All cases of incarcerated uvea should be treated with an adequate steroid along with a broad-spectrum antibiotic. Epithelial wounds heal without scarring; the others leave dense opacities. Corneal wounds are semi-emergencies, in contrast to chemical wounds, which are ophthalmic

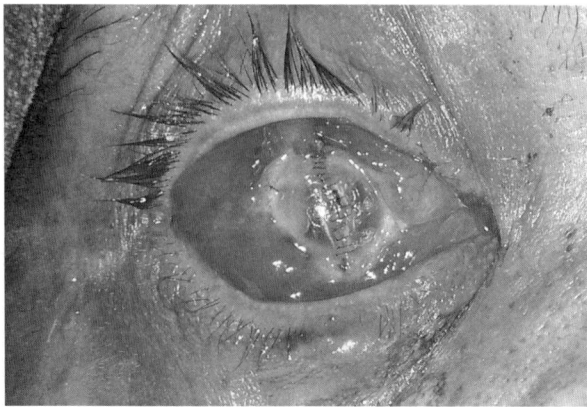

Fig. 10.10: Repaired full thickness corneoscleral wound.
(For color version, see Plate 5)

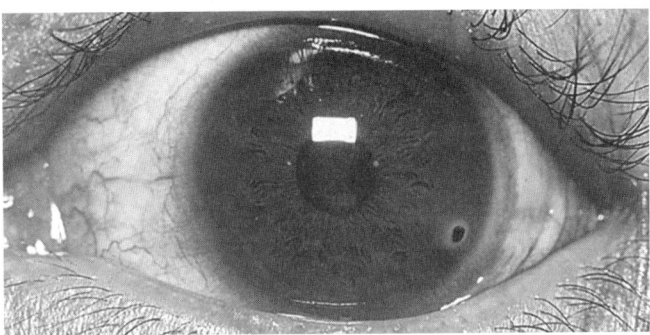

Fig. 10.11: Corneal foreign body with rust ring.

emergencies. The chemical injury may be localised to a part of the cornea or may involve the cornea along with the conjunctiva.

The management of chemical injury begins with primary medical aid consisting of washing the eye with copious amounts of potable water, irrespective of the pH of the chemical. No time should be lost in asserting the pH of the chemical. The wash may last for as long as half an hour. In cases of severe blepharospasm, a local anaesthetic agent helps open the lids. That helps in washing the chemicals. The fornices should be examined for hidden foreign bodies. Alkaline chemicals are more dangerous than acidic ones.

After primary treatment, the patients should be shifted to a hospital to give further treatment. That may be prolonged in the case of an alkaline burn. The severity of the injury depends on the concentration of the chemical.

Artificial Eye

Artificial eyes are non-sighting ocular **prosthesis*** used for cosmetic purposes **(Fig. 10.12)**. They are made of acrylic material to substitute for the missing eye, i.e., an eviscerated or enucleated eye. With modification, they can be used over phthisis bulbae or microphthalmos. A well-fitted artificial eye should look similar to the normal eye and move with the movement of the normal eye. They are removable devices that should be removed every night and cleaned regularly.

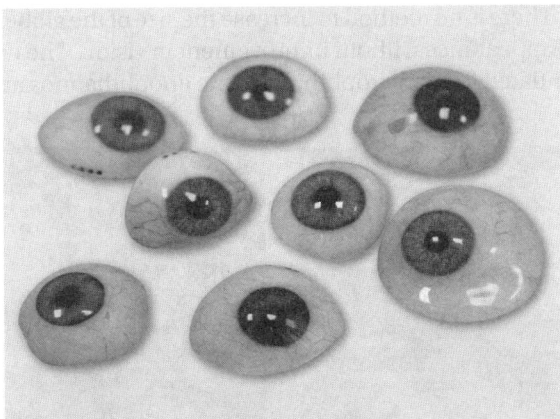

Fig. 10.12: Artificial eyes of different sizes.

***Prosthesis**
A prosthesis is a device designed to replace a missing part of the body or to make a part of the body work better. An artificial eye is an example of a prosthesis.

CHAPTER 11

Disorders of Sclera

The sclera is the largest part of the outer coat of the eyeball; it is opaque without any visual function. Its main function is to protect the intraocular structure, act as an attachment for the extraocular muscle, and serve as a conduit for the nerves and vessels. The sclera has very poor blood supply and sensation. It is white in color; the anterior part is covered by the conjunctiva. The eyeball moves freely in the orbital fat. The average diameter of the adult sclera is 24.00 mm.

The common disorders of the sclera are:
- Congenital
- Inflammation
- Ectasia (bulging)

The sclera shares injuries like any other extraocular structure. It is not capable of new growth. The commonest congenital anomaly of the sclera is microphthalmos.

CONGENITAL ANOMALIES OF SCLERA

Microphthalmos

Microphthalmos is a congenital state of reduced diameter of the sclera all-round, including the cornea. An eye is said to be microphthalmic when its diameter is less than 20.00 mm. It may be as small as a few millimeters and may be unilateral or bilateral (**Figs. 11.1 and 11.2**). The cornea is small with reduced curvature, may be flat, the anterior chamber is shallow, the pupil is small, and may be associated with coloboma. The lens is spherical; all the other structures of the eye are small with normal movement and pseudoptosis. The vision is low to very low; sometimes there may be no perception. There is no method to increase the size of the globe. Corneoscleral contact lenses may restore the appearance without improvement in vision. The two acquired conditions that need to be differentiated from microphthalmos are enophthalmos and phthisis bulbae.

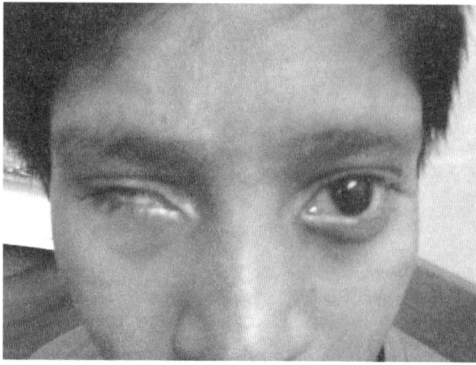

Fig. 11.1: Unilateral microphthalmos.

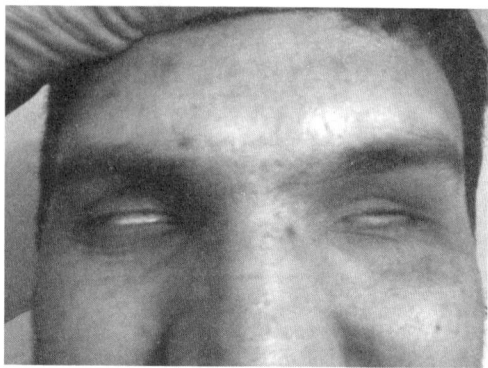

Fig. 11.2: Bilateral microphthalmos.

Enophthalmos

Enophthalmos is an acquired condition where the shape, curvature, and size of the sclera and cornea are normal with normal movement and the eyeball is retracted. The vision may be normal or marginally reduced, which may be improved by glasses. It shares a narrowed interpalpebral aperture with microphthalmos and phthisis. The most common cause of enophthalmos is fractures of the orbital floor. The other causes are Duane's retraction syndrome and Horner's syndrome, following the involvement of the sympathetic chain. No specific treatment is required except correction of vision and management of the fracture floor of the orbit.

Phthisis Bulbae

Phthisis bulbae is the irregular shrinking of the globe on all sides due to the destruction of the ciliary body following inflammation or trauma. Resulting in a total or partial reduction in the formation of aqueous The eyeball is soft and may be tender initially, but that passes off with time. The globe loses its spherical shape and becomes quadrilateral in shape. The places where the recti are depressed. Pseudoptosis is common, and the movements are normal. The vision may be absent or very poor. There is no specific treatment once the eye has gone into the state of phthisis. A timely treatment of severe intraocular inflammation and the management of penetrating wounds reduce the chances of phthisis **(Fig. 11.3)**. A cosmetic sclera corneal contact lens improves the appearance.

INFLAMMATION OF SCLERA

Due to the avascularity of the sclera, it is rarely invaded by microorganisms. Except in cases of embedded infected foreign bodies in the sclera. More common are inflammations of the sclera and episclera. The former is called scleritis, which is rarer than the latter, called episcleritis.

Episcleritis

The exact cause of episcleritis is not known; it is seen in adults, more in females, and is more common in persons suffering from diabetes and inflammation of the joints. It is generally unilateral. It has been divided into two classes, i.e., simple and nodular. Simple episcleritis is almost symptoms less except localized conjunctival congestion away from the limbus **(Fig. 11.4)**. The condition is nontender and self-limiting in most of the occasions. An episcleritis not healing by itself; it responds well with weak solution of steroids. Recurrences are common; the condition does not interfere with vision. The nodular form consists of a well-defined subconjunctival nodule

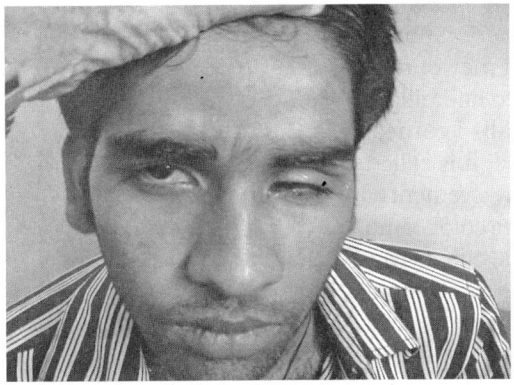

Fig. 11.3: Phthisis bulbae left eye.

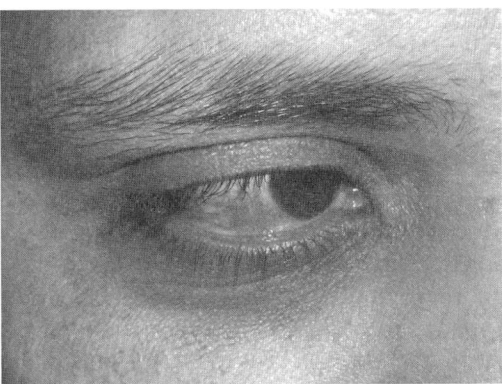

Fig. 11.4: Episcleritis.

similar to conjunctival phlycten, generally on the temporal side; it is nontender. The condition requires treatment by local steroid.

Scleritis

Scleritis is rarer than episcleritis but more serious and difficult to treat, seen equally among adult males and females. The exact cause of the disease is not well understood; the predisposing factors are age, diabetes, rheumatoid arthritis, and other autoimmune diseases.

The nodule is fixed to the sclera and tender. A scleritis nodule near the limbus invariably invades the cornea, causing sclerosing keratitis and sclerouveitis. As per location, it has been divided into two groups: more common anterior scleritis and less common posterior scleritis. The posterior scleritis presents with mild pain in the globe and mild proptosis. It is best diagnosed on a B-scan, USG, or CT scan.

It rarely responds to local steroids. The treatment of choice is a systemic steroid with usual precaution.

ECTASIA (BULGING) OF CORNEA AND SCLERA

An ectasia of the globe can involve the cornea, sclera, or both and is called staphyloma. Clinically, a staphyloma is defined as ecstatic cicatrization of the outer coat of the globe with the uvea incarcerated. The staphylomas develop on anatomical or pathological weak spots on the globe. The weak spots are: center of the cornea, the corneoscleral junction, and the equator. The staphylomas have been divided into two groups, i.e., corneal and scleral. **Flowchart 11.1** shows various types of staphylomas as per location.

Flowchart 11.1: Distribution of staphyloma.

```
                    Staphyloma
           ┌────────────┼────────────┐
      Corneal       Corneoscleral   Scleral
     (Anterior)          │        ┌───┼────────┐
      ┌───┴───┐       Intercalary Ciliary Equatorial Posterior
   Partial  Total
```

Corneal Staphyloma

The most common cause of corneal staphyloma is sloughing corneal ulcers, where the floor of the ulcer after perforation is replaced by fibrous tissue called pseudocornea. It may or may not be lined by the iris when the iris is incarcerated and bulges with normal or raised intraocular tension. It is called corneal staphyloma. If the whole of the cornea is involved, it is called total anterior staphyloma **(Fig. 11.5)**, and partial involvement of the cornea is called partial anterior staphyloma. The color of the anterior staphyloma is white, sprinkled with iris tissue that gives it a gray color. The surface is lobulated. The size of the staphyloma depends on the amount of cornea involved, duration, and intraocular pressure. The total corneal staphylomas are without vision. The symptoms of corneal staphyloma are cosmetic and painful blind eye. Once a staphyloma has developed, it cannot

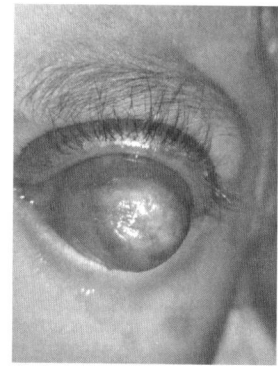

Fig. 11.5: Total corneal staphyloma with degeneration. (*For color version, see Plate 5*)

be reduced. Small, partial anterior staphylomas may be masked by a suitable corneoscleral contact lens. It is best to enucleate the eye with a painful staphyloma. The other causes of corneal staphylomas are keratomalacia and blast injuries.

Scleral Staphyloma

Most of the scleral staphylomas are acquired, except for rare idiopathic scleral staphylomas and posterior staphylomas. Rhinosporidiosis is also known to produce scleral staphylomas. The scleral staphyloma develops on anatomically weak spots after trauma or extensive pro-long scleritis. The staphyloma anterior to the equator is lined by conjunctiva. The posterior staphylomas are surrounded by orbital fat. The sclera at the site of staphyloma is thinned and lined by uvea; so long as the thin sclera can with stand it does not bulge. Once the intraocular pressure is raised, the sclera bulges out. They are called intercalary when present at the corneoscleral junction, ciliary when over the ciliary body, and equatorial when under the attachment of extraocular muscles. The commonest type of scleral staphyloma is ciliary staphyloma, which may be seen in a sector or may encircle the whole of the limbus. In such cases, they are called total staphyloma; generally, they are without vision and likely to rupture. The only treatment for scleral staphyloma is enucleation with an appropriate prosthesis. The most common cause of posterior staphyloma is congenital high myopia. They are not visible in the anterior segment. They are best seen with an indirect ophthalmoscope, USG, and CT. **Figure 11.6** shows various sites of staphylomas and the intraocular structure lining them.

Figures 11.7A to C show various types of scleral staphyloma.

Trauma

Sclera is mostly involved in mechanical injuries like incisions or lacerations. They may be localized to the sclera or associated with a corneal wound. It may be associated with uveal incarceration; the eye with a hidden scleral wound is a soft eye.

The treatment of scleral trauma is stitching the sclera after the uvea has been freed from the wound and covering it with conjunctiva. All cases of scleral wounds should be investigated for retained intraocular foreign bodies.

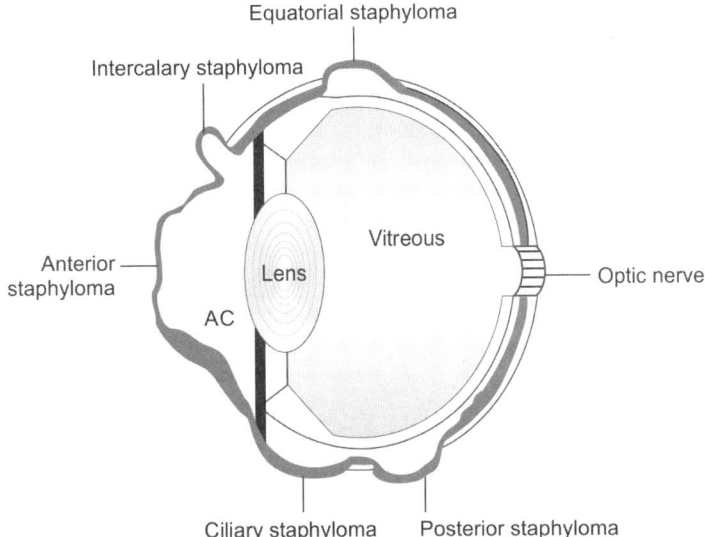

Fig. 11.6: Various types of staphylomas with intraocular structure lining them.

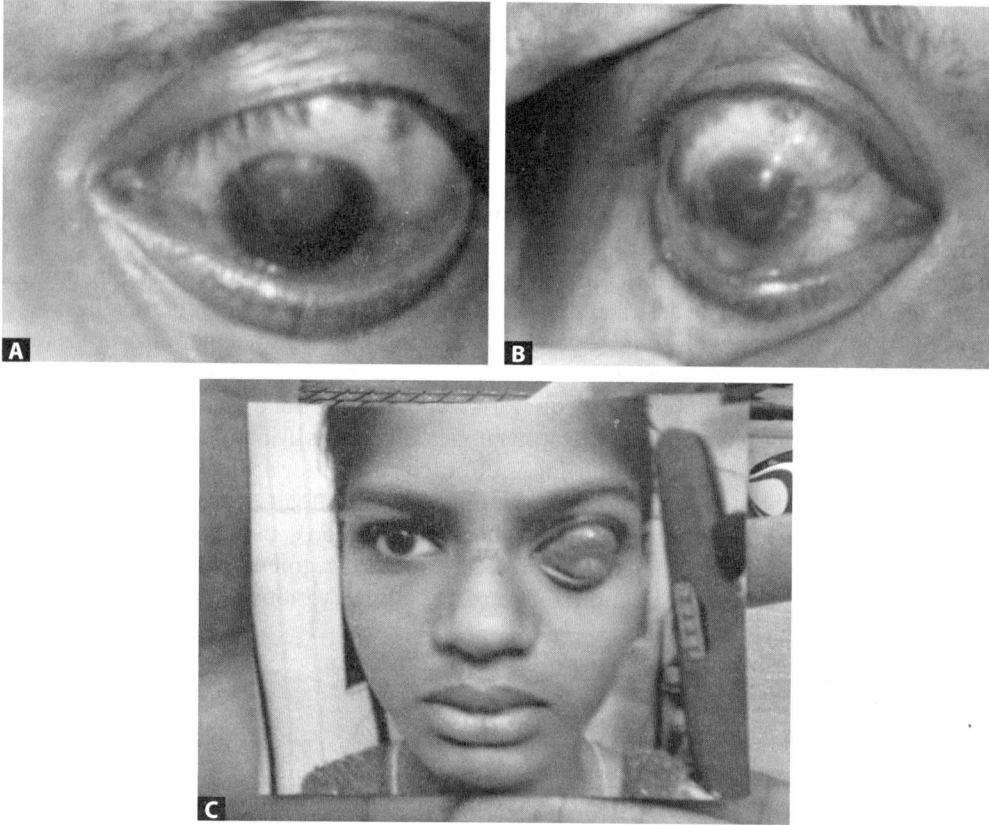

Figs. 11.7A to C: Various types of scleral staphyloma.

CHAPTER 12

Disorders of the Lens

The main function of the lens is optical; it is capable of focusing parallel rays from infinity (60 meters) on divergent rays from a near point. This faculty of focusing divergent rays is called accommodation. The other function is to separate the aqueous chamber from the vitreous chamber; for this, it requires intact zonules all-round and a functioning ciliary body. For its optical purposes, the lens must remain transparent. The lens is an elliptoid, transparent structure that is thick in the middle, gradually decreasing towards the periphery. The central anterior part of the lens is called the anterior pole. While its corresponding area in the posterior part is called the posterior pole, the rounded edge where the two surfaces meet is called the equator of the lens, to which the zonules are attached all-round. The lens is suspended between the posterior surface of the iris and the vitreous, with the pupil in the center, by zonules that extend from the ciliary body to the periphery of the lens. The lens has the following parts: the capsule, epithelium, and lens fibers. Which are again divided into two parts, i.e., the large cortex and the small nucleus. The nucleus is nothing but a compressed cortex; the size of the nucleus increases with age. Initially, both the cortex and nucleus are soft, but as age advances, the nucleus enlarges and hardens.

Disorders of the lens can be congenital or acquired. The latter are more common, and most of them are amenable to treatment. **The disease of the lens can be divided into three groups:**
1. Loss of transparency (cataract)
2. Displacement of the lens (ectopia lentis)
3. Morphological changes (shape and size)

The eye with a lens in place is called a phakic eye, while the eye without a lens is called an aphakia. The replacement of a natural lens with an artificial lens is called pseudophakia.

LOSS OF TRANSPARENCY

A complete or partial loss of transparency is called a cataract. It can be congenital or acquired and may be localized to the cortex, nucleus, or both. An opacity extending from pole to pole and equator all-round is called mature cataract, and an opacity not fully filling the above criteria is called immature cataract.

Flowchart 12.1 shows various possibilities for cataracts.

Flowchart 12.1: Various possibilities for cataracts.

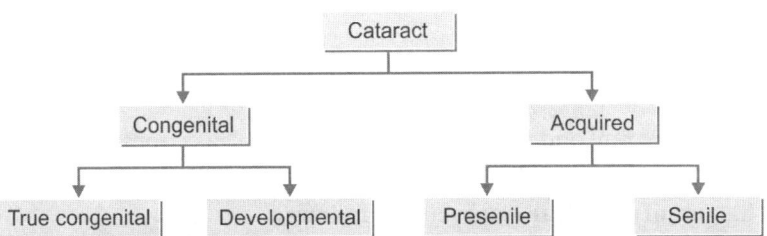

From **Flowchart 12.1**, the cataract can be divided into two age groups, i.e., children and those over 40 years old. The cataracts seen under 40 years are congenital, developmental, traumatic, and secondary to infection, inflammation, and drugs. The types seen above 40 years are senile traumatic, cataract in systemic disease, secondary to intraocular inflammation, and drug-induced.

Cataract in Adult

Senile Cataract

Also known as age-related cataract, is a slow-progressing acquired opacity in the lens after 50 years of age in both sexes all over the world. Some races develop age-related cataracts earlier than others. The condition is bilateral; one eye may develop cataracts earlier than the other. The condition causes slow-progressing diminished vision without pain, redness, or itching. If the eye with cataracts has redness and watering, the cause of them should be found out. According to the position of the opacity, the cataract can be nuclear or cortical. It is not uncommon for both conditions to be present at the same time. Exaggerating clinical picture of the two.

Nuclear Cataract

This is the most common type of cataract, where the opacity starts and progresses slowly in the center of the lens; its progression is slower than the cortical verity. The vision is slowly reduced; the other symptoms are scattering of light and intolerance to light. The vision gets further diminished in bright light. One of the causes of diminished distant vision in nuclear cataracts is induced index myopia. The advantage of this phenomenon is better near vision. A person who was dependent on near correction can see without glasses. This is called second sight. The nuclear cataract rarely becomes total. With the passage of time, the cataract becomes harder. Changing its color from gray to brown resulted in an uncorrectable improvement in vision.

Symptoms

Most of the time, the nuclear cataract is without pain, redness, or raised intraocular pressure. In others, it may be associated with pain and redness that require early management.

The symptoms of cataracts without pain are:
- Gradual fall of distant vision
- Glare and intolerance to light
- Poor vision in bright light (noon)
- Better vision in dim light (evening)
- Polyopia (one thing looks more than two or three)
- Improvement of near vision (patient can read without glasses)

The painful symptoms are:
- Gross loss of distant and near vision
- Redness
- Severe pain in the eyes
- Headache

These symptoms are rare and develop only if the protein leaks from the capsule or there is a rise in intraocular pressure due to protein-induced inflammation.

The natural history of a nuclear cataract is as follows:
Nuclear haze → Nuclear hardening → Brown cataract → Black cataract → Total nuclear cataract

The signs of a nuclear cataract:
- ❖ The eye is normal externally, with whiteness in the pupil that is better seen on dilatation and found to be at the center of the clear cortex.
- ❖ The cornea and anterior chamber are normal.
- ❖ The pupil is central, circular, and reacts briskly, directly and indirectly.
- ❖ The intraocular tension is normal.
- ❖ **Iris shadow*** is present.
- ❖ On retinoscopy, the opacity looks like a black spot in the center of a pink glow.

*__The iris shadow__ is a black crescent-shaped shadow of the iris on the transparent/semitransparent lens seen in oblique illumination. The cause behind the phenomenon is that the iris casts a shadow on the translucent cortex. If the cortex is fully opaque, as in mature cataracts, the shadow is lost (__Figs. 12.1 and 12.2__). The iris shadow is also absent following complete removal of the lens from the pupillary area, as in intracapsular lens extraction. The transparent lens is also devoid of iris shadows.

Treatment

1. There is no medical treatment for any type of cataract.
2. The definitive treatment is surgical. It consists of the removal of the cataract and replacing it with an intraocular lens.
3. The surgery depends on the visual requirements of the individual and not the maturity of the cataract.
4. The surgery can be delayed by following non-surgical methods, i.e., prescribing minus lenses for distance and asking the patient to do the near work without classes. Using an umbrella to ward off the bright light Tinted glasses may help improve distant vision.

Cortical Cataract

In contrast to the nuclear cataract, the opacities develop from the periphery, progressing centrally and expanding laterally. This converts; the cortex the whole of the cortex into a white, opaque mass.

Sometimes, the cortex between the posterior capsule and nucleus is converted into a disc-shaped opacity. The above changes are called the incipient stage of cortical cataract. On retinoscopy, the opaque areas stand out as black cones with a base towards the periphery. As time passes, the cortex is liquefied, and the whole of the lens increases in size. This stage is called intumescence. The increased volume of the lens pushes the iris forward, narrowing the angle of the anterior chamber and causing a rise in intraocular tension.

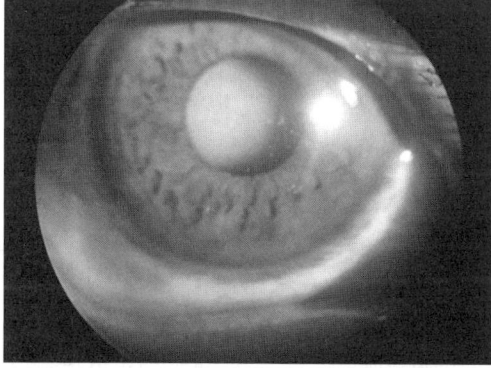

Fig. 12.1: Immature cataract with iris shadow.

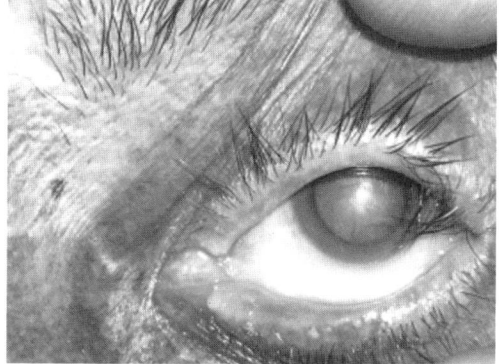

Fig. 12.2: Mature cataract without iris shadow.

Symptoms of Cortical Cataract

The cortical cataract shares diminished vision with the nuclear cataract. The only difference is that a cortical cataract has better vision than a constricted pupil. The patient may have normal vision as long as the opacities do not reach the pupil. The cataract is best seen with a dilated pupil on retinoscopy; the opacities extend from the periphery towards the center in the pink glow. **Figures 12.3A** and **12.4A** show the retinoscopic appearance of the two and **Figures 12.3B and 12.4B** show clinical appearance of immature and mature cataract.

The loss of vision in cortical cataracts is variable; so long as it does not encroach the pupil, the vision may not be effected. In such cases, the opacities are discovered by dilatation of the pupil. The cataract grows faster than in nuclear cataract; hence, loss of vision is faster in cortical cataract. The chance of lens-induced glaucoma is more in cortical cataracts. The only treatment available is the surgical removal of cataracts by phacoemulsification and implanting an intraocular lens.

Posterior Subcapsular Cataract

Posterior subcapsular cataract **(Fig. 12.5)** is a type of cortical cataract with the difference that, unlike spokes of opacity in cortical cataract, the posterior subcapsular cataract is a circular disc between the nucleus and the posterior capsule with a denser centre. It develops earlier than usual.

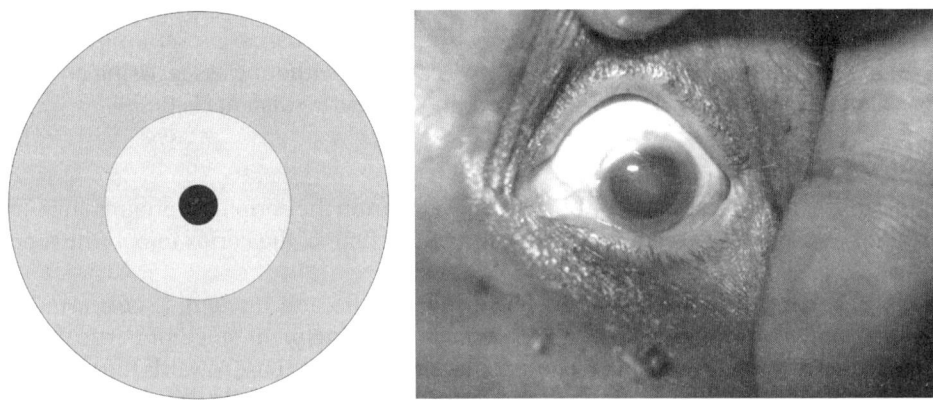

Figs. 12.3A and B: (A) Nuclear cataract as seen on retinoscopy; (B) Clinical picture of nuclear cataract.

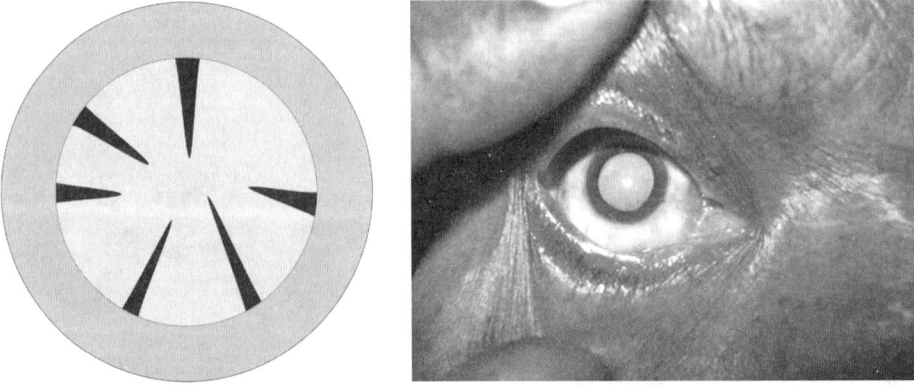

Figs. 12.4A and B: (A) Cortical cataract as seen on retinoscopy; (B) Clinical picture of a mature cortical cataract.

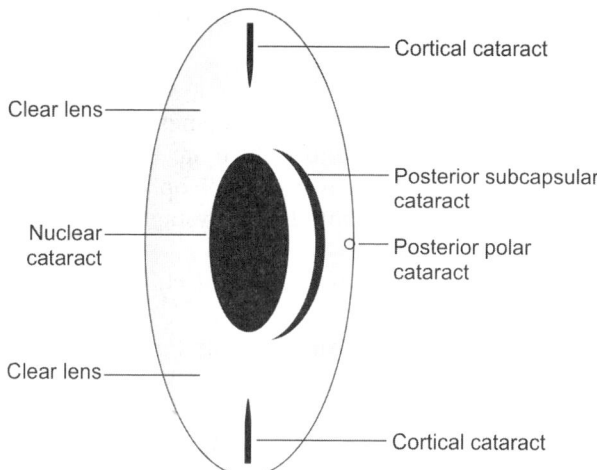

Fig. 12.5: Difference between the positions of the nuclear, cortical, and posterior subcapsular cataracts.

In a cortical cataract, the loss of vision is similar to that of a nuclear cataract. The exact cause of the condition is not known; it may be genetic. The other causes are uveitis in childhood and prolonged use of strong steroids.

Treatment is similar to other cataracts, i.e., a posterior chamber IOL implant. Cases of posterior subcapsular cataracts are more likely to develop posterior capsular opacity, which requires treatment by laser capsulotomy.

Congenital Cataract

Congenital cataracts are lenticular opacities that develop during the early stages of gestation. They can be nuclear, subnuclear, polar, and cortical. The exact causes of congenital cataracts are not well understood. Many of them are hereditary; they may be seen in generations and among siblings and blood relations. In one-third of the cases, no cause can be found. The remaining is due to maternal infection, maternal disorders of metabolism, and malnutrition. Congenital cataracts can be unilateral or bilateral; depending on the area of the lens involved, they can be partial or total. The latter is less common. As per symptoms, congenital cataracts are divided into two groups, i.e., those that predominantly cause diminished vision and those that do not interfere with vision. In the first group, the opacities situated on the visual axis. The anterior polar cataract hardly causes diminished vision in contrast to posterior polar cataracts, which are associated with visual loss.

The congenital cataracts may be associated with other congenital anomalies of the globe like congenital coloboma of iris (**Fig. 12.6**) and systemic metabolic disorders. Though the common symptom of congenital cataract should be diminished vision,

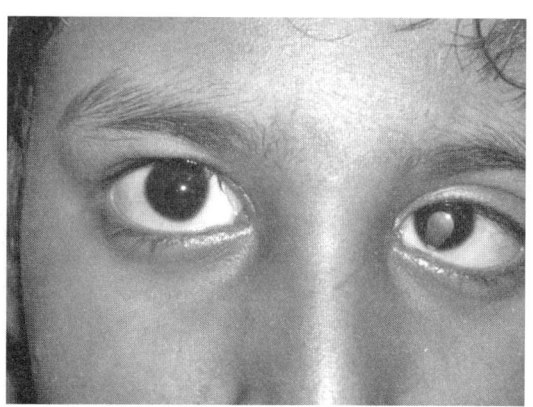

Fig. 12.6: Congenital cataract with coloboma of iris.

diminished vision becomes apparent only when the child grows up and the parent becomes aware of the defect.

The other features are:
- A visible white opacity in the pupillary area that becomes more marked in dim light.
- The late features are nystagmus, squint, and amblyopia.
- Unilaterally dense opacities develop squint and amblyopia more frequently.
- Developmental cataracts are not associated with nystagmus but may cause squints and amblyopia.
- The most common congenital cataract that brings the child for consultation is a complete, dense, white, soft opacity.
- The next frequent congenital cataract is lamellar (zonular) cataract.

Zonular Cataract

About half of the congenital cataracts are zonular, generally bilateral, and develop before birth or may become obvious after birth. They have a specific shape that is a central circular laminated disc with an irregular border and projection towards the center called riders that do not reach the periphery. The rest of the lens is clear; the cataract is best visualized following complete mydriasis, the opacity being central, and the vision is poor with a normal pupil but improves following dilatation **(Figs. 12.7 and 12.8)**.

Treatment

The ideal treatment consists of phacoemulsification with an intraocular lens implant and near vision correction by spectacle. In the absence of surgical facilities, the pupil up to the age of 6 to 8 years should be kept dilated to prevent amblyopia.

Rubella Cataract

Rubella can be prevented by immunizing every girl in her childhood under the national program of immunization. The disorder develops in non-immunized females with an array of malformations, including eye. If the unimmunized mother gets infected by rubella in the first three months of pregnancy, the chances of the child getting a rubella cataract are maximum. The eyes may be involved with/without the involvement of other organs. The organs commonly involved are the heart, lung, brain, and ear. The changes in the eyes vary from microphthalmos with/without cataracts to rubella cataracts and glaucoma. The rubella cataract is a large, complete opacity that contains live viruses. Once rubella has developed, there is no treatment

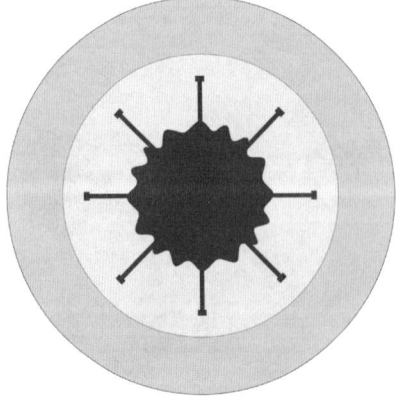

Fig. 12.7: Lamellar cataract on retinoscopy.

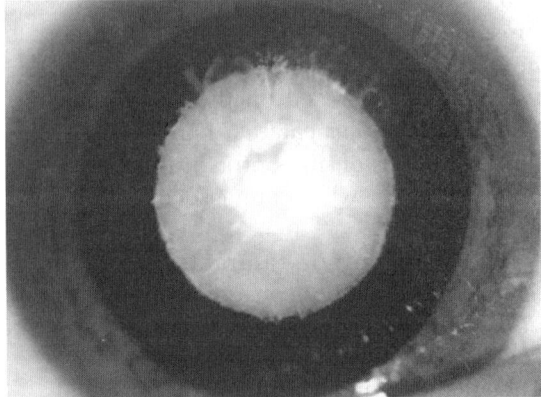

Fig. 12.8: Lamellar cataract on oblique illumination.

for the mother or the child. The effect of rubella cataracts is worsened by other anomalies of the eye and systemic involvement. The treatment for rubella cataracts is surgery in a specialized center. Only one eye should be operated on at a time; postoperative management involves prolonged use of cycloplegics and steroids for months to years. The prognosis is not very satisfactory.

Sutural Cataract

Sutural cataracts are rare congenital cataracts that involve the Y sutures of the fetal nucleus. Are slow to progress with minimal visual loss not requiring any treatment, the associated error of refraction needs to be corrected **(Fig. 12.9)**.

Blue-dot Cataract

Blue-dot cataracts are rare and, when present, are missed too often. They are developmental anomalies of the lens involving both the nucleus and cortex. The conditions can be diagnosed by simple, bright oblique illumination, better seen on a slit lamp. They are asymptomatic and may have errors of refraction. Do not require treatment except correction of the error of refraction by the second decade.

Traumatic Cataract

Traumatic cataracts are seen in all ages, from childhood to adulthood. The most common age groups of persons getting traumatic cataracts correspond with the most active period of life, i.e., between 15 and 50 years. The causes of these cataracts are sports injuries, brawls, and agricultural and industrial injuries. Traumatic cataracts are more common among males; they are generally unilateral, except in blast injuries. The two common types of traumatic cataracts are penetrating injuries (needle, knife, thorn, and projectile) and blunt injuries.

Cataract due to a Penetrating Injury

Any projectile that passes through the full thickness of the cornea is likely to injure the lens. It may be localized to the lens or traverse through the lenticular material. The size of the opacity depends on the extent of the projectile; it may be pinpoint, not allowing aqueous to enter the lens, and is generally stationary. If aqueous enters the cortex, the cortex swells and turns white, involving the whole of the lens. After a few days, the opaque cortical matter comes out of the wound as

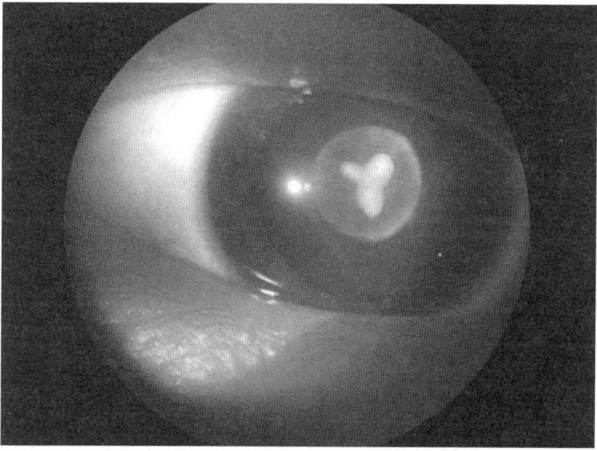

Fig. 12.9: Sutural cataract.

fluffy soft matter in the anterior chamber **(Fig. 12.10)**, which may cause secondary glaucoma. Vision depends on the size and position of the opacities. Small opacities on the periphery may go unnoticed; large opacities cause a fast fall of vision. Some of the cortical matter, if not removed early, gets absorbed partially or totally, leaving the eye aphakic with after cataracts. Traumatic cataracts in children have better chances of cortical absorption. A form of nucleus does not get absorbed, requiring surgical removal. Sometimes the penetrating injury may involve the iris, causing wholeness in the iris, rupture of the pupillary border, or iridodialysis **(Fig. 12.11)**; occasionally, the penetrating injury may leave an intraocular foreign body.

The treatment of a traumatic cataract following a penetrating injury consists of repair of the corneal and corneoscleral wounds, management of prolapsed uvea, and removal of as much of cortical matter as possible, followed by a secondary IOL implant.

Cataract Due to Blunt Injury

Cataract due to blunt injury differs from that caused by penetrating injury in the sense that there is no visible opening in the capsule.

The changes brought about by a blunt injury to the lens are:
- Vossius ring

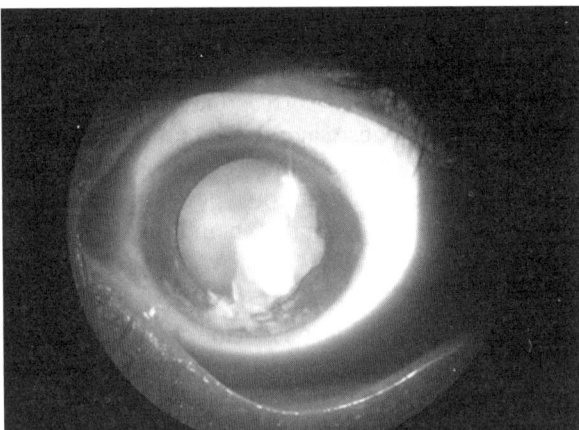

Fig. 12.10: Traumatic cataract with cortical matter in AC.

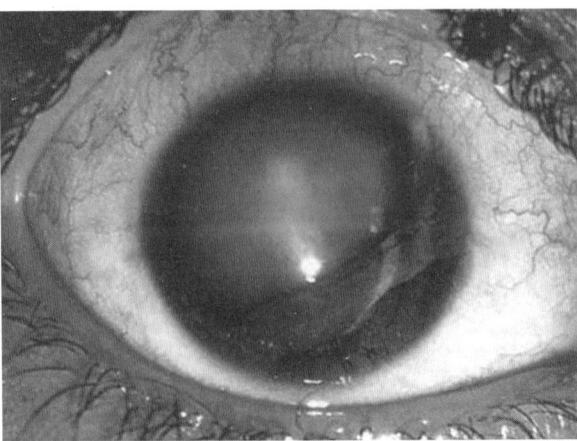

Fig. 12.11: Traumatic cataract with iridodialysis. *(For color version, see Plate 5)*

- Concussion cataract
- Anterior subcapsular opacity
- Posterior subcapsular opacity
- Subluxation or dislocation of the lens
- Changes in the macula in the form of commotion retinae or Berlin's edema.
- There may be associated changes in the iris, like dialysis.

Vossius Ring

This is the deposition of iris pigment on the anterior lens capsule when the posterior surface is forced against the anterior lens capsule in a circular fashion, corresponding to the constricted pupil. The iris pigmentation being away from the visual axis does not cause diminished vision. It is mostly diagnosed following mydriasis. The pigments gradually fade without any treatment. May be associated with concussion cataracts.

Concussion Cataract

Concussion cataracts develop a few days to a few months following a blunt injury to the globe; the effect is most marked in the posterior cortex. The cause of concussion cataracts is supposed to be due to entry of a small amount of aqueous through a microtear in the capsule. It develops as a central opacity from which radiate petal-like opacities similar to bottle brushes **(Fig. 12.12)**. The opacity is best visualized on slit lamp examination. Without magnification, the cataract looks like an irregular, smudged opacity in the posterior cortex **(Fig. 12.13)**. A small concussion cataract may not progress, and a large opacity may grow fast enough to be converted into a complete cortical cataract.

Management of Congenital Cataracts

- There is no medical treatment for congenital cataracts. The rubella cataract can be prevented by compulsory immunization against rubella of girls by nine years of age.
- All congenital cataracts do not require treatment.
- Opacity away from the visual axis may be left without any treatment.
- Central opacities with clear cortex exposed following full mydriasis may also be left without treatment until specialized surgical treatment is available.
- Uniocular cataracts should be operated on as soon as possible.
- The results of unilateral cataract surgery are not very encouraging.

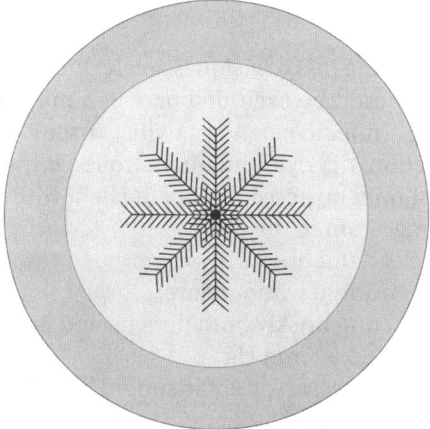

Fig. 12.12: Concussion cataract as seen on retinoscopy.

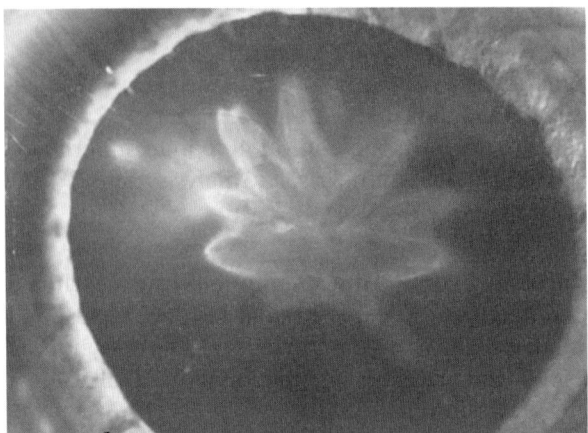

Fig. 12.13: Concussion cataract as seen on oblique illumination.

- A bilateral, dense cataract should be operated on as soon as possible.
- Both eyes should not be operated on in single seating.
- All surgeries should be done under general anesthesia.
- All surgeries should be done under an operating microscope with viscoelastic.
- The best results are obtained by putting on an intraocular lens at a specialized center.

Treatment of Adult Cataracts

All cataracts do not require surgery; there is no medical treatment for cataracts. Optical correction may postpone the surgery for some time. The gold standard of surgery is lens extraction, followed by optical correction. That could be spectacle correction, a contact lens, or an intraocular lens implant. The eye left without a natural lens is called aphakia, and an eye with an intraocular lens is called pseudophakia. The surgery no more depends on the maturity of the cataract; it depends on the visual requirements of the person. Only one eye should be operated on at a time.

Evaluation of the Patient for Lens Extraction

- Find out that the sole cause of diminished vision is cataract only.
- The following conditions may worsen the vision secondary to cataract; they are central corneal opacity, high error of refraction, squint, deep amblyopia, diseases of the posterior segment, and optic nerve.
- Once it has been settled that the loss of vision is solely due to cataracts, the following ocular and systemic conditions should be excluded or, when present, managed before surgery. The ocular conditions are—infective conjunctivitis, chronic dacryocystitis, lid deformity, diminished corneal sensation, dry eye, and uncontrolled intraocular tension.
  - The minimum vision should be perception of the light with accurate projection.
  - There should be no congestion in the eye.
  - The cornea should be clear and bright.
  - The anterior chamber is normal without flare.
  - Pupil central circular reacting briskly both directly and indirectly
  - Intraocular tension under 20.00 mm Hg
  - Negative regurgitation. If necessary, the sac should be syringed.
  - Diabetes, high blood pressure, and other neo-vascular diseases are not contraindications so long as they are under control with usual medical treatment.

The lens can be removed by the following methods—removing the complete lens; the procedure is called intracapsular lens extraction, which is contraindicated in patients under 40 years of age. The other method is called extracapsular lens extraction, which includes sufficient anterior capsulectomy, removal of the lens, and washing out all the cortical material, leaving the posterior capsule intact. The intracapsular lens extraction is no more surgery of choice.

Following both methods, the eye becomes **aphakia***. In the past, it was corrected by plus lenses for distance, on top of which near correction was added either in a separate glass or by bifocal glasses. Elderly aphakics do not tolerate bifocals; they prefer to separate glasses for far and near. Younger persons prefer contact lenses over aphakic correction by spectacles.

*****Aphakia**
*The absence of a lens completely or partially from the pupillary area is called aphakia **(Fig. 12.14)**. It is called partial when only one part of the pupil is devoid of a lens. As seen in subluxation of lens. Aphakia is rarely congenital. The most common cause is the surgical removal of the lens. The next cause is dislocation of the lens where it falls in the vitreous, either due to blunt trauma or a syndrome, such as Marfan syndrome. The sign of aphakia depends on the amount of opacity left following its removal; the more of the cortex left, the greater the opacity. Such opacities are called aftercataracts. Which is common after extracapsular lens extraction. An aphakic eye has a deep anterior chamber and tremulousness of the iris. Post-surgical aphakia invariably has 1–2 iridectomies. The pupil should be central and circular, reacting to light without accommodation. The color of the pupil is jet black following intracapsular lens extraction and dislocation of the lens; it looks grey if there is an after cataract. The after cataract consists of parts of the anterior capsule, the equatorial capsule, the posterior capsule, and cortical matter.*

The most dominant part of the symptoms of aphakia is diminished distant vision and no near vision. The distant vision commonly ranges between 1/60 to 2/60 with good projection. The cause of diminished vision is the absence of a lens. A transparent lens has a power of +17D; thus, an eye without a lens is left with +43D power, which makes the eye highly hypermetropic. Postoperative aphakia is associated with astigmatism ranging between 1 to 2Dcyl at 180°. The absence of a lens is the cause of loss of near vision. The distant vision is corrected by prescribing +10Dsph with +1Dcyl at 180° in spectacle. The near vision is corrected by prescribing +13Dsph and +1Dcyl at 180°. The other possibility is to correct distant vision by contact lens, the power of which will be more than +10Dsph. Difficulty of +10Dsph in spectacle lens is enlargement of the size of the object by 33%. The patient has best vision at the center of the spectacle lens with

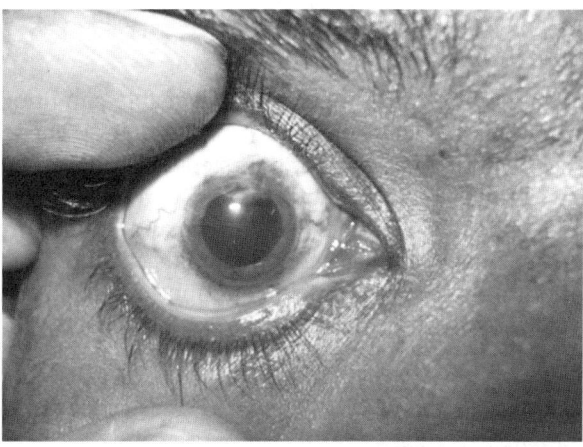

Fig. 12.14: Aphakia.

diminished and distorted vision. On the periphery. The contact lens gives magnification of only 5%; all these are absent following an intraocular lens implant. A patient with IOL generally requires near vision correction provided in spectacle. An eye that was emmetrope before the development of cataracts should have vision 6/6 following correction. There are some conditions where vision does not improve to this level.

The causes of non-improvement of vision following lens extraction are put into two groups. The first group consists of those the surgeon becomes aware of before surgery and must inform the patient about the possibility of non-improvement. The causes are central corneal opacity, high error of refraction, both spherical and cylindrical, squint, amblyopia, chronic uveitis, and advanced glaucoma.

The causes discovered after the surgery are—macular lesions, retinal dystrophy and degeneration, retinopathies, partial optic atrophy, and pre-existing retinal detachment.

The conditions that reduce vision after surgeries are postoperative uveitis, endophthalmitis, corneal edema, posterior capsular opacity, postoperative retinal detachment, aphakic glaucoma, and age-related macular degeneration. Out of the list, the two conditions that require special mention are postoperative endophthalmitis and posterior capsular opacities. The first is an ophthalmic emergency if it develops within 2–3 days. The second is not an emergency; it develops slowly over months and can be treated by laser capsulotomy.

Pseudophakia

Pseudophakia is a condition where the lens has been removed and replaced by an IOL. The surgery to replace the lens is extracapsular lens extraction. The most common practice is to remove the lens by phacoemulsification. Followed by putting an IOL of proper size and power in the bag that consists of an intact posterior capsule, an equatorial capsule, and part of the anterior lens capsule. The other positions where IOLs can be placed are the anterior chamber and the pupil. These are done following intracapsular lens extraction. The practice of putting an IOL in the anterior chamber and pupil has been given up. The PCIOL placed immediately after phacoemulsification is called primary IOL, in contrast to secondary IOL, when IOL is placed after a few months to years following extracapsular lens extraction. The IOL has a central optic that carries the power of the lens and a pair of haptics to keep the lens in place. The calculation of the power of the IOL is decided by a method called biometry that measures the length of the eyeball, corneal curvature, and depth of the anterior chamber. The readings are used in any of the standard formulas for calculating the power of the IOL.

The common power of IOL in an emmetrope eye is roughly +20D.

Postoperative Endophthalmitis

This is an avoidable, preventable, and sometimes manageable condition, provided complete antiseptic and aseptic methods are used before and during surgery. The results of management depend on how soon it has been diagnosed and prompt steps taken. Postoperative endophthalmitis has been divided into two groups, i.e., acute and chronic.

Acute endophthalmitis develops within two days of surgery due to infection by virulent bacteria. The viruses are not known to cause endophthalmitis; fungal endophthalmitis is chronic, developing weeks to months after surgery. Acute endophthalmitis causes pain, unexplained watering, and redness of the eye with vision below the expected level.

On Examination

- ❖ The lids are swollen.
- ❖ The conjunctiva is swollen and red.

- The cornea is hazy.
- There may be pus in the anterior chamber.
- The pink retinal glow is dull on retinoscopy.
- The fundus is not visible.
- The movements of the eye are present.

If not treated in time, the eye passes into the next stage called panophthalmitis, where all the intraocular structures and periocular structures are involved in total loss of vision. The movements of the eye are lost. There is no treatment once panophthalmitis develops. The patient gets relief from pain only after the contents of the eyeball have been removed surgically. The surgery is called evisceration.

Management of an Eye following IOL Surgery

- All surgeries should be performed under an operating microscope with a viscoelastic substance with complete antisepsis and asepsis.
- After the surgery is over, a subconjunctival injection of a combination of gentamicin with dexamethasone is given.
- A drop of cycloplegic is put in the conjunctiva.
- In children, the cycloplegic should be atropine.
- The eye is patched for the next 24 hours.
- The patient is ambulatory.
- The eye is examined the next day under a slit lamp for evidence of a severe reaction. If there is a severe reaction, it is dealt with by a suitable method.
- The patient is asked to put combination of broad-spectrum antibiotics and steroids six times during their waking hours. The steroid drops are tapered as per the practice of the institute.
- A drop of cycloplegia is put in the eye at bedtime for 7–10 days.
- The patients are examined every week for the next 4 weeks and then prescribed glasses as per refraction and near correction.

Posterior Capsular Opacification

This condition develops following phacoemulsification, where most of the cortical material is meticulously removed, leaving the posterior capsule transparent. However, 33% of the eyes following phacoemulsification are prone to developing posterior capsular opacity, which is the deposition of opaque lens fibers on the posterior capsule, making it translucent and reducing vision. The condition develops earlier in younger patients more than adults, more is the ageless are the patients, the greater their chances of developing posterior capsular opacification. The chances of PCO in congenital cataracts are as high as cent percent that require reoperation; this should be explained to the parents before the surgery. The management of PCO is laser capsulotomy, which restores vision to the initial level.

After-Cataract

After-cataract is a more severe form of development of opacity over the posterior capsule, it is more common and severe following extracapsular cataract extraction done without phacoemulsification.

The density of the opacity depends on the amount of cortical matter left. In cases where much of the cortex is left behind, the condition becomes obvious within a few days following surgery, and the opacity looks denser than the original cataract **(Fig. 12.15)**. Younger patients are more likely to develop dense after cataracts; they are more frequent and denser following extracapsular lens extraction done on immature cataracts. The duration of the development of after cataract depends on the amount of cortical matter left; lesser the cortical cataract, the longer is the time to develop after cataract.

The treatment of an after-cataract is called needling, i.e., manually cutting the after-cataract. Laser capsulotomy is not very effective in dense after cataracts.

CONGENITAL ANOMALIES OF THE LENS

The most common congenital anomaly of the lens is congenital cataract. The other anomalies are ectopia, i.e., displacement of the lens from its natural position, complete or partial. Complete ectopia is called dislocation, while incomplete dislocation is called subluxation. Congenitally, the lens may differ in shape and size. They are microphakia, spherophakia, and microspherophakia. In the first condition, the size of the lens remains smaller than the age-related size; in spherophakia, the lens instead of the disc shape assumes a spherical shape. This is generally associated with microphakia and is called microspherophakia (MSP).

Ectopia Lentis

The normal lens is placed behind the posterior surface of the iris in front of the vitreous, suspended all-round by the zonule. The pupil lies in front and center of the pupil. If the lens shifts from its normal position, the condition is called ectopia lentis. If the whole lens is absent from the pupil, the condition is called dislocation. The most common place of dislocation is backward in the vitreous. An incomplete shift of the lens is called subluxation. The subluxated lens divides the pupil into two parts, i.e., the phakic, where the lens is present, and the aphakic part where the lens is absent. The iris on the aphakic part is tremulous, and the depth of the anterior chamber is deeper than the rest of the AC. The lens can shift in any direction that is horizontal, vertical, or oblique.

The aphakic part is hypermetropic, while the phakic part is mostly myopic with irregular astigmatism. The vision in eyes with subluxated lenses depends upon the degree of dislocation. In cases of minimal subluxation, the patient may have normal distant and near vision. With a high degree of subluxation, vision depends on the aphakic area.

The most common congenital cause of ectopia lentis is a deficiency in zonules. The lens moves away from the area of absent zonules, i.e., if the lower zonules are absent, the lens will shift

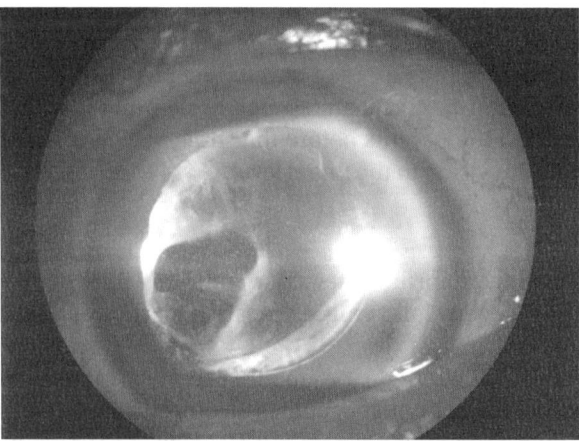

Fig. 12.15: Dense after-cataract in pseudophakia. *(For color version, see Plate 6)*
(Courtesy: Dr Santosh Patel)

upward, and vice versa **(Figs. 12.16 and 12.17).** The congenital ectopia lentis is generally bilateral and similar; a large shift of the lens may be obvious enough to be seen on oblique illumination; small ectopia lentis are diagnosed following full dilatation of the pupil. On examination, there is no redness, pain, or watering. In uniocular ectopia, the eye with dislocation may squint and be amblyopic, and the iris is tremulous over the aphakic part. The AC is shallow over the phakic part in dislocation, and the features of the pupil and iris are similar to those following intracapsular lens extraction without a surgical scar. The anterior chamber is deep, iris tremulous, with a central circular jet black pupil and normal reaction. The eye with dislocation may improve with aphakic correction, provided there is no pathology in the posterior segment.

The ectopia lentis may be an isolated congenital anomaly of the eye or may be associated with multiple ocular and systemic anomalies. The ectopic lens develops age-related cataracts earlier than usual, at the age of fifty or more.

The most common systemic condition is Marfan syndrome, where ectopia is associated with multiple skeletal changes that include a tall, thin body with long arms and fingers.

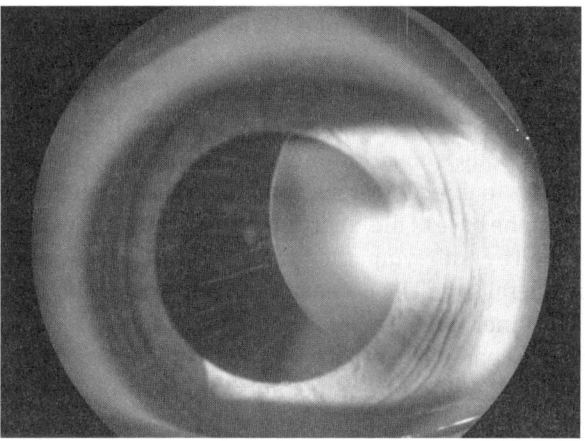

Fig. 12.16: Lens dislocated out and up.

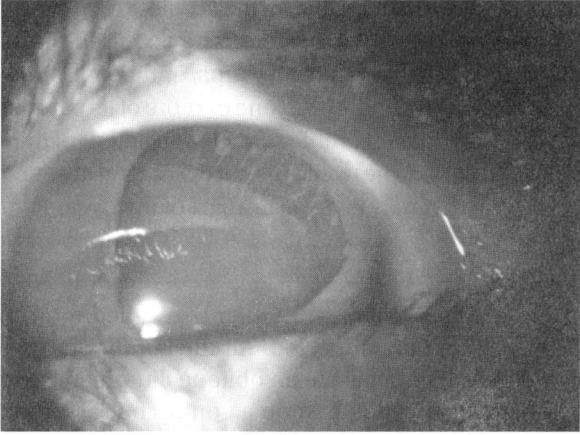

Fig. 12.17: Lens dislocated down and in.
(Courtesy: Dr Santosh Patel)

Disorders of the Iris, Ciliary Body and Choroid

The iris, ciliary body, and choroid are collectively called uvea, each with a definite function. The iris is the anteriormost part of the uvea. It lies parallel to the cornea, with a hole in the center called the pupil. The iris divides the aqueous chamber into anterior and posterior chambers, both communicating with each other through the pupil. The function of the pupil, besides acting as communication between the two chambers, is to regulate light entering the globe. The iris is the least vascular; it has two plane muscles that control the size of the pupil. They are constrictor pupillae and dilator pupillae. The first is supplied by the oculomotor nerve; the second is supplied by the sympathetic nerve. The iris is the thinnest part of the uvea, with a thin root and thick at the pupillary margin. The normal iris does not bleed when cut. The ciliary body is the thickest part of the uvea; it is triangular in shape with the apex backwards. The apex blends with the choroid. The function of the ciliary body is to accommodate and produce aqueous it is highly vascular; it contents striated muscles in three forms, i.e., longitudinal, radial, and circular. It is pigmented and highly vascular. From the base of the ciliary body arise the zonules that keep the lens in place. The ciliary body is supplied by both sympathetic and parasympathetic nerves. The inner end of its base is attached to the scleral spur. The outer surface of the ciliary body lies parallel to the inner surface of the sclera. The inner surface faces the vitreous.

The choroid is the largest part of the uvea, spreading from the apex of the ciliary body up to the border of the optic foramen. It differs from the other two parts of the uvea in the sense that it is devoid of any muscle, it is highly vascular and pigmented. It keeps the interior of the globe dark; it supplies blood to the outer layers of the retina. Its inner surface is in close contact with the retina, and the outer surface lies against the sclera.

The disorders of the uvea may be broadly divided into two parts, i.e., congenital and acquired. The congenital anomalies are mostly in the form of colobomas of the uvea, ranging from colobomas of the iris to colobomas of the choroid. The acquired disorders can be infective/inflammatory vascular, degenerative/dystrophy, trauma, and neoplasm.

The congenital disorders of the uvea may be in one or more of its parts, i.e., the iris, ciliary body, and choroid; they may be in isolation or combination; involvement of the retina is common. The most common congenital anomaly of the uvea is its partial or total absence of iris. Partial absence is called coloboma of the uvea; that may involve any part of the uvea.

ANIRIDIA

Aniridia is a rare congenital absence of iris, though it is called total absence of iris; in fact, complete absence of iris has not been reported. All the conditions of aniridia content small tags of rudimentary iris. Which are not visible on oblique illumination except under a slit lamp biomicroscope under high magnification and on a gonioscope. The zonules and lens are not affected; the lens is prone to subluxation. In oblique illumination, the lens is more spherical and visible with intact zonules. The condition is generally bilateral, present at birth, but diagnosed late when the child is found to have diminished vision and intolerance to light. The condition is hereditary and seen equally in both sexes. The child is brought for consultation due to intolerance to light, diminished vision, squints, and nystagmus. On examination, the child has variable loss of distant vision, which may be with/without squints and nystagmus. The pupil seems to be very large, and on further examination, the iris seems to be absent. The edge of the lens is visible as a bright crescent, similar to that seen in a subluxated lens. The intraocular tension is raised and difficult to manage. The management consists of prescribing colored glasses with power as found out on retinoscopy, keeping intraocular pressure under control, and rehabilitation of the child.

Uveal Coloboma

The term coloboma is used to denote the absence of the uvea, whether congenital or surgical. The congenital colobomas are due to a fault in the closure of the uveal fissure. They are most common at the 6 o'clock position of the uvea. A coloboma at the 6 o'clock meridian is called a typical coloboma; those in other places are atypical. The most common atypical coloboma involves the macula and is called as macular coloboma. The coloboma may be localized to any part of the uvea at the lower part of the globe. The most common coloboma of the uvea is the coloboma of the iris; the coloboma may extend into the choroid, involving the ciliary body in between. The iris coloboma may be as small as a notch **(Figs. 13.1 to 13.3)** and at the pupillary border or extend from the pupillary margin up to the limbus. The less common variety is a hole in between the pupillary margin and the limbus, more often near the limbus. Sometimes the coloboma may

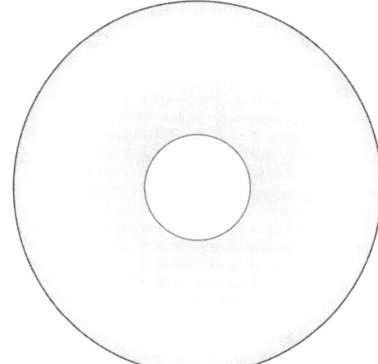

Fig. 13.1: Iris without coloboma.

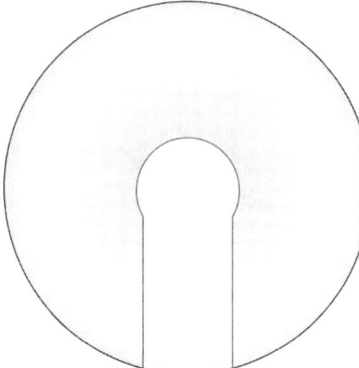

Fig. 13.2: Iris with typical coloboma.

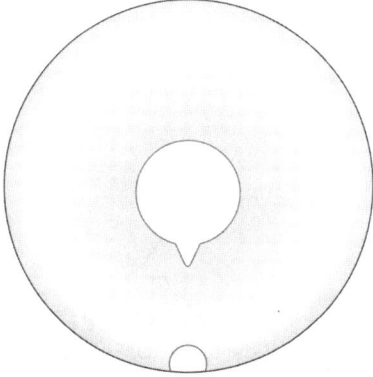

Fig. 13.3: Iris with notch and peripheral coloboma.

be spanned by a tag of iris tissue, and the condition is called bridge coloboma. The eyes with coloboma are smaller than normal with shallow AC, and the pupils react well to light and accommodation. The edge of the lens is visible through the coloboma if the coloboma is large **(Fig. 13.4)**. Vision is a variable that may be the loss of one or two lines on Snellen's chart to as little as a counting figure. The lens behind the coloboma may show opacities.

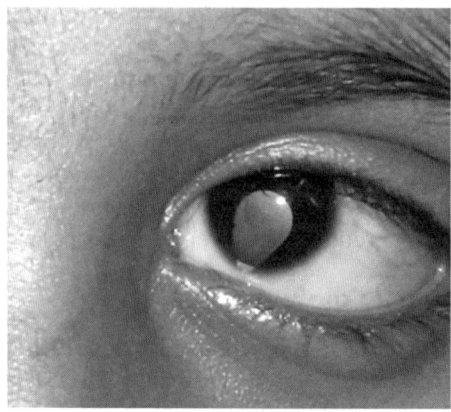

Fig. 13.4: Eye with typical coloboma and advance congenital cataract.

The congenital colobomas should be differentiated from the acquired colobomas, which are due to trauma, accidental, or surgical. The acquired coloboma can be anywhere on the iris, not always at the 6 o'clock meridian. The most common example of traumatic coloboma is iridodialysis, which can be anywhere on the iris, generally at the limbus, distorting the pupil. The pupillary margin towards the dialysis is flat **(Fig. 13.5)**.

The following figure shows various types of surgical iridectomy **(Fig. 13.6A to D)**.

Choroidal Colobomas

Choroidal colobomas, such as other uveal colobomas, are found at the 6 o'clock meridian. They can be part of an extensive ciliochoroidal coloboma or isolated; they may be as small as a small oval white area with an irregular margin anywhere between the lower pole of the disc or as

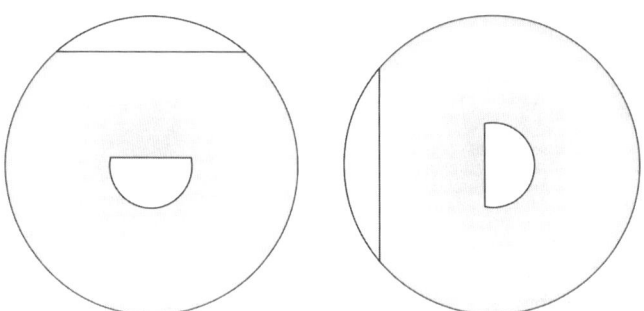

Fig. 13.5: Traumatic iridodialysis.

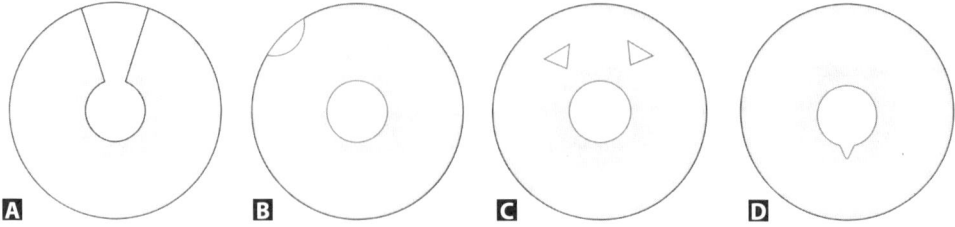

Figs. 13.6A to D: Surgical iridectomy: (A) Broad-based iridectomy; (B) Basal iridectomy; (C) Peripheral iridectomy; (D) Sphincterotomy.
Note: The acquired colobomas do not react either to light or accommodation.

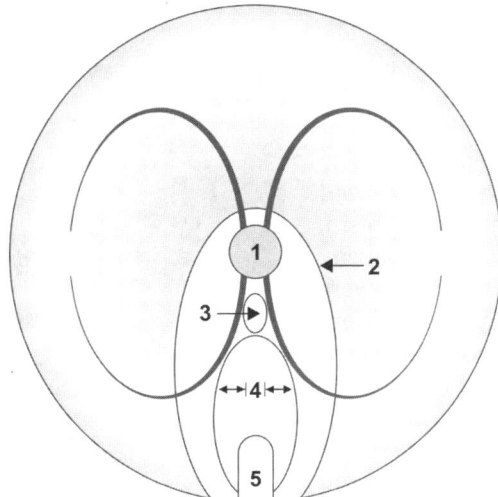

Fig. 13.7: Composite diagram of various types of choroidal coloboma.
Note: (1) Optic disc; (2) Coloboma engulfing the optic disc; (3) Small localized coloboma; (4) Choriociliary coloboma; (5) Coloboma involving the iris, ciliary body, and periphery of the choroid.

extensive as spreading from ora serrata to the disc; more extensive choroidal coloboma may engulf the disc as well **(Fig. 13.7)**. The eyes with extensive choroidal coloboma are generally small in size, with poor vision resulting in squints and amblyopia. The colobomas are generally elongated with a white floor and pigmented, irregular edges. The colobomas are best seen on indirect ophthalmoscopy. On retinoscopy, the colobomatous area gives off a white glow among the pink-red reflexes. The conditions do not require any specific treatment except correction of the error of refraction and management of amblyopia.

Coloboma of Macula

The macular colobomas are rarest; they are called atypical because they are not in the 6 o'clock meridian, and the exact cause of their origin is not known. They are situated two and a half discs away from the optic nerve and cause maximum loss of vision, causing infantile esotropia. The vision cannot be improved by any means.

Persistent Pupillary Membrane

The colobomas are due to a deficiency of tissue, in contrast to the excess tissue seen in the persistent pupillary membrane. To understand their origin, it is necessary to understand the embryogenesis of the anterior chamber and lens. The pupil is absent until late in gestation; the area where the future pupil will develop is covered by uveal tissue and the vascular sheath of the lens. By the time of birth, these tissues disappear, leaving a central, circular, transparent pupil. In cases where the uveal tissue fails to disappear fully at birth, it is left as strings of uveal tissue; these strings are called persistent pupillary membranes. They vary in number, length, and position. The fine strands may be seen as thin threads across the pupil. They may be attached to the lens capsule or float freely in the aqueous. They are very common; large strands may be visible with oblique illumination by a simple torch; fine strands are visible only on slit-lamp examination, appearing from the anterior surface. They do not cause any symptoms; they are diagnosed on routine examination and are known to disappear with age.

Albinism

The color of the uvea is due to melanin. More the pigment darker is the uvea, best seen in iris. Absence of pigment, total or partial, causes albinism **(Fig. 13.8)**. The albinism can be generalized or localized to the eye and is called ocular albinism, which is rarer than generalized albinism. In generalized albinism, the skin is very pale with light-colored hair, eyebrows, and lashes. The iris is bluish white with a pink pupil that is centrally circular and brisk to light and accommodation. The condition is present at birth. The patient has severe photophobia, diminished vision, and nystagmus. There is no treatment except correction of the error of refraction by tinted glasses as per retinoscopy.

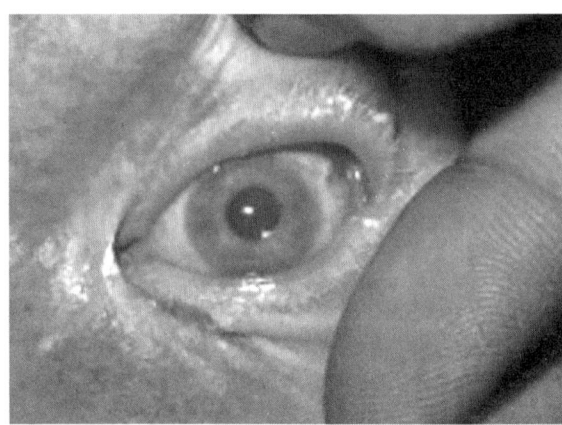

Fig. 13.8: Clinical picture of albinism showing of pigment in the iris and pink pupil. *(For color version, see Plate 6)* *(Courtesy:* Dr Santosh Patel)

Inflammation of the Uvea

Inflammation of the uvea is called uveitis, and it is seen in all ages and in both sexes the world over. It may be unilateral or bilateral, simultaneous or separate, and there may be a gap between involvements of two eyes. It could be acute, chronic, or recurrent; the name of the disorder depends on the part of the uvea involved, i.e., iritis when only the iris is involved. Involvement of the ciliary body is called cyclitis. Choroiditis means involvement of the choroid. Iritis and cyclitis are rarely isolated; they generally present as involvement of the iris and ciliary body and are called iridocyclitis (anterior uveitis), and Choroiditis is generally isolated (posterior uveitis) unless all the uveal structures are involved. Involvement of all the parts of the uveal is called panuveitis; associated involvement of the vitreous is called endophthalmitis; and involvement of the globe along with extraocular muscle and other structures of the orbit is called panophthalmitis. Involvement of Pars plana is called Pars planitis, or intermediate uveitis.

Figure 13.9 summarizes various possible sites of uveitis (anatomical classification).

Table 13.1 shows possible sites of uveitis and involvement of non-uveal tissues.

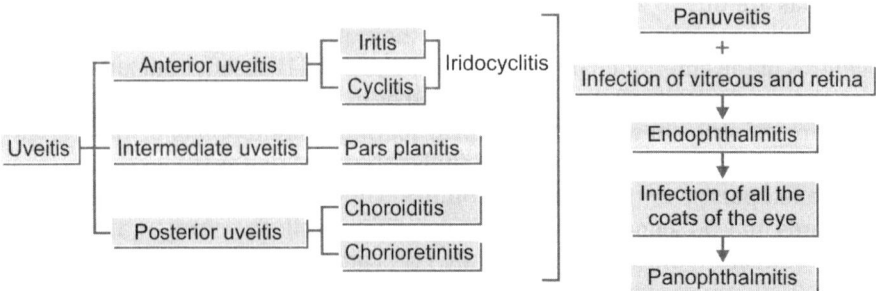

Fig. 13.9: Anatomical classification of uveitis.

Table 13.1: Possible sites of uveitis and involvement of non-uveal tissues.

Uveitis	Part involved	Non-uveal parts involved
Iritis	Iris	Nil
Cyclitis	Anterior part of ciliary body	Nil
Iridocyclitis	Iris and ciliary body	Angle of AC
Pars planitis	Posterior part of ciliary body	Anterior choroid, retina, macula, vitreous
Choroiditis	Choroid	Retina, macula, vitreous
Endophthalmitis	All intraocular structures except lens	Sclera
Panophthalmitis	All intraocular structures	Extraocular muscle and contents of orbit

Iridocyclitis (Iritis + Cyclitis)

Involvement of the iris or ciliary body alone is uncommon due to the continuity of the two structures; hence, both are involved in the process. It is presumed that the iris gets involved first, then the pathology passes to the ciliary body. The disorder involves both structures in a circular fashion; sectorial involvement of the structures has not been reported. The condition is acute in onset, more common among children and young adults, and generally unilateral; the other eye may get involved sometimes later or after the disorder has subsided. The symptoms consist of dull pain in and around the eye that may radiate on the skull of the same side. The patients may complain of tenderness of the globe; the eyes are red due to circumciliary congestion. The lids are mildly swollen; there is photophobia, lacrimation, and diminished vision that may vary from a loss of 1–2 lines on the vision chart to 6/60 with good projection. On examination, the cornea is bright with a mild to moderate circumciliary flush and ciliary tenderness that is elicited by applying gentle pressure over the globe through the lids. Due to the circumciliary tenderness, it may not be possible to evert the upper lid.

The cornea is bright without any stain; the posterior surface shows small white deposits on it. These deposits are called keratic precipitate (KP).

Keratic Precipitates (KPs)

The keratic precipitates mostly arise from the ciliary body, are inflammatory cells of different numbers, shapes, and sizes. They are generally seen in the center of the cornea; in severe cases, they may be scattered all over the endothelium. They may be well-formed and circular, or they may be fine enough to be called dusty KP. The KPs are best seen under high magnification from a slit lamp. Large white KPs are seen in chronic granulomatous iridocyclitis, scattered all over the posterior surface of the cornea and are called mutton fat kps **(Fig. 13.10)**. The most common distribution of KPs in acute iridocyclitis is triangular in the lower part of the cornea, with the apex towards the pupil. The KPs are early to develop and late to disappear; they may be present even when the inflammation has been brought under control.

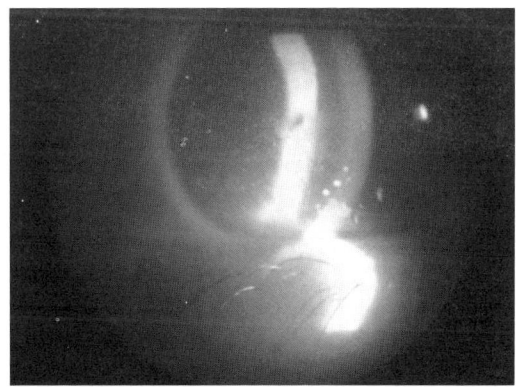

Fig. 13.10: Keratic precipitates (KPs) of various sizes seen on slit lamp.
(*Courtesy*: Dr Santosh Patel)

Flare

The KPs are preceded by flare, caused due to small cells suspended in the aqueous, best seen on a circular small beam of a slit lamp with maximum brightness and high magnification. The presence of a flare is a definite sign of anterior uveal inflammation. They disappear with treatment. The cells suspended in flare are heavier than the other contents of aqueous; they settle down at the most dependent part of the eye. The accumulated cell in the anterior chamber is called the hypopyon.

Hypopyon

Hypopyon is a sign of severe inflammation of the anterior uvea. The hypopyon is a collection of cells (Pus) in the anterior chamber. The hypopyon is white in color, unless tinged with blood. The hypopyon in a fungal infection is yellowish, while in a pseudomonas infection it is greenish. The hypopyon is sterile unless infected by perforation of the cornea. The hypopyon settles down at the most dependent part of the eye. It is fluid and changes its position as per the tilting of the head. If the patient lies down, the hypopyon spreads all over the iris and pupil, giving a false impression of its disappearance, only to appear if the head is erect. The upper edge of the hypopyon in the sitting position is horizontal, parallel to the ground **(Fig. 13.11)**.

Any white matter in the anterior chamber should be considered hypopyon unless proved otherwise. The other white materials in the anterior chamber are called pseudohypopyons. The white material in the upper part is called upside-down or inverse hypopyon **(Fig. 13.12)**. The most common cause is silicone oil in the anterior chamber.

Abnormal contents of anterior chamber
- Hypopyon
- Pseudohypopyon, any gray substance in AC:
    - Upside down hypopyon
    - Lens:
        - Mature cataract
        - Cortical matter
        - Nucleus
    - IOL:
        - AC IOL
        - Dislocated PCIOL
- Blood—hyphema
- Vitreous
- Parasites:
    - Worms—filaria
    - Parasitic cyst—cysticercosis
- Foreign body
- Tumor of iris, ciliary body and retinoblastoma

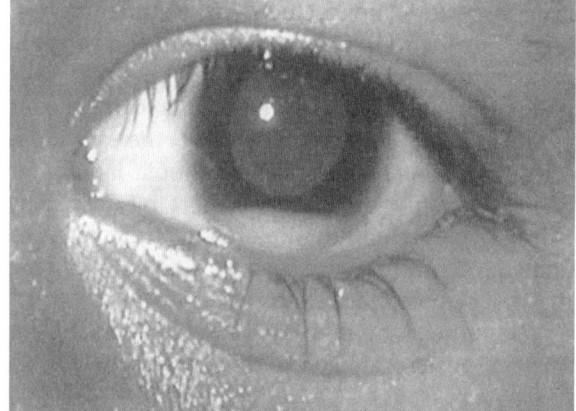

Fig. 13.11: Hypopyon in endophthalmitis.

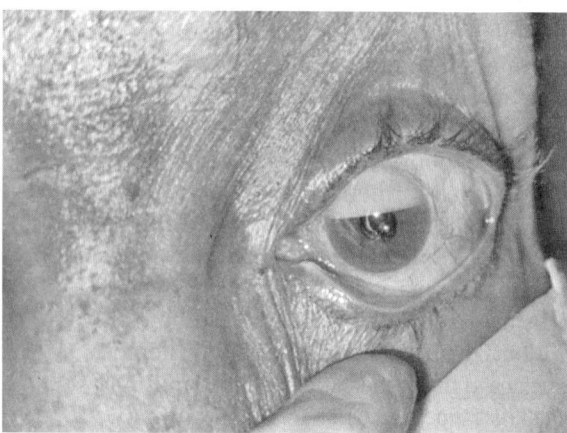

Fig. 13.12: Upside down hypopyon due to silicone oil in anterior chamber.
(*Courtesy:* Dr Santosh Patel)

Treatment of Hypopyon

Hypopyon should always be considered an ophthalmic emergency and treated promptly. The first step is to find out if it is true or false hypopyon by—history, appearance, and position in suspected retinoblastoma, which is an important cause of pseudohypopyon. Ultrasonography is a standard investigation ordered to settle the matter. The treatment of hypopyon is basically the management of severe uveitis (posterior uveitis does not cause hypopyon). The treatment consists of complete cycloplegia with an age-matched dose of atropine not more than two times a day. Steroids with broad-spectrum antibiotic drops are instilled as frequently as six times a day. When there is no corneal ulcer, hypopyon corneal ulcer gets precedence over uveitis by the standard method. If hypopyon without ulcer does not respond to local instillation of drops, the next step is to start subconjunctival injections of antibiotic and steroid combinations once a day with concurrent use of drops.

Pupil in Iridocyclitis

The pupil is generally constricted, irregular, and sluggish to light and accommodation. The irregularity is due to formation of posterior synechiae, The pupil develops a festoon appearance on dilatation and leaves multiple iris pigments on the lens capsule. The iris pigments left on the lens capsule are visible for many weeks to months after the inflammation has been cured (**Figs. 13.13A to D**).

The irregular pupil in iridocyclitis should not be confused with persistent pupillary membrane, traumatic miosis, or rupture of the pupillary margin.

In severe cases of iridocyclitis, the pupil is covered by exudate, and the condition is called occlusio pupillae. The color of the membrane is white, which may be confused with lenticular opacity (**Fig. 13.14**).

If the posterior synechiae are extensive, they encircle the already constricted pupil; this is called ring synechiae, which separate the anterior chamber from the posterior chamber and are called seclusio pupillae. Causing the accumulation of aqueous behind the iris and pushing it forward in a dome shape, the condition is called **iris bombe***.

Iris bombe

In the iris bombe, the anterior chamber is of irregular depth; it is shallowest at the top of the bulging iris between the pupil and the limbus. The peripheral iris may block the angle of the anterior chamber, causing secondary glaucoma (**Figs. 13.15A to D**).

Nodule Formation on the Iris

In chronic iridocyclitis, nodules of various sizes develop on the anterior surface and pupillary margin at certain places. They are translucent yellowish brown, spherical; they do not cause diminished vision; they are best seen on a slit lamp; their presence is diagnostic of iridocyclitis,

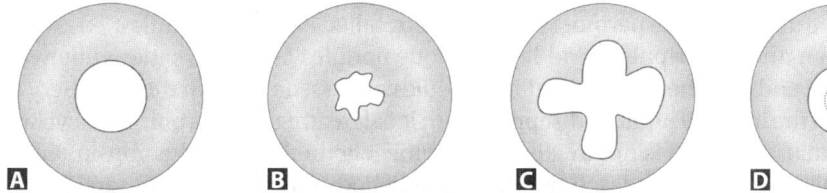

Figs. 13.13A to D: (A) Normal center circular pupil; (B) Constricted pupil in acute iritis; (C) Festoon pupil after dilatation; (D) Iris pigment on the lens capsule after complete mydriasis.

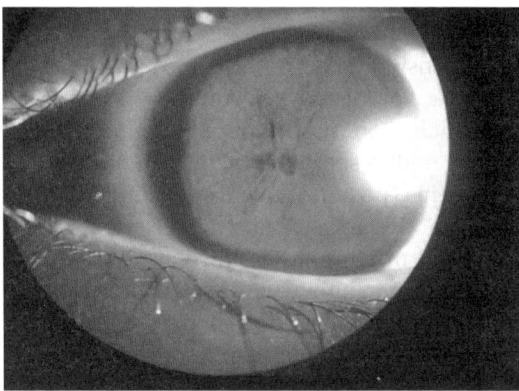

Fig. 13.14: Occlusio pupillae in long standing anterior uveitis.

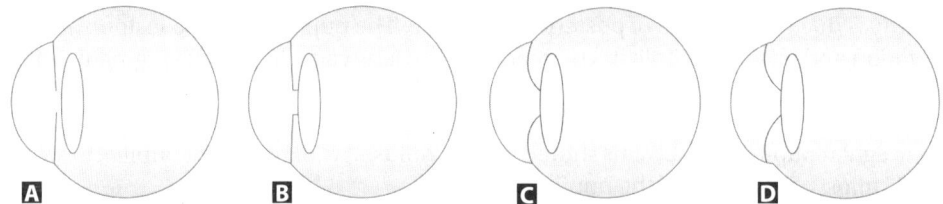

Figs. 13.15A to D: (A) Eye without posterior synechiae; (B) Eye with ring synechiae; (C) Iris bombe; (D) Eye with iris bombe and peripheral anterior synechiae.

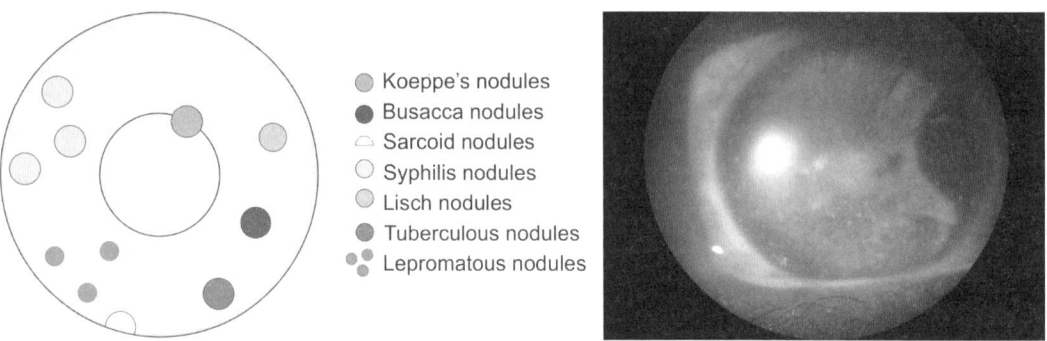

Fig. 13.16: Various types of iris nodules.

both granulomatous and non-granulomatous **(Fig. 13.16).** The common causes of nodules on the iris are tuberculosis, syphilis, and leprosy. The nodules at the pupillary margin are called Koeppe's nodules, and the nodules at the periphery of the iris are called Busacca's nodules. The tubercular nodules are seen on the periphery, and lepromatous nodules are seen scattered between the pupillary margin and periphery. The syphilitic nodule can be seen both on the periphery and on the substance of the iris. The nodules disappear with local treatment of chronic iridocyclitis. May recur if the primary infection is not treated by systemic chemotherapy. The non-inflammatory causes of nodules on the iris are Lisch nodules, foreign body granulomas, and sarcoid nodules. Lisch nodules are seen in neurofibromatosis type 1.

Differential Diagnosis of Acute Iritis

The condition should be differentiated from conjunctivitis, acute congestive glaucoma keratitis, corneal foreign body, and tarsal conjunctivitis. The characteristics of acute iridocyclitis are: generally unilateral with acute onset commonly in the second and third decade with pain, lacrimation, photophobia, moderate loss of vision, ciliary tenderness, ciliary flush, flare, KPs, irregular constricted pupil, rarely hypopyon.

Complications of Iridocyclitis

The first attack of acute iridocyclitis in 50% is self-limited and known to recur or pass into a chronic stage, causing secondary glaucoma, complicated cataracts, band keratopathy, and hypotony, leading to phthisis and loss of vision.

Treatment of Acute Iridocyclitis

- The treatment comprises of dry, hot formation over the closed lids 2–3 times a day.
- Mild analgesics orally
- Specific treatment consists of:
  - Instillation of cycloplegic, initially 3 times a day, by cyclopentolate, tropicamide, and home atropine
  - Simple mydriatics like phenylephrine have no role in the treatment of acute iridocyclitis.
  - If the above cycloplegics fail to dilate the pupil, the eye should be atropinized at an age-matched dose and frequency.
  - Local antibiotic drops have no role in the treatment of iridocyclitis.
  - The sheet anchor of treatment is frequent instillation of steroid in sufficient strength and frequency for long duration and tapering as per the practice of the institution.
  - Atropine is the cycloplegic of choice under 15 years of age, with usual precaution.

Cyclitis

The term cyclitis is used to denote isolated inflammation of the ciliary body. Cyclitis may start in the ciliary body and extend into the iris, called iridocyclitis. The reverse is also possible; if cyclitis spreads into the choroid, it is called peripheral choroiditis or pars planitis. Cyclitis is associated with more KPs than iritis; the anterior part of the vitreous may be dusted by infiltration. Cystitis shares the etiology of iritis. It is more common in adults.

Pars Planitis

Pars planitis is also known as intermediate uveitis or anterior choroiditis. It presents as chronic inflammation of the junction of the ciliary body and peripheral choroid. Generally without any systemic infection. It is more common in the early second decade, with minimal symptoms of floaters and diminished vision. Without circumciliary congestion, photophobia, or pain. On examination, there are few cells in the peripheral part of AC without hypopyon. The anterior vitreous is dusted with inflammatory cells. The condition is best diagnosed by an indirect ophthalmoscope with scleral depression. The condition is often associated with macular edema which is the cause of diminished vision; neovascularization is a common complication that requires treatment by photocoagulation. In most of the cases it is self-limited and prone to recurrence. Prolonged use of a weak steroid solution and weekly use of mild cycloplegic have been found to ward off recurrence.

Posterior Uveitis (Choroiditis)

Posterior uveitis is less common than iridocyclitis. In rare instances, it can be congenital, starting during fatal life due to congenital toxoplasmosis.

The choroiditis is not painful; it is without anterior segment involvement, i.e., circumciliary congestion, ciliary tenderness, KPs, and flare. It may be unilateral or bilateral, more common in adults. Posterior uveitis may be localized only to the choroid or may involve the retina, macula, and optic nerve. Involvement of the macula is called central choroiditis **(Fig. 13.17)**. The rest are called by various terms depending on the ophthalmoscopic picture and location in relation to the macula or optic nerve. The central choroiditis involving the macula has the poorest vision. The rest do not cause diminished vision. The patches of choroiditis produce corresponding field changes.

The **other symptoms** of choroiditis are—floaters, scotomas, or distorted vision. The common causes of choroiditis are—toxoplasmosis, congenital or acquired; syphilis; tuberculosis; rheumatoid arthritis; sarcoidosis; congenital rubella; congenital cytomegalovirus; and HIV/AIDS. Choroiditis can both be granulomatous or non-granulomatous.

Treatment

The choroiditis does not respond to local drops of antibiotics or steroids. The systemic conditions may require specific chemotherapy and systemic steroids. Systemic steroids may be given orally or by posterior subtenon injection.

Panuveitis

The term panuveitis means inflammation of all the parts of the uvea. The condition is generally chronic. Most of the systemic infections and inflammation that cause iridocyclitis may result in panuveitis. Some non-infectious conditions also cause panuveitis. The best example is sympathetic ophthalmia. Panuveitis generally involves the retina and optic nerve as well. Involvement of the vitreous, along with panuveitis, is called endophthalmitis.

Endophthalmitis

Endophthalmitis is inflammation of all the intraocular structures except the lens. Generally unilateral, it has been divided variously, i.e., on the basis of onset—acute/chronic, depending on the mode of infection, i.e., exogenous/endogenous. The exogenous being more common.

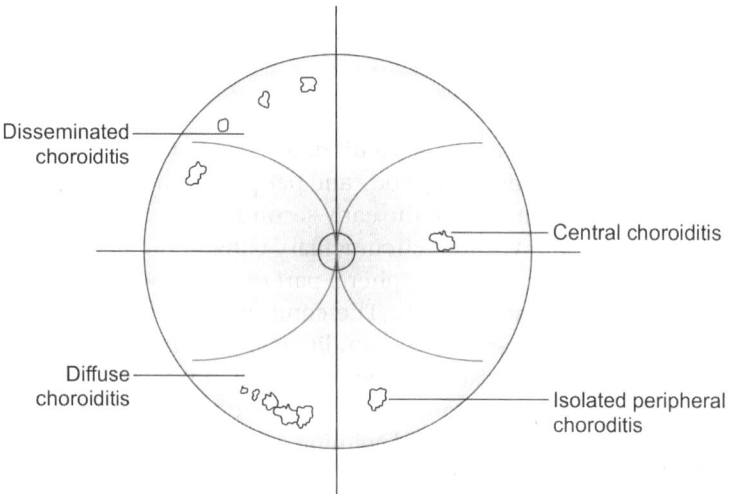

Fig. 13.17: Composite diagram of various types of choroiditis.

The most common cause of exogenous endophthalmitis is perforating injury, whether accidental or surgical. The other cause is perforation of a virulent corneal ulcer. Acute exogenous endophthalmitis is caused due to pus-forming bacteria; viruses do not cause endophthalmitis; and fungal endophthalmitis is always chronic. Acute endophthalmitis develops within 1–2 days of injury. It is common following cataract surgery and is called postoperative endophthalmitis. In acute endophthalmitis, there is always a history of surgery or perforating injury to the globe with or without a retained intraocular foreign body.

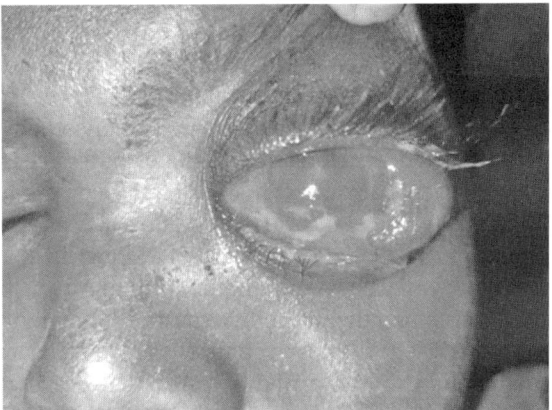

Fig. 13.18: Endophthalmitis.

The common symptoms are fast-developing pain in the eye spreading towards the head on the affected side. A rapid fall in vision that may be as low as perception of light or loss of projection of light is a bad omen. Edema of the lids, redness of the eye, chemosis of the conjunctiva, unexplained watering, and discharge

The signs are: edema of the lids, swelling of the conjunctiva, conjunctival congestion, haziness of the cornea, wound of entry, pus in AC, exudate in the pupillary area, absent retinal glow **(Fig. 13.18)**, and movements are present. Mild proptosis and the presence of movement differentiated it from panophthalmitis, which is the end result of untreated exogenous endophthalmitis.

Endogenous Endophthalmitis

Endogenous endophthalmitis happens when pus-forming organisms spread into the eye from a distant focus of infection that could be bacterial or fungal. It is less common than exogenous endophthalmitis as the cause of the disorders is hematogenous; it generally infects the choroid first, followed by the vitreous, and may be bilateral and difficult to treat. It is seen in general debility, uncontrolled diabetics, and drug addicts.

Panophthalmitis

Panophthalmitis is an extended form of endophthalmitis where the infection has crossed the boundaries of the globe, involving the peribulbar structure **(Fig. 13.19)**. The vitreous is full of pus; there is moderate proptosis; and movements are absent. On examination, there is no perception of light, the lids are swollen, there is mild to moderate proptosis with absent movement, chemosed conjunctiva, and a hazy cornea. In post-cataract surgery, the wound may open, exuding intraocular structures. Generally, the condition is unilateral. The condition does not respond to any medical treatment; the only treatment is the removal of the cornea along with all the intraocular contents, leaving the sclera intact. The procedure is called evisceration.

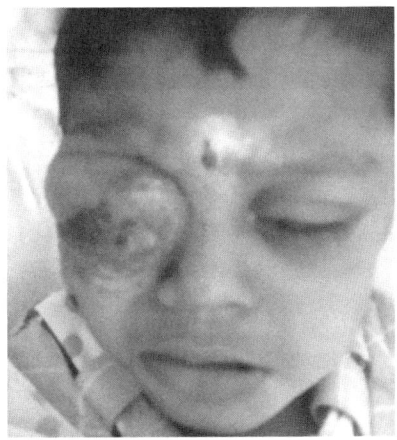

Fig. 13.19: Panophthalmitis in a child following penetrating injury.

Sympathetic Ophthalmitis

This is a form of panuveitis developing in the contralateral eye following a perforating injury involving the ciliary body in the ipsilateral eye. The other eye gets involved 3–4 weeks following the injury to the contralateral eye. The onset may be delayed for months or years. The injured eye is called the exciting eye, while the other eye is called the sympathizing eye. The condition is chronic uveitis; the onset in the sympathetic eye begins with marked photophobia, lacrimation, and blurring of distant and near vision. On examination, there is circumciliary congestion, various types of KPs with flare, and signs of iridocyclitis.

Management of sympathetic ophthalmitis is tricky. It has been divided into two parts, i.e., management of the injured eye and management of sympathizing eye. The management of the injured eye consists of—repair of the wound carefully after separating incarcerated uvea lens matter and vitreous from the wound. The eye is treated on the line of a postoperative wound by instilling atropine with usual precaution, subconjunctival injection of a steroid pad, and bandage. The next day, the bandage is removed, followed by atropine twice a day and strong steroid drops every 2 hours for the first 3 days, thereafter gradually tapering the steroid.

If there is no perception of light in the injured eye, the eye should be enucleated. The other eye is examined for any evidence of uveitis every week for the first one month followed by an examination every month. Then, every six months, the patient should be instructed to report for consultation if he/she develops photophobia, lacrimation, or diminished near and far vision. Once sympathetic ophthalmia has been confirmed, both eyes should be treated as severe forms of chronic panuveitis for months.

Uveal Trauma

Uveal trauma can either be—penetrating injury or a blunt injury.

Penetrating Injury of the Uvea

An injury is supposed to be penetrating when it cuts the full thickness of the cornea or sclera. A combination of the two is also possible. Penetrating wounds of the cornea are generally associated with prolapse of the iris; in severe cases extending beyond the limbus, the ciliary body may be involved **(Fig. 13.20)**. Scleral penetrating injuries are associated with prolapse of the choroid. The lens may be injured, and the penetrating injury may be associated with intraocular foreign bodies. The injuries involving the ciliary body and choroid bleed profusely,

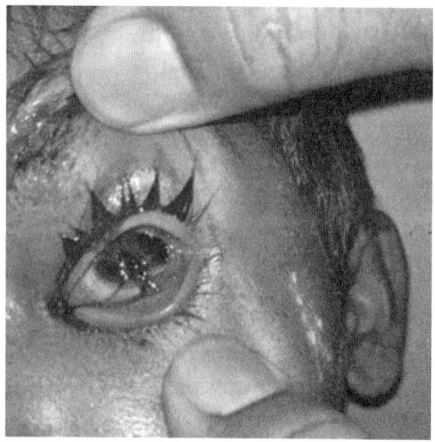

Fig. 13.20: Penetrating corneoscleral injury with large iris prolapse.

while injuries to the iris do not bleed. The management of a penetrating injury consists of the exclusion of an intraocular foreign body by X-ray. Glass and plastic foreign bodies are not seen in ordinary X-rays. X-rays should be taken both in lateral and anteroposterior views by standard methods. USG, CT, and MRI are better options. MRI is contraindicated in suspected metallic foreign bodies. Once the foreign body is excluded, the next step is to stitch the cornea/sclera by 8/0 suture under a microscope with a viscoelastic substance. Care should be taken to include only half the thickness of the cornea. No attempt should be made to put the iris back in the AC. The best option is to cut it. The procedure is called iridectomy. No attempt should be taken to cut either the ciliary body or the choroid because they may bleed profusely. Injured lenses may be removed in the same sitting if the wound is large; otherwise, they should be removed as a secondary procedure, latter by standard phacoemulsification. Prolapsed vitreous is best removed by vitrectomy. Following stitching, the anterior chamber is formed by a bubble of sterile air. A subconjunctival injection of a steroid and broad-spectrum antibiotic is mandatory. The eye is bandaged after the instillation of age-matched atropine. Intraocular foreign bodies are best removed by a vitreoretinal surgeon by the standard method. If there is no perception of light, the eye should be removed by evisceration.

Blunt Injury of the Uvea

Blunt injury to the uvea is that injury that compresses the eyeball by a force acting along any meridian. The most common meridian is anterior posterior; it may be as mild as involving the iris only or extensive enough to disrupt all the parts of the uvea in the line of the acting force. The injuries to the iris consist of traumatic miosis and mydriasis, Vossius ring* rupture of the pupillary margin, and iridodialysis (**Figs. 13.21A to F**).

* Vossius ring

The vossius ring is an irregular ring of iris pigment deposited on the anterior lens capsule following blunt injury to the iris. It corresponds to the pupil at the time of injury, which is invariably constricted. It may be complete or incomplete and does not need any treatment. It passes off over months without involving the vision.

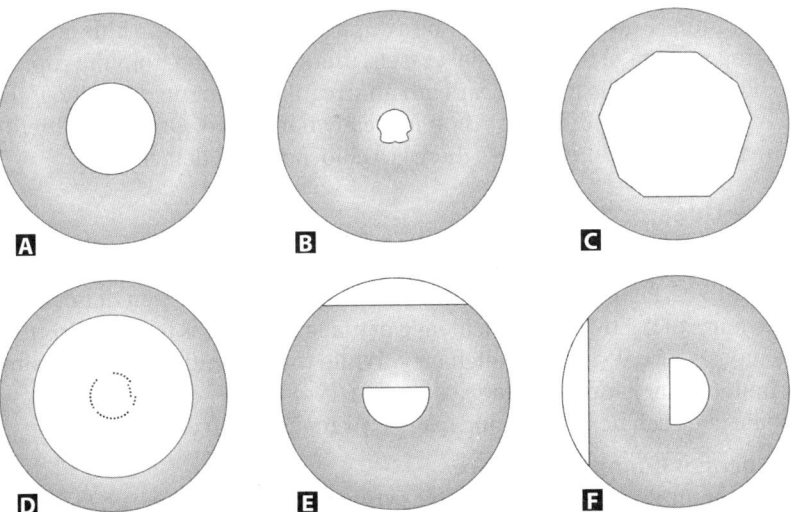

Figs. 13.21A to F: Diagram showing various effect of blunt injury to the iris: (A) Normal central circular pupil; (B) Traumatic miosis; (C) Traumatic mydriasis; (D) Vossius ring; (E) Iridodialysis upper part; (F) Iridodialysis lateral side.

Hyphema

Hyphema is a common result of blunt injury to the eye, causing disinsertion of the iris from its root. If the ciliary body is injured, it bleeds profusely, causing the accumulation of blood in the anterior chamber. Hyphema may only be in traces or may fill the anterior chamber. The color of hyphema is bright red that passes to a dark shade and gradually disappears. The blood settles down at the most dependent part of the eye. It has a horizontal upper border; it is measured in millimeters from the limbus or its relation to the pupillary margin. The normal iris does not bleed even following an iridectomy, unless it is diseased, such as chronic anterior uveitis or neovascularization of the iris. The hyphema per se does not require any treatment; it fades away gradually without leaving any trace. If the hyphema is complete and remains so for more than a week, it causes raised intraocular pressure. In such a condition, the blood in the anterior chamber damages the endothelium of the cornea, causing a yellowish coloration of the iris. This condition is called blood staining of the cornea. That requires the evacuation of blood by the usual method, along with anti-glaucoma drugs.

Blunt Injury to the Ciliary Body

The injury may rupture the ciliary body; the direction of the rupture is parallel to the anteroposterior axis of the ciliary body. Unlike the iris, the ciliary body bleeds profusely following a blunt injury. The blunt injury may detach the ciliary body from its attachment. The condition is called traumatic cyclodialysis and is associated with a lowering of intraocular tension. The tear may extend deep into the substance of the ciliary body and damage the trabecular meshwork. This is called a recession of angel of anterior chamber that causes a late rise in intraocular tension, causing glaucoma, which develops after a few weeks to months and is confused with wide-angle glaucoma.

Blunt Injury to the Choroid

Blunt injury to the choroid results in rupture of the choroid. The choroidal rupture is seen away from the disc margin like a crescent with concavity towards the disc; the distance of the rupture from the disc and its length varies, depending on the force of trauma and its direction. Generally, there is a single rupture; however, there may be a duplication of the first, a little away from the first. Initially, following rupture of the choroidal vessels, there is bleeding from the ruptured choroid. Which gradually passes off, leaving a scar with an irregular pigmented border. If the rupture is between the macula and the disc, the vision is greatly hampered. Otherwise, there is no visual loss, and no treatment is required unless there is a ciliochoroidal detachment.

Tumors of the Uvea

Tumors of the uvea are rare. They can be benign or malignant, pigmented or no pigmented flat or raised from the surface. Pigmented tumors are most common. The benign tumors are nevus, seen on all the three parts of the uvea. The incidence of malignancy rises from the iris to the choroid; the iris is the most unusual site for malignancy. While the choroid is the most common site of malignancy, both primary and metastatic.

Tumors of the uvea can be benign (non cancer) or malignant (cancer).

The common benign tumors of uvea are:
- **Iris:** Nevus, hemangioma, neurofibroma, congenital cysts, parasitic cysts, foreign body granuloma.
- **Ciliary body:** Hemangiomas, medulloepithelioma*
- **Choroid:** Hemangioma, neurofibroma, benign melanoma (nevus)

The malignant tumors of the uvea are mostly pigmented. They are mostly malignant melanomas. They can arise from pre-existing nevus or may arise as primary growth. The most common.

* **Medulloepithelioma**

Medulloepithelioma arises from a non-pigmented epithelium of the ciliary body that resembles the primitive retina. It is supposed to be congenital that becomes obvious between four and twelve years. Initially, they are symptomless, but they draw attention on routine fundus examinations for errors of refraction. The child is brought in for consultation regarding diminished vision. The next symptom is pain in the eye. The condition is unilateral, slow, progressive, thought to be benign; it spreads slowly but does not metastasize. It may grow forward, tilting the lens and causing diminished vision, and be seen as a dark dome on the periphery of the pink retinoscopic glow; its extension in the canal may cause secondary glaucoma. The tumor is diagnosed on ultrasonography, CT, and MRI.

The management consists of observing and, if found to be causing pain and uncorrectable diminished vision, enucleation. On histopathology, the section shows a rosette similar to that seen in retinoblastoma.

Malignant Melanoma of the Choroid

The choroid is a common site of primary and secondary tumors. The most common malignant tumor of the choroid is melanoma. It is the most common intraocular malignancy seen in adults. It is seen in persons over the age of 50 years. It is an unilateral tumor which is single to begin with. It is commonly seen in lateral side of the choroid, may be well defined or diffuse, and does not spread by seedling, which is common in retinoblastoma. Initially, the tumor is symptomless, than the patient develops diminished near and distant vision due to ensuing axial hypermetropia caused due to elevation of the retina. The near vision is also effected both requiring frequent changes of glasses. The other symptom is loss of corresponding field. As the tumor enlarges, it may fill the large part of the globe may infiltrate in the angle, causing secondary glaucoma and pain. The tumor may perforate the globe and invade the orbit. Causing proptosis with its usual complications once the tumor invades the orbit, it spreads to distant organs by blood and lymphatics. The most common site of metastasis is the liver.

The treatment of the intraocular stage is enucleation, small intraocular tumor are treated by radiotherapy of laser. Once the tumor invades the orbit, the treatment is exenteration* of the orbit. Followed by chemotherapy. The tumor does not responds well either to radiation or chemotherapy. The extraocular spread is best managed by oncologists.

*****Exenteration**
Exenteration consists of removal all the contents of the orbit along with the lid and periorbita.

CHAPTER 14

Disorders of Retina

Retina is one of the most important part of vision. It is responsible for central vision, peripheral vision, night vision, and partly color vision. It may be considered a part of the central nervous system. It is mostly neural, with an abandonment of blood supply and glial tissue. It is devoid of any muscle; it gets its nutrition from two sources, i.e., choroidal and retinal circulation.

Development of retina is summarized below:
- The retina develops from two layers of secondary optic vesicles.
- The inner layer gives rise to nine layers of sensory retina.
- The ganglion cells of the retina grow backward in the optic nerve.
- The outer layer gives rise to the pigment epithelium of the retina.
- There is a narrow space between the two layers called subretinal space. The two layers can get separated if fluid accumulates in between. The condition is called detachment of the retina.
- The macula is a specialized area in the retina with different stages of development.

The differences are:
- The sensory retina at the future macula is thicker than the rest of the retina up to 8 months of pregnancy.
- The thickness is reduced to form the depression of the macula.
- The macula is not completely developed at birth.
- It continues to develop after birth for up to 5 years.

Clinical Features of Retinal Disorders

The clinical features depend on the part of the retina involved, i.e., central or peripheral.

The disorders of the central retina, which include the macula and paramacula, result in diminished distant vision and a defective central field in the form of a central scotoma. Diminished photopic vision and distorted vision (metamorphopsia).

The disorders of peripheral retina do not cause diminished distant vision but cause diminished night vision, peripheral field loss and flashes of light.

The disorders of retina can be congenital or acquired. The acquired causes consist of infection/inflammation, dystrophies/degenerations, trauma, vascular accident, retinopathies detachment and new growth.

Most of the disorders of the retina can be revealed by examination of fundus. This is divided in two parts, i.e., examination of retina and examination of optic nerve head. The fundus cannot be visualized by oblique illumination. It requires special devices to examine the fundus.

The retina is examined by the following instruments:
- **Ophthalmoscopes**: Direct and indirect

❖ **Slit-lamp with special attachment**: Minus lens (Hruby lens)/plus lens (+78D to +90D)
❖ Three mirror gonioscope

Special methods used to examine the retina are:
❖ Fundus fluorescein angiography
❖ **Ultrasonography:**
  ◆ A scan
  ◆ B scan
❖ **CT:** Computed tomography
❖ **MRI:** Magnetic resonance imaging
❖ **OCT:** Optical coherence tomography

Out of all the instruments mentioned above, the most commonly used is the direct ophthalmoscope. It is a small, easy-to-handle, easy-to-use, and cheap instrument. Its optics and power supply are incorporated into the instrument itself. It gives a vertical, erect, and fifteen-time magnified image. The image is formed behind the retina and not laterally reversed **(Fig. 14.1)**. The pictures show to sides of a standard direct ophthalmoscope.

The disadvantages of the instrument are:
 i. It shows only a small area at a time **(Fig. 14.4)**
 ii. The illumination is poor.
 iii. The periphery is not visible with the instrument.
 iv. There is no depth sense.

Indirect Ophthalmoscope

An indirect ophthalmoscope is the most useful optical device to see the periphery with stereopsis. It has three components, i.e., a power supply, an optical part, and a magnifier. Unlike the power supply of a direct ophthalmoscope, which is built into the handle of the ophthalmoscope, the power of an indirect ophthalmoscope is provided by a separate unit that works on electricity. The optical system converts images formed by two eyes into a single image. The magnifier, also known as the condenser, is held in the right hand of the examiner. The power of the magnifier varies, i.e., +15D, +20D, and +30D. Lower the power, better the magnification, but smaller the field. The examiner wears the viewing system on the head and adjusts it to bring two separate images into one. The patient lies down on the examination table, fixing a spot on the ceiling with a maximally dilated pupil. The light from the illuminating system is reflected back as diverging rays, which are condensed by a condenser held in the right hand of the examiner within two inches of the eyes of the patient. The condenser also provides the required magnification. **Table 14.1** shows the effect of various types of condensers on magnification and field.

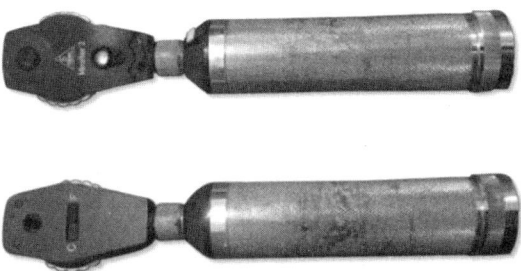

Fig. 14.1: Two sides of a direct ophthalmoscope.

Table 14.1: Comparison between various diopters of condensing lenses.

Feature	+15D	+20D	+30D
Distance from the eye	3 inches	2 inches	1.5 inches
Magnification	4x	3x	2x
Field	30°	50°	60°
Stereopsis	Normal	¾ normal	½ normal
Illumination	Low	Medium	Bright

The +15D gives four times magnification, the +20D has three times magnification, and the +30D has only two times magnification but the largest field.

The indirect ophthalmoscope **(Fig. 14.2)** gives a real, inverted, and magnified image of the fundus in front of the patient. It is laterally reversed.

The findings of indirect ophthalmoscopy are drawn on a special chart with a specific color code **(Fig. 14.3)**.

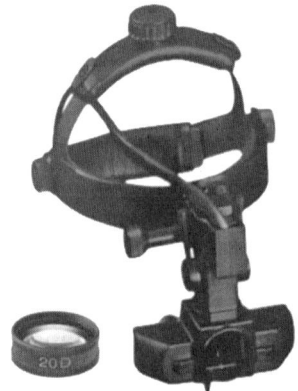

Fig. 14.2: Indirect ophthalmoscope and commonly used +20D condenser (magnifier). (*Courtesy*: Appasamy Associates)

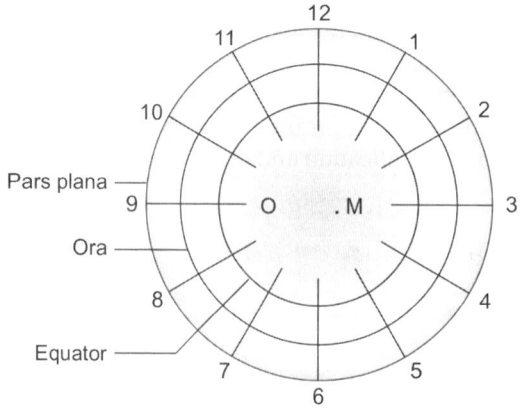

O = Optic nerve, M = Macula
Note: The equator is represented by the innermost circle, pars plana by the outer most circle, with ora serrata in between

Fig. 14.3: Various parts of a standard chart to record the findings of indirect ophthalmoscopy.

The disadvantages of an indirect ophthalmoscope consist of:
- It takes a longer time to learn to operate the instrument.
- Magnification is far less than that of a direct ophthalmoscope.
- The image is laterally reversed.
- The cost of the instrument is more than the direct ophthalmoscope.

Table 14.2 shows the comparison between direct and indirect ophthalmoscope.

Table 14.2: Comparison between direct and indirect ophthalmoscope.		
Features	Direct	Indirect
Image	Virtual, erect, magnified 15x behind the eye	Real, inverted laterally reversed, magnified ranging between 2x, 3x and 4x
Brightness	Less bright	Very bright
Stereopsis	Nil	Good
Resolution	Poor	Better
Field*	Small 10°	Large 37°
Peripheral view	Not possible	Well seen
Working distance	Very short	Long
Scleral indentation	Not possible	Possible

*Comparative fields seen by direct and indirect ophthalmoscope

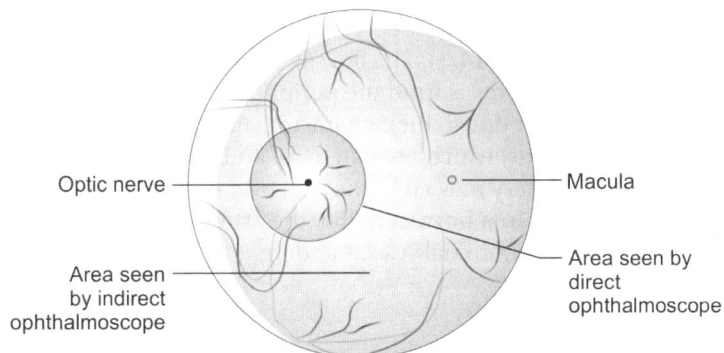

Fig. 14.4: Comparative fields as seen by direct and indirect ophthalmoscope. The smallest circle represents area seen by direct ophthalmoscope.

Ophthalmoscopic Appearance of a Normal Fundus

- The area seen by any ophthalmoscope is circular.
- The disc is taken as the center of the fundus while doing direct ophthalmoscopy.
- The macula is taken as the center of the fundus while doing indirect ophthalmoscopic.
- The fundus is examined under the following heads, i.e., media, retina, and disc.

MEDIA

The opacities in the media stand out as black spots. When seen through the direct ophthalmoscope from a distance of 33.00 cm.

Retina

The retina is examined under two heads: the central retina and the peripheral retina. The peripheral retina is examined for its color, transparency, blood vessels, hemorrhage, exudate, pigment, and elevation.

The normal retina is transparent with a pink hue, which is due to the underlying choroid. A retina is said to be tessellated when the large choroidal vessels are visible in the fundus. This is a normal feature in many eyes.

The retina is pale from anemia, central retinal artery obstruction, generalized edema and detachment of the retina.

The following are responsible for loss of transparency of retina:
- Retinal edema
- Opaque nerve fibers
- Exudate
- Hemorrhage
- Retinal detachment
- Retinal tumor

Blood Vessels

The central retinal artery divides into two main branches at the lamina, the temporal and nasal; each again divides into superior and inferior branches, each sweeping away from the disc towards the periphery with concavity towards the macula. They divide and re-divide two times to be reduced in length and breadth. The main branch is the artery, which is divided into arterioles and capillaries. Each artery has its corresponding vein, which starts as a capillary and changes into a venule and vein **(Fig. 14.5)**. The flow of blood in the artery is from the disc to the periphery, while the flow in the veins is from the periphery to the disc. The arteries and veins are differentiated from each other due to their characteristic appearance. The arteries are thin, rounded, and paler than the veins, which are flat, dark, and broad. The normal ratio between the artery and vein is 2:3. The artery may cross the vein over or under; the two elements have a common sheath at the crossing. In a normal retina, the arteries and veins do not anastomose either among themselves or with choroidal vessels underneath; the development of anastomosis in any case is abnormal.

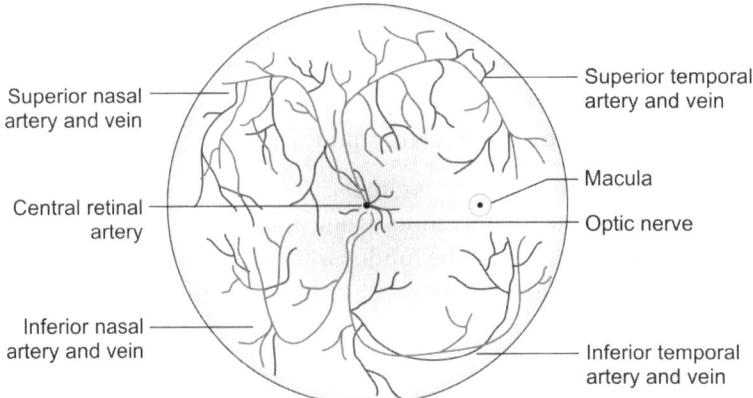

Fig. 14.5: Appearance of normal retinal vessels as seen by indirect ophthalmoscope.
(For color version, see Plate 6)

Chapter 14: Disorders of Retina

The vessel of the retina is examined under the following head:
Caliber, changes in the vessel wall, tortuosity, irregularity, anastomosis, aneurysm, neovascularization, exudates, and hemorrhages.

More important is the presence of the following—hemorrhage, exudate, and neovascularization.

Hemorrhage

Retinal hemorrhages are caused by the leak of blood from the vessels. The hemorrhages can be preretinal, intraretinal, subretinal, or combined.

Preretinal hemorrhages, when large, are called subhyaloid hemorrhages; they develop between the retina and the vitreous. Common causes of subhyaloid hemorrhage are diabetic retinopathy, central vein obstruction, trauma, and retinal vasculitis.

Intraretinal hemorrhages are capillary hemorrhages; there are two types of them, i.e., superficial and deep; in severe cases, both may coexist. The superficial hemorrhages are called flame-shaped hemorrhages. The hemorrhages differ in number, shape, size, and location. It is not unusual for them to be accompanied by exudates. The common causes of superficial hemorrhages are hypertension, venous thrombosis, papilledema, papillitis, and retinitis. The deep hemorrhages are mostly seen in the posterior pole, arising from deeper layers of the retina as small, bright pinpoint spots either alone or in cluster. They may be associated with deep exudates. They are seen in diabetic retinopathy.

Subretinal hemorrhages are generally localized, dark, raised, and circular of different sizes; they develop between the pigment epithelium of the retina and choroid. The retinal vessels cross them on the surface. The most common cause is neovascularization of the choroid. The common causes are age-related macular degeneration and choroidal rupture.

Exudate

They are due to the escape of blood from the diseased retinal wall; the common causes are retinitis, hypertension, and degeneration. According to the level of the exudate in the retina, they are called superficial and deep. Both may exist in the same eye, with/without hemorrhages. The superficial exudates are called cotton wool or soft exudates. They are present in the nerve fiber layer. Deep exudates are called hard exudates. They are small with a clear cut border, waxy yellow in color, circular in shape, and situated deep in the retina. They are mostly seen in diabetic retinopathy.

Examination of the Macula

The macula is best seen with a direct ophthalmoscope, as it gives 15 x magnifications. It can be otherwise seen by indirect ophthalmoscope with less magnification but better stereopsis in relation to other structures, by slit lamp either with +76D lens or by Hruby lens with -55D. The other method to evaluate macula is OCT and fluorescein angiography.

The macula is examined for its central bright reflex, edema, hemorrhage, exudate, and scars in and round the macula. The central reflex is called the fovea, which is the seat of central vision. Any dullness of the fovea results in diminished distant vision.

The causes of dull foveal reflexes are:
(1) Hypoplasia of macula; (2) Edema (swelling) of the macula; (3) Exudates on the macula; (4) Hemorrhage on the macula; (5) Central serous retinopathy; (6) Membrane formation on the macula; (7) Detachment of the macula; (8) Macular degeneration; (9) Scar on macula.

Disorders of the Retina

Retinal disorders can be unilateral or bilateral. The unilateral causes are generally ocular; in systemic conditions, they are bilateral but may start in one eye first; the disorders can be acute or chronic. The disorders of the retina do not cause pain, redness, or watering from the eyes. The main symptoms of retinal diseases are diminished distant vision, diminished color sense, loss of central/peripheral field, or there may be sectorial loss of vision, and diminished night vision.

The causes can be divided into two broad groups, i.e., congenital and acquired. The acquired conditions may be superimposed on the congenital anomaly. Congenital anomalies are generally associated with congenital anomalies of the uvea.

Coloboma

The most common congenital anomalies are the colobomas, which are always associated with colobomas of the choroid, hence seen in the 6 o'clock meridian below the disc **(Fig. 14.6)**. Both the choroid and retina are absent in the coloboma; the floor of the coloboma is formed by the sclera, hence white in color. The retinal vessels are not affected by the coloboma; they travel over the coloboma. The edges of the coloboma may be sharp without pigmentation or with pigmentation. A large coloboma may be seen as a white reflex on a plane mirror retinoscope.

The second congenital anomaly of the retina is opaque nerve fiber, also called medullated nerve fibers, which should better be called a neuroretinal anomaly. In normal eyes, the retinal nerves are transparent up to the edge of the optic disc; once they enter the optic nerve, they lose their transparency and become opaque. The opacity is due to medullation of the nerve fibers. The medullation starts from the end of the nerve nearer the brain and stops at the lamina. In cases where this medullation fails to stop at the lamina and progresses towards the periphery, involving the retinal nerve fibers, they replace transparent nerve fibers with opaque fiber. Generally, the opaque nerve fibers are continuous with the margin of the disc, generally sectorial, but on rare occasions, they may encircle the whole disc. The typical opaque nerve fiber is a flame-shaped white opacity with a base at the optic disc extending towards the periphery. The edge of the opaque nerve fibers is feathery; they overlap the retinal vessels.

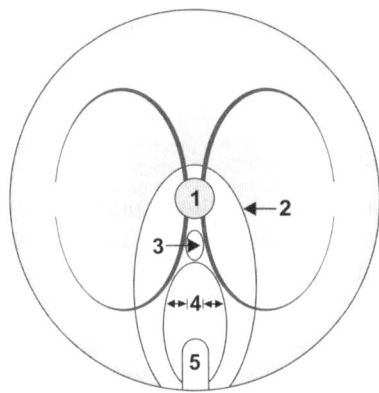

1. Optic disc
2. Coloboma engulfing the optic disc
3. Small localized coloboma
4. Choriociliary coloboma
5. Coloboma involving the iris, ciliary body, and periphery of the choroid

Fig. 14.6: Composite diagram of various types retinochoroidal colobomas.

They are symptomless; large defects cause corresponding field loss. The most common field change is the enlargement of the disc. They do not require any treatment.

Congenital Retinal Pigmentation

They are not true developmental anomalies but effects of maternal infection, such as rubella, syphilis, influenza, and toxoplasmosis. The toxoplasmosis involves predominantly the macular area. The others cause small, black, granular spots intermingled with white spots in between. The condition is called pepper-salt fundus. They are symptomless and diagnosed on routine fundus examinations, not to be confused with retinitis pigmentosa. The salt pepper fundus does not cause any field change either and does not require any treatment.

The other congenital anomalies of the retina are the congenital septum of the retina, also called the congenital retinal fold, and congenital hypertrophy of the retinal pigment epithelium.

Inflammation of the Retina

The inflammation of the retina is called retinitis; the word should be exclusively for infection of the retina and not for other degenerative and vascular retinopathies. The retina is infected by the following organisms—viruses, bacteria, fungi, and parasites. The bacteria can cause both purulent and non-purulent retinitis. The sources can be exogenous (following penetration) or endogenous. The endogenous causes are the blood, choroid, vitreous, and optic nerves. The infection may be limited to the retina without other intraocular structures such as the choroid, optic nerve, or vitreous. Retinitis can be acute, subacute, or chronic; it may be central or peripheral. When other structures are involved, they are called according to the part involved, i.e., chorioretinitis, neuroretinitis (NR), and retinal vasculitis. The symptoms of retinitis depend on the part of the retina and other structures involved. Involvement of the peripheral retina does not cause diminished vision. The loss of vision follows involvement of the macula and optic nerve. Peripheral retinitis generally does not cause diminished vision but causes flashes of light and corresponding field loss.

Many viruses are capable of causing retinitis, mostly congenital. The most common are rubella, cytomegalovirus, and HIV.

Rubella Retinitis

Retina is involved during pregnancy if the mother is infected by rubella during the first three months of pregnancy. The retinal involvement is a form of mild peripheral retinitis causing pepper and salt fundus without causing any visual disturbance or night blindness. In severe form, the child may have many birth defects, such as heart, brain, ear, and eyes. The involvement of these has been discussed in previous chapters.

Cytomegalovirus

Cytomegalovirus can cause both congenital and acquired retinitis. In congenital retinitis, the infection is passed to the fetus from the infected mother. The acquired form is seen in two forms, i.e., in newborns and adults. The newborn gets the infection during delivery from the infected passage. This is less common than the congenital type. The adult gets infected by persons already infected via droplets, sex, or blood transfusion. The condition can be mild, and the patient may not know about it, or it may be as serious as involving the whole retina in patches. The condition may involve the macula only to cause central chorioretinitis. The cytomegalovirus retinitis becomes worse when present in a person with AIDS.

HIV Retinitis

The condition is caused by a virus, better known as a human immune deficiency virus; it can infect any part of the body. The term AIDS stands for acquired immune deficiency syndrome. The body, including the eye, is involved in two different ways. The first is direct invasion by HIV; the second is involvement of the eye by opportunistic microorganisms, which are organisms that generally do not cause any disease as long as immunity is present. They may be commensals. The retinal involvement is bilateral, presenting with cotton wool spots, deep and superficial hemorrhage, microaneurysms, and retinal vasculitis.

The above features may be isolated or in various combinations. The condition is best treated by persons trained in the management of AIDS.

Bacterial Retinitis

Almost any bacteria can cause retinitis, generally reaching the retina through blood or from the choroid and optic nerve. The pus-forming organism may present as acute retinitis or subacute retinitis. Acute retinitis presents with swelling of the retina, superficial and deep hemorrhages, and exudates. Involvement of the macula causes a rapid form of central vision. The retinitis does not cause involvement of the anterior segment; hence, it is not painful. Acute retinitis should be treated as an emergency; otherwise, it may pass into the state of endophthalmitis.

Subacute Bacterial Retinitis

Subacute bacterial retinitis is the haematological spread of pus-forming organisms, mostly cocci. It involves mostly the fine capillaries. The typical presentation is the formation of Roth's spot. This has the specific appearance of a round, flame-shaped hemorrhage with a white center in the posterior pole. The most common cause in children is subacute bacterial endocarditis. Where infected embolus from the valves of the heart are lodged in capillaries. The other causes are leukemia (blood cancer) and purpura.

Parasitic Retinitis

The most common parasite to infect the retina is *Toxoplasmosis gondii*. The parasite is found in many animals, of which cats are the most important. Human beings get infected by consuming food contaminated by the stools of cats, from which the organisms reach various parts of the body. The ocular infection could be acquired or congenital. The acquired disease is mild and non-fatal unless the patient suffers from ADIS or is pregnant. In pregnant women, the organism reaches the fetus from the placenta to infect many organs, including the brain and eye of the fetus. In the eyes, the retina is frequently involved, and central involvement is more common than peripheral involvement. Macular involvement is bilateral and always congenital. As the macula is involved, the child is born with diminished vision, which prevents the development of binocular single vision, causing squinting. The most common type of squint is a high degree of esotropia, which brings the child for examination and is found to have a large central patch of chorioretinitis involving the macula. Other lesions produced by toxoplasmosis are repeated iridocyclitis and generalized chorioretinitis. The vitreous is also affected.

Retinal Vasculitis

Retinal vasculitis is generally bilateral and may begin in one eye; both the arteries and veins are involved in the inflammatory process. It is not a true infection but most probably an autoimmunity disorder. The infection starts at the periphery in finer branches, spreading towards the center. The causes can either be ocular or systemic; there are many cases where no definite cause can be found out. The ocular causes are retinitis, pars planitis, and choroiditis. In the past, systemic infections caused by tuberculosis and syphilis were thought to be the main causes; other infections were thought to be the cause, such as herpes zoster and cytomegalovirus. Idiopathic vasculitis is better known as **Eales' disease***.

*Eales' disease

Eales' disease used to be a major cause of bilateral retinal perivasculitis. One eye may be more involved than the other without causing any symptoms. It was found to be involved more than the symptomatic contralateral eye. The disease is commonly seen in healthy males in the third or fourth decades. Involvement of women is far less than that of men; patients seek medical examination for sudden painless loss of vision in one eye. The loss of vision may be as small as a few lines on the vision chart or as grave as hand movement, depending on the amount of hemorrhage and the part of the retina involved. On examination, the eye does not show involvement of the anterior segment. The vision is diminished by a brisk pupillary reaction; the real finding lies in the fundus. This consists of no visible hemorrhage in the anterior vitreous under oblique illumination or may be large enough to be seen as a bright red blotch behind the retina. Obscuring the fundal glow. The changes in the fundus are divided into two parts, i.e., retinal and vitreal. The retinal changes in Eales' disease consist of peripheral vessels showing evidence of perivasculitis with sheathing, resulting in superficial hemorrhages and the formation of new vessels. Formation—initially, the new vessels are confined to the surface of the retina; later, they grow in the vitreous. The vitreal changes consist of a few new vessels growing in the substance of the retina. There may be a frank hemorrhage in the vitreous that settles down as typical subhyaloid hemorrhage or may be large enough to involve the whole of the vitreous. In the long run, vitreoretinal bands develop that may cause traction detachment of the retina. In cases of suspected Eales' disease, the funds should be examined by an indirect ophthalmoscope with a large visible field. It is mandatory for the other so-called asymptomatic normal eye to have evidence of Eales' disease, which may be found to have more advanced periphlebitis on the periphery, not involving the macula. Generally, the first episode of hemorrhage clears without treatment, and vision returns to the pre-hemorrhage state only to reappear within months. Such a cycle of diminished vision and improvement may become a regular affair, with a prolonged period of diminished vision appearing with more frequency. Ultimately, a stage of non-improvement is reached. The causes of non-improvement of vision in Eales' disease are large unabsorbed hemorrhages called hemophthalmos, traction detachment of the retina, complicated cataracts, and neovascular glaucoma.

The diagnosis of Eales' disease is easy if the following points are kept in mind:
- **Age:** Between 20 and 40 years
- **Sex:** Male
- **Symptoms:** Sudden painless loss of vision in one eye without redness of the eye.
- No history of diabetes, sickle cell anemia, or hypertension
- Satisfactory projection of light from all quadrants
- Normal pupil
- Intraocular tension within normal limits
- Fundus changes of retinal vasculitis

Differential Diagnosis

Differential diagnosis consists of other causes of retinal hemorrhages, which are as follows:
- Diabetic retinopathy
- Hypertensive retinopathy
- Sickle cell anemia
- Central retinal vein occlusion
- Branch retinal vein occlusion
- Trauma
- High myopia
- Congenital anomalies of retinal vessels

Management

The first step is to exclude any systemic cause and treat it. If no cause is found, the case is confirmed as Eales' disease.

Treatment

Following the first episode, the patient remains ambulatory with restricted physical activity. With rest, the blood settles down, improving the vision with a false sensation of cure; this is short-lived, recurrence is rule an attempt should be made to treat vasculitis by oral corticosteroid with usual precaution as per practice of the institute. The next step is to photocoagulate the newly formed vessels. The last step is vitrectomy with repair of traction retinal detachment.

Retinal Degeneration and Dystrophies

Before discussing the conditions, it is better to know the difference between the two the two are often used as inter changeable terms, the differences are as follows:

The dystrophies are genetic may be seen in many members of the family, present at birth, or manifest later in life. They are generally bilateral and progressive, without evidence of other ocular diseases. The common dystrophies of the eye, besides the retina, are corneal dystrophies. There is no treatment for retinal dystrophies; in contrast, corneal dystrophies are amenable to keratoplasty.

The degenerations are acquired may be unilateral, non-genetic, do not run in the family, generally do not progress, are secondary to ocular diseases. The management consists of timely treatment of the primary disease.

Retinal Dystrophies

Retinal dystrophies are divided into two groups: namely, central and peripheral. The central dystrophies are referred to as macular dystrophies. The two types differ in clinical presentation. The macular dystrophies involve cones mostly, are generally bilateral, slow progressive with diminished uncorrectable distant vision, the loss of vision varies from a few lines on the optotype to <6/60, poor vision in bright light, better vision in dim light, reduced color sense, distorted vision, temporal pallor of the disc, without vascular changes.

The common macular dystrophies are Best's disease, Stargardt's disease, cone dystrophy, and Sorsby macular dystrophy.

The peripheral dystrophies involve mostly rods; hence, the most obvious feature is diminished night vision, with better vision in bright light, generally not associated with loss of central vision. The conditions are associated with peripheral field loss.

Most common form of retinal dystrophy is retinitis pigmentosa.

Retinitis Pigmentosa

Retinitis pigmentosa involves photoreceptor and pigment epithelium associated with changes in blood vessels. The most common symptom is night blindness. The condition is divided into two types, i.e., typical retinitis pigmentosa and atypical retinitis pigmentosa.

Typical Retinitis Pigmentosa

Typical retinitis pigmentosa is a hereditary disease in which generally more than one member of the family is involved. It is more common in males and is bilateral and progressive. The patient first becomes aware of diminished night vision in teens, which becomes worse with time. Central vision remains good for many years, only to be lost by the fourth or fifth decade. The patient has loss of peripheral vision, which begins on the superiotemporal side, which makes the patient move their head from side to side to see on the periphery. Ultimately, the field becomes tubular **(Fig. 14.7)**, still retaining useful central vision. The diagnosis is revealed on a fundus examination, best seen with an indirect ophthalmoscope. The fundus shows floaters in the vitreous, the disc is waxy pale, and the vessels are thin with typical black star-like pigments around the vessels **(Fig. 14.8)**, between the macula and ora. The eye loses central vision if the macula is involved, the most common involvement being macular edema. The other causes of diminished central vision are high myopia, posterior subcapsular cataracts, and chronic glaucoma.

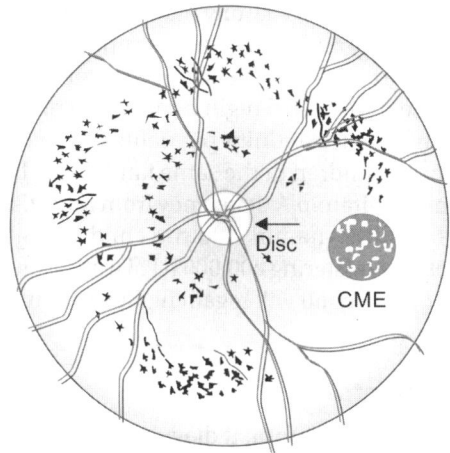

Fig. 14.7: Retinitis pigmentosa with cystoid macular edema (CME).

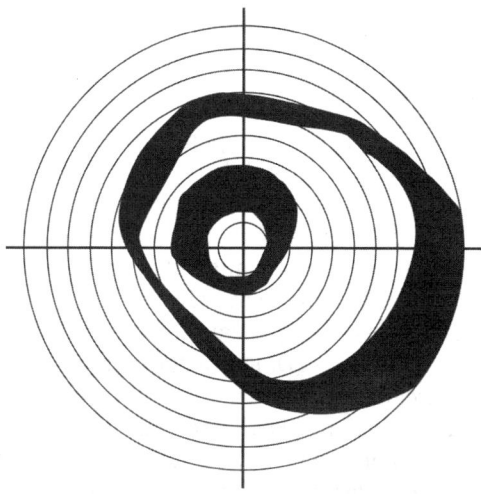

Fig. 14.8: Ring scotomas in retinitis pigmentosa.

Atypical Retinitis Pigmentosa

The incidence of atypical retinitis pigmentosa is less than that of typical retinitis pigmentosa. The typicality may be in the pigmentation, specially in its distribution and varied field changes. Atypical retinitis pigmentosa may be associated with systemic disorders. The atypical retinitis pigmentosa may be present in one eye only, with usual fundus changes, or the pigmentation may be seen in one sector, causing sectorial field changes; in a still rare form, there is no visible pigmentation, but the condition has other features of retinitis pigmentation, i.e., diminished night vision, thin retinal vessels, and typical peripheral field changes. The condition is called as Retinitis pigmentosa sine pigmento.

Systemic conditions associated with retinitis pigmentosa are seen in children who are obese with more than five fingers and toes, non-development of genitals, and mental retardation.

The diagnosis off typical retinitis pigmentosa is not difficult with diminished progressive night blindness and a good central-field, positive family history. The common conditions that should be excluded are vitamin A deficiency and choroidal dystrophies.

Diminished night vision due to vitamin A deficiency requires special mention in relation to retinitis pigmentosa; both cause diminished night blindness. The progress of night blindness in vitamin A deficiency is faster than typical retinitis pigmentosa, there is no hereditary back ground in vitamin A deficiency but many children in the same family may be affected.

The simple rule to differentiate vitamin A deficiency from retinitis pigmentosa is a therapeutic trial by administering water-soluble vitamin A to the child brought with complaints of night blindness. The trial consists of administering 200,000 IU of water-soluble vitamin A intramuscular. In cases of vitamin A deficiency, the child will regain night vision within 48 hours, which will not be seen in typical retinitis pigmentosa.

Treatment of Retinitis Pigmentosa

There is no treatment for retinitis pigmentosa. If diagnosed in teens, the child should be treated as any visually impaired child. The usual low-vision aids are of hardly any use to a child suffering from retinitis pigmentosa because none of them will treat the night blindness or restricted field.

COMMON MACULAR DISORDERS

Beside macular dystrophies, the macula is prone to developing the following disorders—central serous retinopathy, age-related macular degeneration, and cystoid macular edema.

Central Serous Retinopathy (CSR)

The condition is also called central chorioretinopathy. In this condition, there is a leak under the retinal pigment epithelium that is best visible on fluorescein angiography. In some cases, the leak is away from the fovea. CSR is unilateral; in one-third of cases, the disorder in the other eye may develop; the disease after months or years. The most common symptom is a circular scotoma in front of the eye with diminished distant and near vision. The vision does not improve with a pinhole. The loss of vision is not more than a few lines on the vision chart; the cause of this phenomenon is acquired axial hypermetropia caused by elevated retina. The vision improves with plus lenses ranging between +1D to +2D. The hypermetropia diminishes with a reduction in macular edema with/without treatment. The other visual symptom is distorted vision. Which is best noted on the Amsler grid. The patient takes longer time to recover from glare; on retinoscopy, the area is more hypermetropic than the rest of the retina. On fundus examination, there is an elevated circular area over the macula with absent or dull fovea; the circular area is many times larger than the normal optic disc without any new vessels, hemorrhage, or exudate. The elevation may be as much as 1-2 diopters. Best seen in OCT. On fluorescein angiography, there is a leak in the pigment epithelium; occasionally, the leak may be away from the fovea, forming a mushroom-shaped leak.

Management

The condition is self-limiting, clearing in 2-3 weeks initially without any scar; in 75% of cases, there may be a recurrence that may repeat every second to third month with prolonged recovery time. Each recurrence has a shorter recurrence time and a longer recovery period. Repeated attacks leave the macula scared. The role of steroids is debatable; photocoagulation is indicated in repeated attacks; intravitreal anti-VEGF injection has been found to be effective in repeated attacks.

Age-related Macular Degeneration

This was previously known as senile macular degeneration. It is a very common cause of bilateral loss of central vision in both sexes after sixty years of age. The incidence increases with age, and the two eyes may not be involved equally at a time. It is not preventable and treatable; the treatment used presently only reduces the progress of the condition. The symptoms are non-correctable diminished central vision with fair peripheral vision and satisfactory near vision without loss of color sense or loss of stereopsis. The Amsler grid shows distorted vision; there are two clinical types of age-related macular degeneration, i.e., dry and wet. The former is more common and less troublesome due to the development of drusen in the macula and atrophy of the pigment epithelium. The condition is not treatable; the patient may be helped by the use of low-vision devices. The wet type is less common, the incidence of which is increasing due to an increased life span. Only 10% of ARMDs are wet in nature, but 90% of persons suffering from wet AMRD will have severe loss of vision. It is more common in women; wet ARMD is also called exudative or neovascular ARMD. It has been observed that persons with dry ARMD are more likely to get converted into wet ARMD than those without dry ARMD. The main cause lies in the underline choroid, which develops neovessels, leading to submacular bleeding, exudative retinal detachment, and scar formation*. It is best seen in fluorescein angiography and OCT. The condition is difficult to treat and generally does not respond to laser therapy. Anti-VEGF is administered to reduce progress.

Other causes of choroidal neovascularization are high myopia, rupture of the choroid, and drusen of the optic nerve head.

Cystoid Macular Edema

Cystoid macular edema (CME) is one of the major causes of non-improvement of vision following intracapsular lens extraction or even phacoemulsification.

The other causes of CME are:
- Diabetic retinopathy
- Central retinal vein thrombosis
- Posterior uveitis
- Retinal dystrophies
- Local and systemic drugs
- Idiopathic

The condition is caused due to accumulation of fluid under the outer plexiform and inner nuclear layers of the retina under the macula. The main symptoms are diminished central vision, fast falls in central vision, and distorted vision. The condition itself is painless without involving the anterior segment. The condition is confirmed by fundus fluorescein angiography and OCT. The management consists of treatment of the causative factors such as diabetic retinopathy, central vein occlusion, etc.

The commonly used drugs to manage CME are:
- **Local:** Non-steroidal anti-inflammatory drugs twice a day for many weeks.
- Intraocular triamcinolone acetonide, too, has been found to be effective, but it does not prevent recurrence.
- The recent trend to manage postoperative CME is intravitreal anti-VEGF injections. The prognosis is not equally satisfactory by any of the above methods.

Vascular Disorders of the Retina

Retina being highly vascular, it is but natural that it will be exposed to many disorders of the vessels. The common vascular disorders are:
- **Vascular retinopathies**
    - Diabetic retinopathy
    - Hypertensive retinopathy
    - Retinopathy of pregnancy
    - Retinopathy of prematurity
- **Vascular obstructive disorder of retina**
    - Retinal artery occlusion
    - Retinal vein occlusion

VASCULAR RETINOPATHIES

Diabetic Retinopathy

Diabetic retinopathy is a common cause of uncorrectable diminished vision and a major cause of blindness worldwide. It is caused either by a lack of insulin in the body or an inability to use available insulin. Its magnitude can be assessed by the enormous number of people suffering from the disease. About 10% of the general population all over the world suffers from diabetic retinopathy, mostly due to ignorance of the complications of diabetes or half-hearted treatment of the condition. The incidence of diabetes and its complications in general and retinopathy in particular is increasing by many fold in developing countries. There are two types of diabetes, classified according to age and ability to use insulin. The first is called type 1 diabetes, or insulin-dependent diabetes, seen under 20 years of age. Though diabetic retinopathy is less common in this group, the other non-ocular complications are more common. The condition is mostly treated by insulin. The second is called type 2 diabetes, seen in elderly persons with a positive family history and diabetes for >15 years.

Other factors that predispose diabetic retinopathies are uncontrolled or poorly controlled diabetes, diabetes present for >15 years, genetic predisposition, the presence of hypertension, raised lipids in the blood, and pregnancy.

Diabetic retinopathy has been classified variously from time to time. The simplest way is to divide it into two clinical groups, i.e., background retinopathy and proliferative retinopathy. The background retinopathy develops in the posterior pole with deep hemorrhages and deep exudates, with occasional flame-shaped hemorrhages and sometimes clinically significant macular edema. The background retinopathy, if not managed well, will progress to the next stage of proliferative retinopathy. The fundus changes are superficial and deep hemorrhages all over the fundus, superimposed on already present back ground retinopathy with new vessels on the periphery and even the optic disc. The macula is generally edematous, with a circle of exudates all-round. The new vessels are unsupported with a tendency to bleed; the bleeding may extend in the vitreous, which, in the long run, causes band formations which when extended on the retina, cause traction detachment of the retina. The retinopathy is worsened by the presence of hypertension, increased lipid, anemia and pregnancy. Proliferative retinopathy develops less frequently in type 1 diabetics.

Management of Diabetic Retinopathy

The management of diabetic retinopathy depends on the following factors—type of diabetes, duration of diabetes, biochemical control of diabetes, associated hypertension, hyperlipidemia, and anemia. All these conditions produce hypoxia in the retina, releasing vasoproliferative factors.

Well-controlled diabetes delays the onset of diabetic retinopathy. The management of diabetic retinopathy is divided into two groups.

Management of Background Diabetic Retinopathy

- ❖ All cases of background diabetic retinopathy do not require treatment. Many times, the patient is not aware of it until they develop diminished vision. Hence, all patients suffering from diabetes of any type should regularly undergo a detailed fund examination, preferably by indirect ophthalmoscope, and if found to have retinopathy, should undergo a fluorescein fund examination every six months.
- ❖ There is no medical treatment for diabetic retinopathy.
- ❖ To prevent the development and progress of retinopathy, strict biochemical control of diabetes is mandatory under the supervision of an internist.
- ❖ Hypertension, hyperlipidemia, and anemia should be kept under control.
- ❖ The gold standard of treatment for diabetic retinopathy is photocoagulation.
- ❖ Photocoagulation converts hypoxic retina into anoxic retina, which in turn reduces the production of vasoproliferative factor, the sole cause of the formation of new vessels.
- ❖ The type of photocoagulation is better left to a person trained in the medical disease of the retina.

Management of Proliferative Retinopathy

Management of proliferative diabetic retinopathy is tricky and difficult; the treatment is patient-specific. Proliferative diabetic retinopathy requires extensive photocoagulation by a suitable laser. A patient may require multiple sessions of laser treatment. If vitreous bands are present, they are cut to prevent the future development of traction retinal detachment. If traction retinal detachment is present, it requires extensive vitrectomy along with repair of the detachment. The overall results are not very rewarding.

Hypertensive Retinopathy

About 10% of the population suffers from hypertension, the incidence of which is increasing; it is equally divided among both sexes. The term hypertension is used to denote increased pressure of blood in the arteries. Retinopathy is basically the result of changes in the arterial wall due to increased intraluminal pressure in the circulating blood. The changes are seen on ophthalmoscopic examination. There are many classifications of hypertensive retinopathy, which basically revolve around two factors, i.e., the presence or absence of sclerosis of the arteries.

Hypertensive changes with sclerosis are generally seen in older persons with a moderate rise in blood pressure over many months.

The changes are:
- The vessels look tense, straight, and pale.
- The arteries press the veins, which are dilated beyond the crossing of the vein by the hard arteries.
- The color of the artery shifts towards brown, and the arteries look as if they are made of copper; this condition is called copper wire appearance.
- Some flame-shaped hemorrhages and cotton wool exudates

The hypertensive changes without sclerosis are generally seen in persons with high blood pressure of short duration.

The changes are:
- Increased tone of arteries
- Veins are concealed (hidden) by arteries
- Retinal edema
- Flame-shaped hemorrhages and cotton wool exudates
- Silver wire appearance of retinal arteries
- Blurring of the disc margin

Note: The fundus changes reflect the vascular changes present in the brain, heart, and kidneys. The fundus changes are worsened by the presence of diabetic retinopathy.

Retinopathy of Pregnancy

- This is also called retinopathy of toxemia in pregnancy.
- Toxemia in pregnancy is a late feature of pregnancy where there is high blood pressure, swelling of limbs, and fits, and the patient passes albumin in urine.
- The fundus changes are bilateral, and the condition is brought to notice due to a fall in vision.

The retinal changes consist of:
- Narrowing of arteries
- Swelling of retina
- Superficial hemorrhages and exudates
- Exudative retinal detachment.

The causes of diminished vision are retinal edema and exudative retinal detachment.

The detachment subsides with termination of pregnancy normal or artificial and vision returns to normal.

Retinopathy of Prematurity

The condition was previously known as retrolental fibroplasias which is better used for vitreous bands in adults. The incidence of retinopathy of prematurity in increasing due to longevity of newborns. It occurs in preterm babies, birth weight less than 1200 g and exposure to oxygen for long time. The condition is bilateral. There are two types one that terminates automatically without treatment and the second that progresses requiring extensive treatment. The cause of the disorders is not well understood, because it has been observed even in children born full term, with birth weight more than 1200 g and short exposure to oxygen.

The most commonly believed theory is as follows:
- The retinal vessels are not fully developed before eight months of gestation.
- Do not reach the periphery.
- It takes another four months to reach the periphery.

- If the pregnancy terminates before eight months and the newborn is exposed to prolonged concentrated oxygen, the vessels that have not reached the periphery start sprouting; these new vessels are unsupported and prone to bleed.
- There are some vasoproliferative factors that are stimulated in the presence of oxygen.
- The unsupported vessels grow in the vitreous as well, causing traction detachment.

The disease has been divided in two forms:
1. Common regressive disease that do not require treatment and do not cause much visual damage.
2. The progressive type that is less common than the former and requires treatment. They if not treated will proceed a stage of extensive neovascularization, vitreous band formation, and traction detachment leading ultimately to blindness. The treatment is photocoagulation of new vessels, vitrectomy and surgical treatment of traction detachment. Intravitreal injection of anti-VEGF too has been tried without equal success in all cases.

VASCULAR OBSTRUCTIVE DISORDER OF RETINA

There are two types of vascular obstruction of the retinal circulation, i.e., retinal artery and retinal venous obstruction. The two conditions neither occur simultaneously nor do they follow each other. Venous obstruction is more common than arterial obstruction. The chance of retaining some vision is seen in venous obstruction. The clinical picture depends on the part of the vessel involved. Both are unilateral; the venous obstruction, if not treated, is likely to cause neovascularization of the peripheral retina and even invade the eye to cause neovascular glaucoma. Both conditions are painless to begin with until neovascularization and glaucoma set in. The condition may be localized in branches of the vessels with less visual loss or involve the central retinal vessels to cause more loss of vision. **Flowchart 14.1** shows the types of vascular obstruction.

Retinal Artery Obstruction

The condition is generally seen in elderly person suffering from arteriosclerosis, frank hypertension, diabetes, or an obstructive disease of the main blood supply to the brain, i.e., an internal carotid artery, or chronic simple glaucoma. The mechanism of central retinal artery obstruction is as follows—an embolism in a predisposing person from a distant organ gets lodged in either the main retinal artery or its branches. The first is called central retinal artery obstruction, and the later as branch obstruction. There are three types of emboli, i.e., cholesterol, calcium, platelets, and fibrin. The calcium emboli arise from the valves of the heart; the remaining arise from the atheromatous carotid artery. The condition is a unilateral, single episode. The typical presentation is a unilateral, sudden, painless loss of vision. The loss of vision

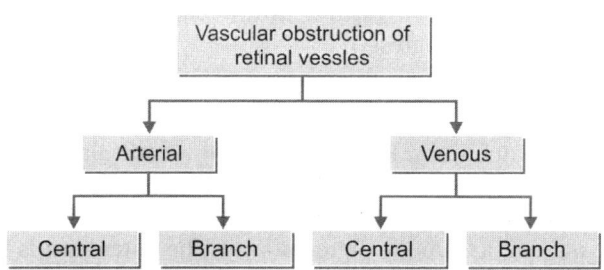

Flowchart 14.1: Division of vascular obstruction of retinal veins.

depends on the position of the obstruction and the time lost following the accident. Loss of vision in central retinal obstruction may be as much as loss of perception of light. In cases of branch obstruction, the loss of vision may be partial.

Clinical features of central retinal artery occlusion (CRAO) are:
- There is no redness, pain, or watering from the eye involved.
- The only finding is a dilated, sluggish pupil.
- There is a relative afferent pupillary reaction.
- Fundus examinations are:
  - Retina is pale white.
  - The arteries are extremely thin, with a loss of vascular reflex.
  - There are no exudates or hemorrhages except for existing features of hypertension or diabetes.
  - The macula stands out prominently as a red spot called a cherry red spot in the middle of the white retina.
  - The disc is pale.
  - In cases of branch obstruction, the findings are sectorial in the area supplied by the effected branch with corresponding field loss; the vision may not be affected if the obstruction is away from the macula. In some cases, where the eye has a papillomacular branch that originates away from the obstruction of the central retinal artery, some vision may be present. The vessel is visible as a non-occluded artery between the papilla and the macula.

There is no effective treatment for CRAO. Patients suffering from central retinal artery occlusion are prone to suffer from cerebrovascular accidents in the coming months and years.

Retinal Vein Obstruction

The vascular accidents of the retinal vein are more common than their counterpart, i.e., CRAO. The condition may affect the central vein or its branch; it is unilateral and presents with sudden painlessness, loss of vision in a white eye, and a sluggish pupillary reaction. The loss of vision is not as profound as seen in CRAO; it is generally hand movement with good projection of light. It is seen commonly in persons with hypertension, arteriosclerosis, hyperlipidemia, increased coagulation of blood, suspected thrombosis of the ipsilateral carotid, and valvular heart disease. The fundus picture of typical central retinal vein obstruction is as follows:
- The veins are dilated and congested.
- Whole of the retina is splashed with large patches of bright hemorrhage.
- The disc is congested with blurred borders.
- The details of the fundus are not visible.

There is no effective treatment for venous obstruction.

One of the complications of central retinal vein thrombosis is the development of thrombotic glaucoma (neovascular glaucoma) after 2–3 months.

The palliative treatment is pan-retinal photocoagulation of the retina to prevent neovascularization or reduce its progress.

Retinal Detachment

To understand retinal detachment, it is necessary to recapitulate the development of the retina.

The name detachment of the retina is a misnomer; it is better called retinal separation, i.e., separation of the neural retina from the pigment layer. The outer layer is firmly attached to the

Bruch's membrane of the choroid and cannot be separated from it. The inner layer is loosely attached to the outer layer with a thin space in between, devoid of any fluid or solid. If some fluid or solid gets access to this space, the two layers are separated, which is clinically referred to as retinal detachment. Retinal detachment is partly preventable and treatable. The retinal detachment can occur at any age, in both sexes and all races. It is bilateral in about 10% of cases, with another 20% at risk of development in their lifetime.

The predisposing factors in the development of detachment are: positive family history, myopia, aphakia, repeated needling in children, pseudophakia, blunt injury, vitreous degeneration, vitreoretinal bands, and **lattice degeneration*** of the retina. It will be noted that myopia, vitreous degeneration, and peripheral retinal degeneration too have genetic predispositions, increasing the chances of retinal detachment.

The retinal detachments for clinical and therapeutic purposes have been divided into three following types.
1. Retinal detachment with a hole (rhegmatogenous)
2. Retinal detachment due to a pull on the sensory retina (traction detachment)
3. Exudative retinal detachment

***Lattice degeneration**

Lattice degeneration is the most common peripheral retinal degeneration seen in 8% of persons of both sexes; one-third of them are at a high risk of rhegmatogenous retinal degeneration. Lattice degeneration is more common in myopic eyes. It is genetically predisposed; it consists of a lattice formation of white strings on the periphery of the retina, parallel to the equator. The surrounding retina, which is thin, may have small round holes that increase the chances of retinal detachment.

Rhegmatogenous

Rhegmatogenous retinal detachment is the most common type of detachment seen in all ages and is more common in young, myopic persons. The word rhegma means a tear or discontinuity in the retina. The defect could be a hole, a rupture, or a tear. The rhegmas have been named variously due to their shape, i.e., round defects are called circular, triangular defects are called arrow heads, and horseshoe tears, both types if they have an attached band, are called operculated. The separation of the retina from the periphery is called retinal dialysis, which is the largest tear that produces rhegmatogenous detachment. It is possible to have various numbers of retinal tears at various places in the same eye. The contralateral eye, without symptoms too, may have retinal tears without symptoms. This makes it mandatory to examine both eyes with an indirect ophthalmoscope with scleral indentation. The various types of retinal tears are shown in **Figure 14.9**.

A traction detachment is secondary to a vitreoretinal band either attached to the operculum or to the retinal surface, exerting traction on the retina and tearing it away from the pigment layer, causing a break in the retina. The break thus produced behaves such as any retinal tear; the symptoms depend on the size of the traction and its position.

Exudative detachment does not have a hole or traction band on the retinal surface. It is caused by exudative fluid accumulating between the sensory and pigment epithelium, the most common source of fluid from the inflamed underline choroid. The detached retina has a smooth surface without a wavy surface on its surface, in contrast to the other two types of detachment, i.e., rhegmatogenous and traction. The detachment settles down once the exudates have disappeared, either through treatment or without.

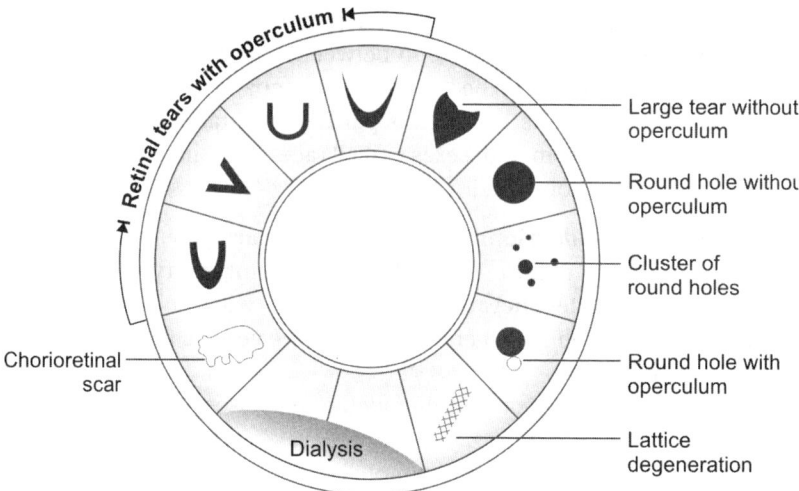

Fig. 14.9: Various types of retinal holes, lattice degeneration and chorioretinal scar.

Symptoms of Retinal Detachment

- The shallow detachments in the lower periphery may be asymptomatic.
- More common symptoms are flashes of light, black spots in front of the eye with/without diminished vision, and corresponding field defects, which seem to be a curtain falling from above.
- **Sudden, painless loss of vision:** This happens when the detachment extends into the posterior pole. Near proximity to the macula causes more loss of vision. Nearer the macula is the loss; ultimately, involvement of the macula causes obliteration of the vision, which may be just counting finger or hand movement with a loss of projection from the involved area.
- Upper detachment causes more visual loss than lower.
- Temporal detachment attracts diminished vision and loss of field earlier than nasal.
- On a long run, untreated or failed treatment may lead to chronic uveitis, complicated cataracts, secondary glaucoma, and loss of vision.

Diagnosis

The diagnosis of well-established retinal detachment is not difficult. The difficulty arises in locating the cause of the disorders that is a retinal tear. Finding out the tear/tears is most important in the management of retinal detachment. Specially in hazy media and aphakia. This shortcoming is mitigated by using an indirect ophthalmoscope with a wide field along with scleral indentation. It is mandatory that the pupil be dilated at the maximum. The detached retina on the indirect ophthalmoscope looks white; with an uneven surface, the vessels travel over the detached retina, and the vessels over the detached retina are darker than normal. The holes are more red than the detached retina. Sometimes bands may be seen to be attached to the operculum of the hole.

Management

Prophylaxis

- All persons with history of ocular trauma, intraocular surgery myopia, and positive family history should get their retinal periphery examined by a trained retinologist who will examine the fundus with indirect ophthalmoscope every year.

- ❖ Whenever there is a retinal detachment in one eye, the other eye should be examined by indirect ophthalmoscope.
- ❖ If holes are detected even without detachment, they should be closed by laser photocoagulation.

Treatment

- ❖ There is no medical treatment for retinal detachment except for exudative detachment, which is treated as per the conditions, which are generally in the choroid and treated with large doses of steroids.
- ❖ The principle of surgical treatment consists of:
  - Search for the hole/holes
  - Locate the hole/holes
  - Find out the size of the hole and any traction to it.
  - Close the hole
  - Drain the fluid under the sensory retina
  - Close all the holes
  - Keep the two layers pressed against each other

In the past, the retinal holes were closed either by a local external plomb or encircling the whole of the retina with an encircling band. Followed by drainage of subretinal fluid. The edges of the tear were sealed either by diathermy or cryo. The present practice is to do a vitrectomy, close treating the edges of the tear by laser and creating a tamponade either by air, gas, or silicon oil.

Retinal Trauma

Trauma to the retina is a common factor that reduces retinal function; traumas involving the macula are more devastating than those on the periphery. The injury on the periphery may be without any symptoms, only to become symptomatic later. Retinal injuries can be unilateral or bilateral; bilateral injuries result when the injuring force affects both eyes, such as a blast injury. The retinal trauma can be mechanical, chemical, or radiation-induced. Out of these, mechanical injury is the most common. The mechanical injury can either be blunt or penetrating.

The blunt injuries are caused by objects with a diameter larger than the orbital rim. The common injuries are sports injuries or scuffles; a patient may bang against a round, hard body as well to get a blunt retinal trauma. A blunt injury is always associated with an injury to the lids, cornea, or sclera. The effects of blunt injuries are retinal edema, retinal hemorrhage, and retinal tear. The retinal edema is caused by a blunt injury of variable hardness ranging from a tennis ball, shuttlecock, cricket ball, fist, or elbow.

The object compresses the eyeball, transferring the force from the anterior to posterior direction, including the retina, just opposite the points of contact of the offending object on the lid, and transmitting it to the cornea or sclera alone or in combination. This is called a Contrecoup injury. The effect is an edema of the retina anywhere on the surface called commotio retinae. The term commotio retinae is presently exclusively used for macular injury and is called Berlin's edema. The lesion has a typical appearance of a slightly raised white area with a pink center. The raised pale represents edema. The pink area represents fovea that is non-edematous. The pink color of the fovea is due to the absence of nerve fibers and its incapability to swell. The other cause is the thinness of the retina at the macula; hence, the choriocapillaris under it are seen as bright pink spots. The symptoms of Berlin's edema may not be obvious for the first few hours, only to become symptomatic thereafter. The main symptom of Berlin's edema is diminished distant vision; the loss of vision is mild to moderate, i.e., not more than 6/18. The vision gradually improves to pre-injury levels. Rarely, the loss is permanent due to pigmentation following hemorrhage during the injury.

The other causes of red spot in the macula are:
- Central retinal artery occlusion (severe loss of central vision, generally seen in elderly)
- Tay-Sachs disease rare, not seen in India
- Hemorrhage on the macula
- Macular hole

Causes of Macular Hemorrhage
- Trauma
- High myopia
- Age-related macular degeneration

Retinal Tears and Ruptures

A disruption in the sensory retina is called a retinal tear, in contrast to the involvement of the full-thickness retina along with the choroid, which is called a retinal rupture. The condition behaves, such as choroidal rupture and presents with signs and symptoms similar to those of choroidal rupture.

Retinal dialysis is the most severe form of retinal tear; it may be traumatic or any other cause that results in retinal tear can cause it. This is also called retinal disinsertion; the traumatic dialysis is secondary to a blunt injury that is directed to the ora serrata. The dialysis can happen anywhere on the retinal periphery. Both cause retinal detachment; the dialysis in the lower part causes less and late detachment, while the upper dialysis causes large and fast-growing retinal detachment. The trauma besides dialysis, can cause retinal tears anywhere on the periphery, making it one of the most common causes of rhegmatogenous retinal degeneration. The retinal dialysis is best seen by indirect ophthalmoscopy and treated by the usual retinal surgical procedure meant for retinal detachment.

Traumatic Retinal Hemorrhage

Isolated retinal hemorrhage due to blunt injury is uncommon; it is generally seen in retinal edema, choroidal rupture dialysis. The pre-existing retinal hemorrhages caused by various vascular retinopathies are worsened by blunt injury. These hemorrhages are generally pre-retinal. Rarely, the hemorrhage may develop in the substance of the retina or may be behind the retina; this is in fact a choroidal hemorrhage and is occasionally referred to as a choroidal hematoma.

Macular Holes

Macular holes differ from other retinal tears in that they are central. They develop over the macula. Most of the time, no cause can be found that results in hole formation; they are mostly sporadic. The size varies from pinpoint to as large as the disc. There is no operculum. The hole is circular with a clear cut margin; the floor stands out as a bright red spot in the midst of the attached retina. There are two types of macular holes, i.e., partial and total. The partial holes may be converted to full-thickness holes. The predisposing factors are age; they are generally seen after the fifth decade and are more frequent among females and myopes. Vitreous suppression is a precursor to macular holes. The holes can be due to blunt injury too; in spite of their size, they cause detachment less frequently than peripheral tears. The incidence of retinal detachment in the macular hole varies from 1 to 5%.

The symptoms are diminished central vision that may be as much as counting fingers from 33.00 cm with fairly good peripheral vision; a unilateral lesion may not cause much difficulty in movement. The loss of central vision is associated with a positive scotoma, whose size corresponds to the size of the hole. Bilateral lesions cause more difficulty in movement, even in known surroundings. The incidence of macular holes is increasing with an increase in longevity. The macular holes are treated by extensive vitrectomy, followed by intraocular injections of air, gas-like substances such as sulfur hexafluoride (SF6), perfluoroethane (C2F6), perfluoropropane (C3F8), and silicone oil.

Penetrating injuries of the retina are always associated with penetrating injuries of the globe, piercing the globe and the choroid. It is associated with wounds in the sclera and choroid. The choroid may/may not prolapse through the wound in the sclera; such wounds may be associated with intraocular foreign bodies. Penetrating injuries to the retina are serious conditions that require repairs in a specialized vitreoretinal unit. The penetrating injury may require multiple surgeries, such as vitrectomy, removal of foreign bodies, and management of retinal detachment. The overall prognosis is poor.

TUMORS OF RETINA

The retina is an extension of the brain and shares many of the tumors of the brain. The retinal tumor can be congenital and may be obvious at birth or manifest in later life. Such tumors are retinal hemangiomas, both capillary and cavernous, as seen in Wyburn-Mason syndrome. They may be uniocular or binocular, single or multiple, benign or malignant. The most common malignant tumor of the retina is retinoblastoma, which is a tumor of children generally not seen after five years of age. It can be unilateral or bilateral.

It is seen in both sexes equally. The most common age presentation is three years. It becomes rare after six years of age.

There are two types of retinoblastoma:
1. Sporadic (without family history)
2. Heritable (with family history).

About 90% are sporadic and only ten percent are heritable. Sporadic cases are unilateral and thirty percent of heritable cases are bilateral.

The retinoblastoma can be divided into two main groups:
1. Without visible white reflex in pupillary area
2. White reflex in pupillary area

The second group passes into following stages if not treated:
1. Stage of glaucoma
2. Stage of extraocular extensive (the tumor comes out of sclera)
3. Metastasis: The tumor spread to other parts of the body.

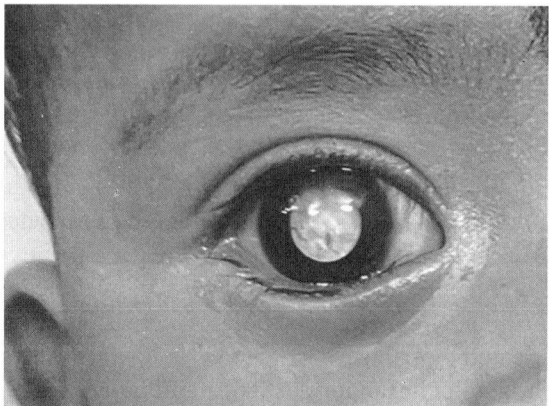

Fig. 14.10: Retinoblastoma: White reflex in the pupillary area in a blind eye.
(For color version, see Plate 7)

Symptoms and Signs of Retinoblastoma

Symptoms depend on the stage of the disease. In the stage of no visible white reflex, the only symptom may be squint or diminished vision, for which the child is brought to an ophthalmologist, and on fundus examination, a white, raised mass is detected in the posterior pole.

The second symptom is that when the child moves the eye, a white reflex is visible in the pupil.

In the stage of white reflex in the pupillary area, the most important finding is a white reflex in the pupillary area even when the child is looking straight but there is no pain or redness. The vision is diminished, and the eye may squint **(Fig. 14.10)**.

In the next stage, the white reflex is present, but the eye is red and painful. The pupil is dilated and fixed. There is a gross loss of vision.

In the next stage, the eye bulges forward (proptosis) with all the findings of the previous stage.

In the stage of metastasis, there are symptoms of involvement of other organs.

Differential Diagnosis of Retinoblastoma

These are the conditions that present with a white reflex in the pupillary area but are not retinoblastoma. Some of them cause blindness, but none cause death.

They are:
- Congenital cataract
- Traumatic cataract
- **Chronic iridocyclitis**
  - Exudate over the lens
  - Exudate behind the lens
- Retrolental fibroplasia
- Intraocular parasitic cyst

All cases with white reflex on the pupillary area should undergo following tests:
- Recording of vision
- Refraction under cycloplegia
- **Fundus examination by**
  - Direct ophthalmoscope
  - Indirect ophthalmoscope

Chapter 14: Disorders of Retina

- Ultrasonography
- CT and MRI

Treatment

In stage 1: White reflex without pain or redness is treated by removal of the eye by cutting the extraocular muscle and optic nerve without puncturing the globe. This process is called enucleation.

In stage 2: Eye is red and painful, treated by enucleation and chemotherapy.

In stage 3: When the tumor comes out of the globe. The condition is treated by chemotherapy and radiation. (Treatment by anticancer drug is called chemotherapy).

CHAPTER 15

Disorders of the Optic Nerve

The optic nerve, commonly referred to as the second cranial nerve, is actually not a true nerve. It is a tract that joins the retina to the brain and does not have a formed nucleus, which causes primary disorders of the brain and its covering effect on the optic nerve.

It is responsible for vision, color vision, field of vision, and contrast. It also carries pupillary fibers. The optic nerve joins the retina to the brain. The optic nerve is a backward extension of retinal ganglion cells, up to the chiasma. The ganglion cells in the retina are transparent and not visible with an ophthalmoscope. Once they reach the disc, they become medullated (myelinated), becoming white and visible by ophthalmoscope. The optic nerve is covered by the dura, arachnoid, and pia from the back of the globe to the optic foramen. The optic nerve constitutes the anterior part of the visual path. It is topographically divided into intrascleral, intraorbital, intracanalicular, and the part that joins the anterior horn of the chiasma. The optic chiasma contains fibers from the two eyes. From the posterior angle of the chiasma arises the optic tract, which ends in the lateral geniculate body. The remaining part fans out posteriorly, ending at the optic tract, and is called optic radiation.

The part of the optic nerve visible by the ophthalmoscope is called the optic nerve head, or optic papilla. The rest of the optic nerve is not visible with an ophthalmoscope and is called the retrobulbar optic nerve.

VISUAL PATH

The visual path starts from the head of the optic nerve up to the visual cortex; the part between the posterior angle of the chiasma and the lateral geniculate body is the optic tract, and the rest constitutes optic radiation. The visual path between the lateral geniculate body and the optic papilla contains both visual and pupillary fibers. Hence, lesions at this level will affect both the visual and pupillary reactions. The optic nerve gets its blood supply from the central retinal artery and pial plexus. In addition to this, the disc also gets blood from the ciliary circulation.

Disorders of the optic nerve can be congenital or acquired. The later can be seen at any age. The acquired disorders can either be hereditary or non-hereditary. The later are—inflammation (optic neuritis), trauma, vascular, and tumors. The swelling of the disc is a special entity that is partly vascular due to raised intracranial pressure and is called papilledema. The term optic atrophy refers to the end result of all disorders of the disc. Disorders of the part of the nerve beyond the globe are called retrobulbar lesions. Which are not visible by the ophthalmoscope. The most common lesion is retrobulbar optic neuritis. All the lesions from the disc to the cortex have some degree of diminished distant vision and characteristic field defects.

The field changes from the back of the globe to the optic radiation are shown in **Figure 15.1**.

Chapter 15: Disorders of the Optic Nerve

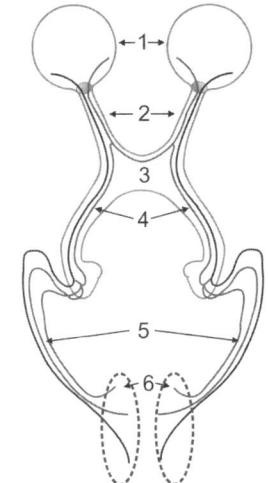

1. Papilloretinal lesion

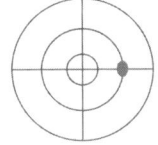 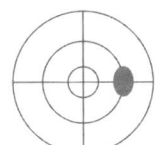 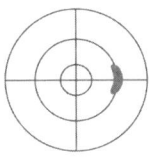 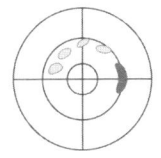

Normal blind spot   Enlarged blind spot   Seidel scotoma   Seidel scotoma with scattered in Bjerrum area

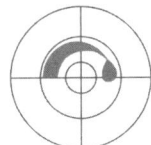 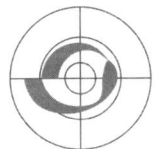 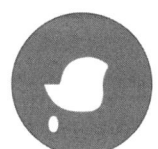

Bjerrum scotoma   Double Bjerrum scotoma with Roenne's step   Extensive scotoma with tubular vision and island of vision

2. Shows lesions in optic nerve

Lesion of left optic nerve

3. Shows mid chiasma lesion

Lesion of mind chiasma

4. Shows lesion in the optic tract

Lesion at posterior end of tract, LBG and anterior radiation

5. Shows lesion in the optic radiation

6. Shows lesion in the visual cortex

Sparing of macula lesion at posterior part of radiation

Fig. 15.1: Field changes at various levels of optic pathway.

The visual features of optic nerve disorders can include pupillary changes and visual changes. The pupillary changes are defective direct pupillary reactions and faulty indirect pupillary reactions. The term relative afferent pupillary defect is used to denote a pupillary reaction when one eye is exposed to light. It is caused by unilateral or asymmetrical disease in one retina or optic nerve up to the lateral geniculate body.

The visual features are diminished central vision, color vision, brightness, and defects in the central field. The optic nerve is best examined by a direct ophthalmoscope. Other instruments used are the indirect ophthalmoscope, Hruby lens, and 78 to +90D lens, fundus fluorescein angiography, and OCT. The ophthalmoscopic examination of the disc comprises its shape, size, border, color, optic cup, vessels, and new growths. The normal size of a disc is 1.82 mm; a normal disc is slightly larger vertically with a clear cut margin. With a light pink hue, the pink color is directly proportionate to the number of capillaries present; the fewer the capillaries, greater the pallor. The presence of hemorrhage or exudate is pathological. The optic cup is a depression in the midst of the disc. It is not always in the center of the disc. From the center of the cup arises the central retinal artery. The color of the cup is lighter than the rest of the disc, and the floor of the disc is like a saucer with a sieve-like bottom; it is called the lamina cribrosa. The color of the cup is light blue. The dots at the bottom represent the deficiency in the sclera, through which the optic nerve passes. Filling of the cup abnormal but not always pathological, i.e., in hypermetropia, pseudoneuritis, and aplasia of the disc. The cup is either very shallow or absent. The depth and elevation of the cup and disc substances are measured by a direct ophthalmoscope, slit lamp, and OCT.

The special methods used to see the funds are:
- Fundus fluorescein angiography
- **Ultrasonography:**
  - A scan
  - B scan
- **CT:** Computed tomography
- **MRI:** Magnetic resonance imaging
- **OCT:** Optical coherence tomography

The optic cup is obliterated in optic neuritis, papillitis pseudoneuritis, and drusen of the disc, high hypermetropia, and aplasia of the disc.

The causes of deep cupping are congenital coloboma of the disc, glaucoma, and high myopia.

The causes of the redness of the disc are:
- Inflammation of the disc (optic neuritis)
- Swollen disc (papilledema)
- A congenital anomaly (pseudoneuritis)
- New vessels on the disc, i.e., diabetic retinopathy
- Central retinal vein obstruction

The causes of pallor in the disc are:
- Anemia
- Optic atrophy
- Central retinal artery occlusion

Causes of swelling of the disc are:
The swollen disc that is also called a choked disc, where the surface of the disc is raised from the retinal surface, the cup is full, the lamina is not visible with blurred margin.

The causes of a swollen disc are:
- Papilledema

- Optic neuritis
- Pseudo-optic neuritis
- Drusen of the disc
- Tumors

Congenital Anomalies of the Disc

The common congenital anomalies of the disc are:
- Opaque nerve fiber
- Pseudoneuritis
- Hypoplasia of the optic disc
- Coloboma of the optic disc
- Drusen of the optic disc

Opaque Nerve Fibers

The ganglion cells that form the main bulk of the optic nerve are not myelinated; hence, they are not visible on ophthalmoscopy. The myelinations start in the intracranial part of the nerve, ending at the disc. If this process continues, some of the retinal fibers will also become myelinated and white. They are seen in patches most commonly at the edge of the disc in a flame shape with a base at the disc of varied shape and size. Rarely, they may be seen away from the disc. They are best visible by ophthalmoscope; when present near the disc, they cause enlargement of the blind spots on field examination. They are asymptomatic, discovered by routine ophthalmoscopy examination, and do not require any treatment.

Pseudoneuritis

All so referred to as pseudopapilledema, the anomaly is caused by the small posterior scleral foramina through which the fibers of the nerve pass. Actually, the passage is too narrow for a normal number of nerve fibers. This causes spilling of the fibers anteriorly, giving the appearance of a swollen disc. The margins are blood, and the cup is obliterated. The condition is generally confused with fully developed optic neuritis or early papilledema without any symptoms. The condition is diagnosed on routine fundus examinations. The condition is bilateral and, most of the time, symmetrical. The condition may be inherited as an autosomal trait. The eyes with pseudoneuritis are generally hypermetropes. The condition is stationary without any complications, not requiring any specific treatment except management of hypermetropia when present.

Hypoplasia of the Optic Disc

This congenital condition is less common than the two discussed above; in 75% of cases, the disorder is bilateral and seen equally in both sexes. The disc is very small due to the paucity of the substance of the nerve. It may be associated with other congenital anomalies of the disc, including diminished vision; the vision can be as low as perception of light to 6/6; and nystagmus is common. There is no specific treatment except correction of the error of refraction and prevention of amblyopia.

Coloboma of the Optic Disc

This rare congenital anomaly is generally associated with extensive uveoretinal coloboma; in less common cases, the coloboma is localised to the nerve, seen at the lower part of the disc. The condition is often mistaken for pathological myopia or an extreme degree of glaucomatous optic vision. The eyes have poor, uncorrectable vision. No specific treatment is available except correction of the error of refraction.

Drusen of the Optic Disc

Drusen of optic nerves are generally familial, without a clear-cut genetic preponderance. Many family members have asymptomatic drusen discovered or routine ophthalmoscope. Children with a family history of drusen optic nerve are ten times more likely to have the condition. The pathology behind the condition is not well understood, but the common theory is that it is an accumulation of protein particles to which calcium has been added. The combinations of the two form a spherical mass in the substance of the optic nerve. Which gradually extends to fill the optic cup and presents as pseudoneuritis/pseudopapilledema. The condition is diagnosed on routine fundus examinations without any visual impairment. There is no treatment required except a yearly examination, lest the child have real papilledema.

Hereditary Optic Neuropathies

Hereditary optic neuropathies are seen in all ages; some are more common in children and young adults, others exclusively in older persons. The most common hereditary optic neuropathy is a heredofamilial neuropathy called Leber's optic neuropathy, which starts between 15 and 25 years in healthy males with sudden painless, fast-deteriorating bilateral loss of vision. The condition starts in one eye to be followed by the other within a few weeks. The condition is generally confused with optic neuritis and treated as such. Generally, involvement of the optic nerve is associated with a defective pupillary reaction and is taken as an important sign of optic neuritis. In the case of Leber's optic neuropathy, the pupillary light reflex is retained till the condition has advanced. The disorder is a mitochondrial defect passed to a male child from an unaffected mother. There is no treatment for the condition the person inflicted, which is better managed by a visually handicapped person.

Inflammation of the Optic Nerve

Inflammation of the optic nerve is called optic neuritis, which could be infectious or non-infectious. Presently, the infectious causes have almost all been eliminated due to the advent of specific chemotherapy. The most common non-infectious cause is demyelination of the optic nerve. As seen in multiple sclerosis. The condition may be limited to the optic nerve or may be associated with myelitis. Which involves the spinal, called optic neuritis, can be acute, chronic, or recurrent. According to the part of the nerve involved, it is divided into papillitis and retrobulbar neuritis. In the first, the changes are visible on ophthalmoscopic examination and are associated with pupillary changes. In retrobulbar neuritis, the disc on ophthalmoscopy shows hardly any change. Papillitis is more common in young adults; in children, it may occur following immunisation against many organisms. It is more common following a viral infection than a bacterial one.

The clinical picture consists of:
- **Diminished distant vision:** The fall of vision follows a definite pattern that consists of a rapid fall of vision from normal to hand movement within an hour. The vision remains at this lower level for 10 to 15 days; the diminished vision is not correctable by glasses. After this period of low vision, the vision starts improving, and the vision may return to the previous level with the possibility of recurrence. After a few months, the time of recurrence gets shorter.
- Central, paracentral and centrocecal scotoma (**Fig. 15.2**)
- Tenderness of the globe

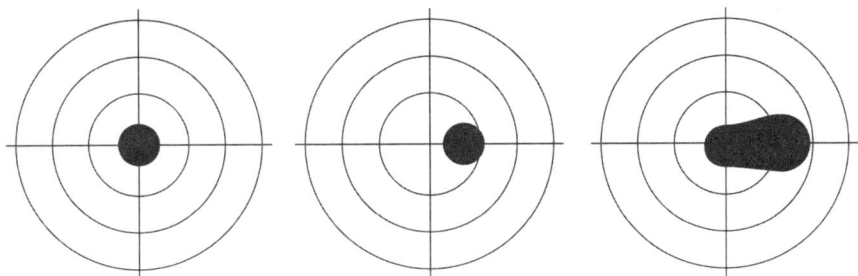

Fig. 15.2: Central, paracentral and centrocecal scotomas.

- Diminished color sense
- There is no redness or watering from the eye
- Moderately dilated sluggish pupil
- The real findings are seen in fundus examination. They consists of hyperemia of the disc, non-visualization of the lamina, filling of the cup, blurring of the disc margin, moderate swelling of the disc not more than +3D as seen on ophthalmoscope.

The exact cause of the disease is not well understood. In 30% of eyes, no cause can be found. The most common cause is suspected to be autoimmune disease. The systemic infections are no longer of any importance. Though some viral infections may be associated with optic neuritis, it is not uncommon to develop optic neuritis following a viral infection. Sometimes infection from the paranasal sinuses may be responsible for the disorders.

Treatment

- In 30% of cases, no cause can be detected. The condition may stop recurring after a few episodes without treatment.
- There is no specific treatment unless the person has definite evidence of an infectious disease, such as tuberculosis or syphilis. In such cases, the patients should get the complete recommended dose of a specific antibiotic for the prescribed period.
- Systemic steroids are the most common group of drugs used to treat optic neuritis. The result of steroid treatment is not always as good as expected. One advantage of steroid therapy is that it reduces severity, improves vision, and delays recurrence.

Retrobulbar Neuritis

Retrobulbar neuritis is an inflammation of the optic nerve that is not visible by an ophthalmoscope. The signs, symptoms, etiology and management of the condition are similar to those of papillitis.

Retrobulbar neuritis is rarely acute; it is more often chronic in nature.

Chronic Retrobulbar Neuritis

This is also called toxic amblyopia. This is due to the effects of external toxins and chemicals taken by the patient, i.e., alcohol and tobacco. Many drugs also cause chronic retrobulbar neuritis. The disease is most of the time due to the death of the ganglion cells in the retina and less commonly due to a direct effect on the optic nerve. The most common toxic substances are tobacco and alcohol. Both ethyl and methyl alcohols can cause retrobulbar neuritis. Methyl alcohol causes acute lesions of the retina and causes severe irreversible blindness and primary optic atrophy. Methyl alcohol poisoning can cause death as well. Ethyl alcohol, along with tobacco consumption, causes chronic retrobulbar neuritis. There is a gradual, painless loss of vision with a central scotoma in both eyes. There is no specific treatment. Stopping consumption of alcohol and tobacco may stop further progress.

Non-inflammatory Disorders of the Optic Nerve

The two conditions that need to be discussed are papilledema and optic atrophy.

Papilledema

Papilledema is also called a swollen or choked disc. It is a non-inflammatory, non-degenerative condition of the disc due to a rise in intracranial pressure. The intracranial pressure is the pressure of cerebrospinal fluid that is produced in the brain and circulates in the ventricles and round the spinal cord. It is an essential fluid. That is produced in the choroidal plexus of the ventricle and flows into the ventricles and subarachnoid space. The presumed function of the CSF is to provide protection to the brain, supply nutrition, and remove base products. It is constantly produced and absorbed to maintain a physiological pressure ranging between 200 and 250 mm of water.

The brain has three coverings—the dura arachnoid and pia. The spaces between them are respectively called subdural and subarachnoid spaces. The pia is firmly attached to the optic nerve; hence, there is no subpial space. The above two spaces are continuous around the optic nerve up to the back of the disc. The CSF circulates in these two spaces, and the pressure, when raised, reflects in these spaces. A raised subarachnoid presses the central retinal vein. It slows the venous flow backward, causing swelling of the disc. The most common cause of papilledema is space-occupying lesions. The most common among them is brain tumor; other causes are brain abscess, meningitis, and hypertension. The condition is painless without tenderness around the globe and without congestion. The patient may be symptomless or may have headaches, vomiting, and other neurological signs and symptoms. The most important findings seen on the ophthalmoscope include—hyperemia of the disc; swelling of the disc, which is more than +3D; obliteration of the cup; blurring of the margin; exudate and hemorrhage on the disc; and exudates over and round the macula. The vision remains fairly good until late. The causes of reduced vision are macular involvement and the progression of the edema to post-papilloedematous optic atrophy. Early papilledema should be differentiated from severe papillitis, pseudopapillitis, and drusen of the optic nerve head. The vision may improve by removing the cause through surgery. The blind spot is enlarged all round.

Optic Atrophy

Optic atrophy is the end result of damage to some of the fibers of the optic nerve, resulting in loss of vision and field changes. The loss of vision is a late feature; it ranges from mild to moderate to severe. The end result is the onset of secondary optic atrophy with complete loss of vision. The pathology consists of degeneration of optic nerve fibers with obliteration of the blood vessels, resulting in pallor of the disc that may just be mild pale to chalk white. The color of optic atrophy depends on the number of capillaries and fibrocytes present on the disc. Optic atrophy is never acute; it is always preceded by other intracranial or local causes, such as optic neuritis, retrobulbar neuritis, advanced glaucoma, and the end result of central retinal artery obstruction. The optic atrophy has been divided into the following types—primary, secondary, and glaucomatous.

Primary Optic Atrophy

Primary optic atrophy is generally bilateral, slow-progressing, painless, and associated with various grades of diminished vision. It can be unilateral following injury and obliteration of the central retinal artery. The most common cause of primary optic atrophy is neurosyphilis. The diagnosis is confirmed by fundus examination, which consists of a pale disc with visible lamina and a visible cup. The margin of the cup is sharp. The vessels are thin; there is no exudate or hemorrhage in the fundus. The overall prognosis is bad.

Secondary Optic Atrophy

If a cause can be found for the paleness of the disc, it is called secondary optic atrophy. The causes can include papilledema, optic neuritis, central retinal artery obstruction, and acute ischemic optic neuropathy*.

*Acute ischemic optic neuropathy

Acute ischemic optic neuropathy is seen generally in persons past sixty years with hypertension, arteriosclerosis, and diabetes; it generally begins in one eye, and the other eye may follow. The cause is obstruction of the posterior ciliary arteries. The onset is a painless, sudden loss of vision with a sectoral loss of the lower hemi field. There are two types, i.e., arteritic and non-arteritic. The former is diminished blood supply to the optic nerve without inflammation in the vessels, like systemic vasculitis or giant cell arteritis.

The **diagnosis** of secondary optic atrophy is based on fundus findings of the disc, retina, and choroid. The color of the disc is yellowish white, the lamina is not visible, and the cup has full and blurred margins. The vessels may have sheathing; no evidence of hemorrhages is seen in the fundus, which always has evidence of degeneration or healed hemorrhage. The prognosis is bad.

The term consecutive optic atrophy refers to inflammation or degeneration of the retina.

The common causes are—retinitis pigmentosa, choroidal dystrophy, and extensive choroiditis.

Glaucomatous Optic Atrophy

Glaucomatous optic atrophy follows prolonged, raised intraocular pressure. The condition is associated with loss of vision and field. The characteristic features of glaucomatous optic atrophy are a pale to chalky white disc with a deep cup almost filling the whole disc. The lamina is visible; the depth of the cup is increased, best seen in OCT. The vessels disappear under the edge of the cup, only to reappear at the border of the cup.

Tumor of the Optic Nerve

Any tissue of the optic nerve can be involved in new growth. The two common types of tumor of the optic nerve are glioma of the optic nerve and meningioma of the optic nerve.

Glioma of the Optic Nerve

Optic nerves glioma is seen in children and are unilateral, slow-growing, developing in the orbital part of the optic nerve, which generally grows forward, causing slow-progressing axial proptosis with gradual loss of vision. The loss of vision precedes the development of proptosis. When it grows backwards, it causes enlargement of the optic foramen. Which is visible on X-ray, the tumor can be seen on USG and CT. The treatment is best left to the neurosurgeon. The glioma does not change into malignancy.

Meningioma of the Optic Nerve

This is seen in persons over 50 years old, and it is more common in women. It arises from the meninges covering the optic cup; it is a slow-growing tumor that causes proptosis, which is preceded by loss of vision. There is a low level of satisfactory treatment. The tumor is non-malignant.

Trauma to the Optic Nerve

The optic nerve is well protected in the orbit from all sides by extraocular muscles, retrobulbar fat, and the optic bony canal. It lies loose in the orbit, so it can be stretched to some extent without harm.

The optic nerve can be injured by:
1. Direct trauma to the nerve by sharp, penetrating objects
2. Indirect trauma

Indirect trauma leads to stretching of the optic nerve, tearing of small vessels, obliterating supply to the optic nerve, and the formation of a hematoma of the optic nerve. These are associated with loss of vision and afferent pupillary reactions. It is difficult to treat an injury to the optic nerve.

16 CHAPTER

Glaucoma

Glaucoma is not a single disease of the eye; it is a syndrome complex, the main feature of which is raised intraocular pressure. About 2% of persons above 40 years of age in both sexes suffer from glaucoma of some type or another. It is one of the most common causes of blindness worldwide. The condition is treatable but not preventable, except for some secondary glaucoma. The treatment prevents further damage to the vision but fails to restore lost vision. Other features of glaucoma are diminished vision, field loss, glaucomatous optic atrophy, diminished vision in dim light, and ultimate blindness if not treated.

Raised intraocular pressure is the most important cause of glaucoma. It is better to recapitulate the applied anatomy and physiology related to glaucoma. The raised intraocular pressure damages the neuroretinal fibers and reduces blood supply to the optic nerve, the two causes of loss of field, glaucomatous cupping of the disc, and diminished vision.

APPLIED ANATOMY OF GLAUCOMA

The lens suspended between the iris and vitreous divides the eye into two chambers:
1. Aqueous chamber
2. Vitreous chamber

Aqueous Chamber

It is far smaller than the vitreous chamber and is responsible for the production, circulation, and absorption of aqueous. The aqueous chamber is divided into two unequal chambers, i.e., a large anterior chamber and a small posterior chamber by the iris. The two chambers communicate with each other through the pupil **(Fig. 16.1)**. Obstruction of the pupil disrupts this communication, preventing aqueous from passing from the posterior chamber to the anterior chamber and

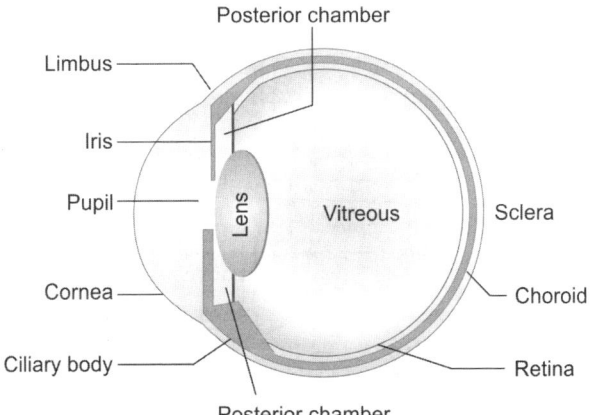

Fig. 16.1: Various chambers of the eye.

causing the accumulation of aqueous in the posterior chamber, leading to a narrowing of the angle of the anterior chamber and the rise of intraocular tension.

The anterior chamber is a planoconvex space bounded anteriorly by the posterior surface of the cornea and posteriorly by the iris and lens. In pathological conditions, such as aphakia, the lens is replaced by vitreous. In pseudophakia, it is replaced by a posterior chamber intraocular lens. The iris lens complex forms the posterior flat surface of the anterior chamber. The curvature of the cornea constitutes the convex anterior surface of the anterior chamber.

This makes the depth of the AC unequal. It is deepest in front of the pupil and almost absent at the periphery, i.e., the junction of the cornea and iris. The junction is called the angle of the anterior chamber. It is the most important structure related to glaucoma. The structure of the angle is complex. It contains tissues from the cornea, sclera, and iris. The angle is divided into trabecular meshwork that opens in Schlemm's canal and directly communicates with episcleral veins. In the eye without glaucoma, the peripheral cornea and iris form an angle of 45°. In some cases of glaucoma, it may be reduced to zero due to formation of adhesion of the iris to the cornea; this is called narrow-angle glaucoma. The angle left following such adhesion is called the pseudo-angle, which is always pathological. In aphakia and pseudophakia, the angle is wider than normal.

The anterior chamber is filled by a crystal-clear fluid called aqueous humor that is responsible for the intraocular pressure. The intraocular pressure is the lateral pressure exerted by the intraocular structure on the outer coat of the eye. The most important among them is aqueous humor. The others are the lens, vitreous, and choroid. The functions of the aqueous, besides maintaining intraocular tension, are—optical; it supplies nutrition to the lens; and it removes metabolic waste products. The aqueous forms in the ciliary epithelium, projecting into the posterior chamber at a constant rate. From the posterior chamber, the aqueous passes into the anterior chamber through the pupil and circulates in the anterior chamber, only to leave the chamber through the angle **(Fig. 16.2)**.

The rate of exit of aqueous is also at a constant rate, a little less than the rate of formation. Any obstruction in the outflow channel will raise intraocular pressure. Similarly, diminished production of aqueous causes a lowering of the intraocular pressure. About 90% of aqueous drains through trabecular meshwork; the remaining is via sclera; this channel is called the uveoscleral outflow channel.

The abnormal contents of the anterior chamber are hypopyon, hyphema, whole lens, cortical matter, nucleus, anterior chamber, IOL, anterior dislocated, posterior chamber IOL, parasitic cyst, parasite, and malignant cells.

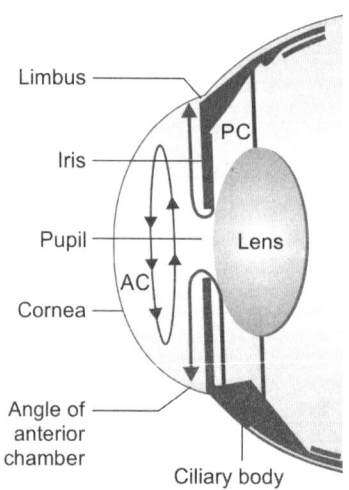

Fig. 16.2: Circulation of aqueous humor.

The anterior chamber is deep in—high myopia, buphthalmos, keratoconus, aphakia, and pseudophakia.

The anterior chamber is shallow in—high hypermetropia, nanophthalmos, pars plana, soft eye, and narrow-angle glaucoma.

APPLIED PHYSIOLOGY OF GLAUCOMA

Formation of Aqueous Humor

The formation, circulation, and exit of aqueous humor have been discussed in the paragraph above. The functions of the aqueous are:

- **Optical:** Aqueous, along with the cornea anteriorly and the lens posteriorly, form a single optical unit of +60D. Out of which +42D is due to cornea, +17D is due to lens, and the rest is due to aqueous.
- **Nutrition:** It supplied nutrition to the lens and cornea.
- **Intraocular pressure:** The aqueous solution creates a pressure higher than outside. This maintains the shape and firmness of the globe.
- It removes waste products from the eye.

The normal intraocular tension varies between 15.00 mm Hg to 20.00 mm Hg. A tension higher than 20.00 mm Hg is considered abnormal. The tension in two eyes is not equal; generally, one eye has 4–5 millimeters higher intraocular pressure in non-glaucomatous patients. A difference of >2 is strongly suggestive of glaucoma in the eye with raised intraocular tension. The tension in the eyes is not uniform during the day and night. A difference of more than 7.00 mm between day and night is suggestive of chronic simple glaucoma.

The two causes of raised intraocular pressure are glaucoma and ocular hypertension.

The intraocular tension is measured by a group of instruments called tonometers. Which can be indentation or applanation. The first example is the Schiotz tonometer, the most commonly used device to measure intraocular tension **(Fig. 16.3)**. It is a small, handy, and sturdy instrument that does not require any external illumination, can be dismantled and reassembled following cleaning, can be sterilized easily, and does not have a long learning curve. It indents the cornea; the indentation is directly proportionate to the intraocular tension. It is a relatively cheap instrument.

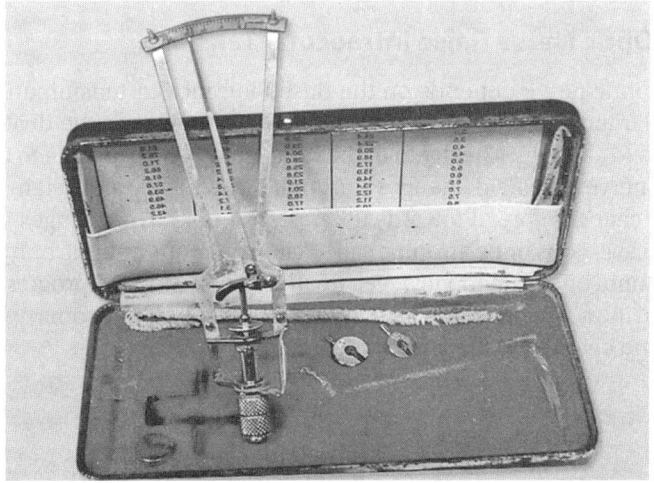

Fig. 16.3: Schiotz tonometer.

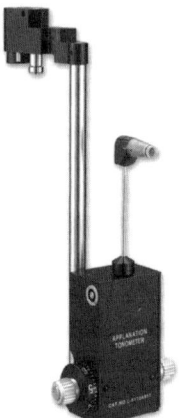

Fig. 16.4: Applanation tonometer.
(*Courtesy*: Appasamy associates)

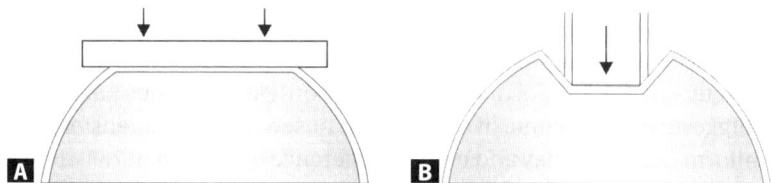

Figs. 16.5A and B: Principle of applanation and indentation tonometer:
(A) Applanation tonometry; (B) Indentation tonometry.

The **applanation tonometer** flattens the surface of the cornea, and the intraocular pressure is proportionate to the area flattening. It is expensive, and most of them require a slit lamp to make it work. It requires fluorescein to stain the tear film and a cobalt blue filter to visualise the stained cornea **(Fig. 16.4)**. It is difficult to sterilize, and the learning period is longer. The intraocular tension recorded by the applanation tonometer is not influenced by scleral rigidity, which is a disadvantage of the indentation tonometer. **Figures 16.5A and B** depict the difference between the principles of the applanation and indentation tonometers.

Changes in the Optic Nerve Raise Intraocular Tension

The change in the optic nerve depends on the raised intraocular tension and the duration of the raised intraocular tension. The raised intraocular tension causes the death of nerve fibers, leading to specific field changes. The death of the intraocular tension is due to diminished blood supply to the optic nerve. The field changes start on the periphery and retain good vision until late, when the field changes spread towards the posterior pole. The changes in the optic nerve are associated with cavernous optic atrophy, called glaucomatous optic atrophy. The vision once lost by glaucoma cannot be regained; however, treatment may stop the progress. The end results of persistently raised intraocular tension lead to a state of absolute glaucoma, which is associated with loss of vision and changes in the anterior segment.

GLAUCOMA

Glaucoma is a state of persistently raised intraocular tension that is not compatible with physiological tension. It is accompanied by field loss and glaucomatous optic atrophy. In the long run, vision is also proportionately lost. About 2% of adults of both sexes and all races suffer from some type of glaucoma.

It is difficult to classify glaucoma. The two most commonly used classifications are congenital and acquired glaucoma. Both of them can be primary or secondary. A glaucoma is said to be primary when no cause except raised intraocular tension with its train of changes is found. This is in contrast to secondary glaucoma, where there is a positive factor directly related to raised intraocular tension. The third classification depends on the width of the anterior chamber, i.e., wide-angle and narrow-angle glaucoma.

Ocular hypertension is an ill-defined, uncertain etiology where the only finding is a raised intraocular tension of long standing beyond physiological limits. It does not show changes in the disc and field. The vision when found to be less is due to pre-existing pathology, such as era of refraction and macular disorders. The condition is seen after 40 years of age, and it has been observed that a percentage of cases with ocular hypertension will convert into primary glaucoma. **Flowchart 16.1** shows various types of glaucoma.

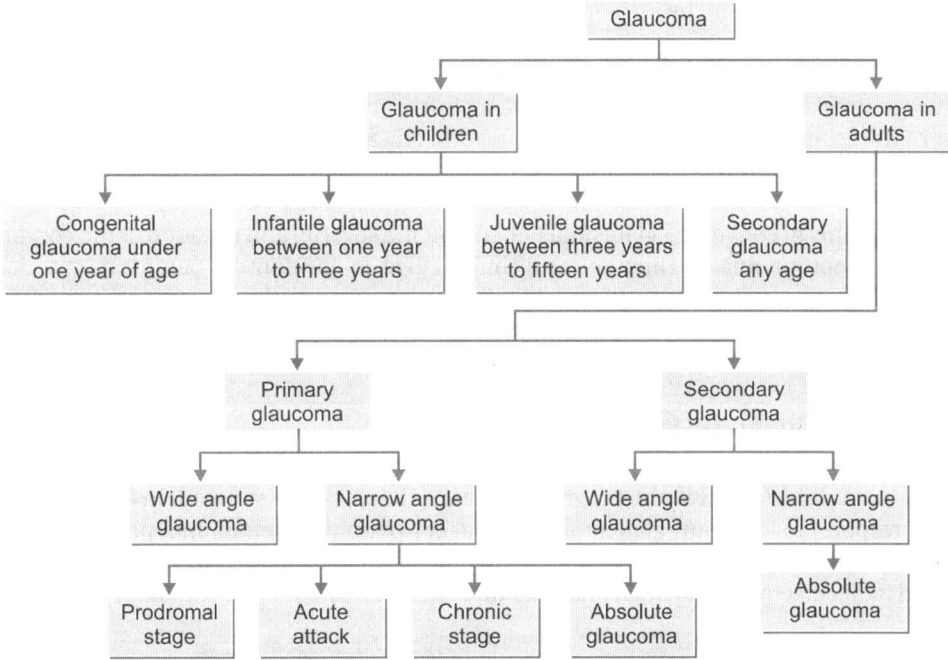

Flowchart 16.1: Various types of glaucoma.

Note: Absolute glaucoma: This is an end result of all glaucomas that results in very high intraocular tension with great loss of vision that may be as much as no perception. The eye shows prominent episcleral vessels, sometimes circumciliary congestion, an edematous cornea, and a fixed, dilated pupil that is invariably associated with complicated cataracts. The condition is painful, and there is no treatment to regain vision. Local and systemic anti-glaucoma drugs can lower the tension, resulting in diminished vision but not improved vision. Surgical treatments are not always successful.

Congenital Glaucoma

Conjunctival glaucoma is a rare but severe condition that may lead to legal blindness even with treatment unless managed before extensive damage has taken place. Due to the all-round expansion of the globe, it is also called buphthalmos. It can be unilateral or bilateral; the latter is more common than the former, when bilateral asymmetry is common. As per the age of development of glaucoma, it can be intrauterine, detected in the first year, or infantile, seen between 1 and 3 years. Glaucoma detected between three and fifteen years old is called juvenile glaucoma.

In the intrauterine type, the disease starts in the uterus with enlargement of the eye and a defect in the outflow facility, causing a rise in tension. Such cases have as high an incidence as 25% of all congenital glaucoma. In the rest of the cases, the presence of the disorders is felt between 1 and 3 years; beyond 3 years and under 15 years, the condition is referred to as juvenile glaucoma, which is more akin to adult chronic simple glaucoma than classical congenital glaucoma. The exact mechanism of production of congenial glaucoma is not well stabilized.

Primary congenital glaucoma is the result of isolated abnormal development of the anterior chamber angle structures.

The most commonly accepted theory is the maldevelopment of the anterior chamber and trabecular meshwork. The eye with congenitally raised intraocular pressure has the following characteristics—the globe is enlarged in all dimensions, including the cornea. The size of the cornea, >13.00 mm, may be as large as 16.00 mm in very advanced cases. The cornea is relatively thin, edematous, and may show bullae on the surface. The anterior chamber is deep, and the pupil is large and sluggish. The intraocular pressure as measured by the applanation tonometer under general anesthesia is >30.00 mm Hg and may be as high as 60.00 mm Hg. The cause of haziness in the cornea is a rupture in the Descemet membrane. The ruptured lines, when healed, leave white streaks called Haab's striae, which are horizontally placed curved lines mostly in the center of the cornea. The similar striae placed vertically are due to the birth stroma. The optic nerve shows glaucomatous optic atrophy. All the above factors lead to painful, diminished vision.

The symptoms of congenital glaucoma depend on the severity and duration of the condition. It consists of photophobia, lacrimation, and conjunctival congestion; the parents may notice an enlarged, hazy cornea **(Fig. 16.6)**. The vision cannot be tested in the early months; by the first year, the mothers realised that the child's vision is less than expected. The child is irritable and likes to stay in dim light.

Treatment of Congenital Glaucoma

Management is difficult and less rewarding, but it is logical that if the tension is lowered and kept under physiological level, the progress of the condition can be stopped. In fact, the tension does not respond to local anti-glaucoma drops; acetazolamide given in therapeutic doses may reduce the tension but cannot be used for a long time. The best treatment available is surgical. The usual trabeculectomy has a high rate of failure. The artificial glaucoma drainage device gadget

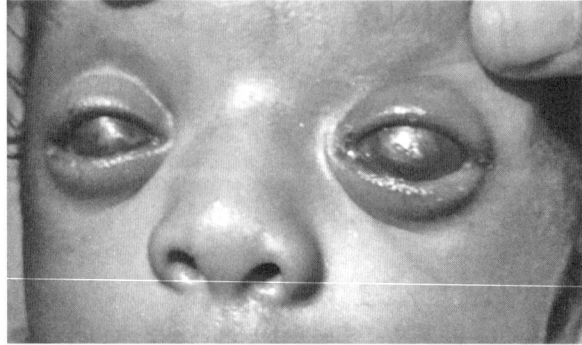

Fig. 16.6: Bilateral advanced congenital glaucoma.
(Courtesy: Dr ML Garg)

has a better result. In spite of controlled tension, the child is left with permanent diminished vision, which makes the child visually handicapped and requires suitable rehabilitation.

Glaucoma in Adults

Glaucoma in adults amount for 2% of irreversible loss of vision worldwide; the incidence of glaucoma increases with age. It is generally bilaterally equal in both sexes; the glaucoma is said to be primary if no cause is detected in the eye that could be held responsible for raised intraocular tension. Glaucomas with detectable causes are called secondary glaucomas. The incidence of secondary glaucoma is higher than that of primary glaucoma.

The glaucoma in adults has been put into two groups depending on the gonioscopic appearance of the angle. Glaucoma with an angle more than 40° is called wide-angle or chronic simple glaucoma. A glaucoma with an angle less than 20° is called a narrow angle. The narrow-angle glaucoma can either have an acute attack or may have a subacute course.

CHRONIC SIMPLE GLAUCOMA (WIDE-ANGLE GLAUCOMA)

Chronic simple glaucoma does not have any symptoms for years; it develops so slowly that a patient is not aware of its presence. The eye with chronic simple glaucoma does neither have redness, watering, or colored halos. By the time patients realise its presence, the condition has much progressed, causing loss of peripheral field and uncorrectable vision. Patients with peripheral loss may complain that they have to move their heads horizontally to see things approaching from the side. He may find difficulty in dim vision. The condition at this stage may be mistaken as age-related cataracts by non-ophthalmic attendants. Age-related cataracts are a common accompaniment of chronic simple glaucoma. This fact is important because vision loss due to cataracts is reversible following modern surgery, while vision lost due to chronic simple glaucoma is irreversible.

Symptoms

The symptoms of chronic simple glaucoma are deceptive; they may be present for quite some time without patients realizing their presence. Frequent changes of glasses in a non-diabetic without any opacity may bring the patient for examination, and on examination, he may have:
- Externally normal eye except slight sluggishness pupil
- On fundus examination, even with an undilated pupil, the fundus shows a large, pale cup with a notch at the lower pole of the neuroretinal rim.
- An estimation of intraocular pressure reveals it to be in the range of 30.00 mm or above.
- The field shows various stages of glaucomatous change.

Signs

The following are the signs of chronic simple glaucoma, which may be mild enough to be missed as errors of refraction and age-related cataracts. The first sign to be noticed is a relatively large bilaterally sluggish pupil. The other signs are:
- Diminished, distant vision is not corrected by glasses.
- Faulty projection of light—this is a late feature.
- Normal anterior chamber
- Raised intraocular pressure
- Normal gonioscopic appearance

❖ Glaucomatous fundus changes: They may be as mild as an enlarge cup to fully developed glaucomatous optic atrophy.
❖ Progressive loss of peripheral field
❖ Positive diurnal variation of intraocular tension
❖ Positive provocative test for glaucoma

The angle of the anterior chamber is examined by an instrument called a gonioscope. The normal angle of the anterior chamber is not visible by oblique illumination or a slit lamp because the ray arising from the angles fails to exit the eye through the cornea. The corneas, due to their curvature, reflect the ray to the other side **(Figs. 16.7A to C)**. The light arising from the angle can be diverted only if the cornea is eliminated from the refractive component. This can be achieved by two methods, i.e., direct and indirect. The indirect method is used more frequently as an office procedure, while the direct method is used mostly in the operating room with the child under anesthesia.

The differences between the two types of gonioscope are given in **Table 16.1**.

The disadvantage of the indirect ophthalmoscope is that it is upside down, i.e., the upper angle is imaged at the lower part of the field. Both types of gonioscopes have various types for different uses. The most popular indirect gonioscope is the Goldmann gonioscope, i.e., available as a single-mirror or three-mirror gonioscope. The three-mirror Goldmann gonioscope has not only mirrors to examine the angle but also the ciliary body and peripheral retina. In addition to three mirrors, it has a minus lens that partly neutralises the corneal refractive power and provides an upright picture of the posterior pole.

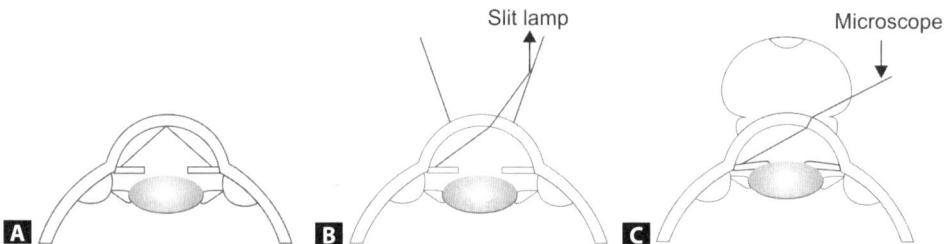

Figs. 16.7A to C: Corneas and their curvature. (A) Rays arising from one angle are reflected to their opposite side without going out of the eye; (B) Optic or indirect gonioscope where a ray from an angle exits the cornea to reach a suitably placed and angled plane mirror or a prism to direct the ray towards the slit lamp; (C) Path of rays in a direct gonioscope. The rays arising from angle instead of reaching the opposite angle as in Figure A, exit out of the cornea due to the combined action of the tear film and direct gonio lens to be picked up by the operating microscope.

Table 16.1: Indirect and direct gonioscope.

Feature	Indirect	Direct
Position of the patients	Sitting	Supine
Viewing system	Slit lamp microscope	Operating or handheld microscope
Source of light	Slit lamp	Fiberoptic Berken light
Image	Inverted image of angle; both eyes cannot be examined	Panoramic, erect; both eyes can be examined at a time
Indentation gonioscopy	Possible	Not possible
Use in surgery	Not possible	Possible

Ophthalmoscopy in Chronic Simple Glaucoma

Glaucoma per se does not cause opacity in the media. The specific changes are seen in the optic disc and blood vessels. The fundus is best seen with a direct ophthalmoscope that gives a magnification of 15 times. **Figures 16.7A to C** show gradual fundus changes in chronic simple glaucoma. **Figure 16.7A** represents a normal disc and cup disc ratio of 0.3, while **Figure 16.7B** shows an advanced glaucomatous cupping nasal shift of blood vessels and a cup disc ratio >0.6. **Figure 16.7C** shows fundus changes in absolute glaucoma where the cup almost fills the whole of the rim of the cup, the cup is very deep and chalky white, and the vessels disappear at the edge of the overhanging margin only to reappear at the border of the disc. The glaucoma does neither not produce any change in the caliber of the vessels nor any hemorrhage or exudate. The macula is not affected. The peripheral retina is normal.

The fundus changes in chronic simple glaucoma are as follows—the changes involve both disc and neuroretinal fibers (**Figs. 16.8A to E**), show various progressive fundus changes in chronic simple glaucoma. **Figure 16.8A** shows a normal disc, **Figure 16.8B** shows a notch at the lower pole, **Figure 16.8C** shows vertical enlargement of the cup, **Figure 16.8D** shows enlargement of the disc in advanced chronic simple glaucoma, and **Figure 16.8E** shows fundus changes in absolute glaucoma with the disappearance of vessels at the cup margin.

Field Changes

Field changes **(Fig. 16.9)** in chronic simple glaucoma are characteristic. They begin with vertical enlargement of the blind spot, followed by scattered scotomas in the Bjerrum area, followed by

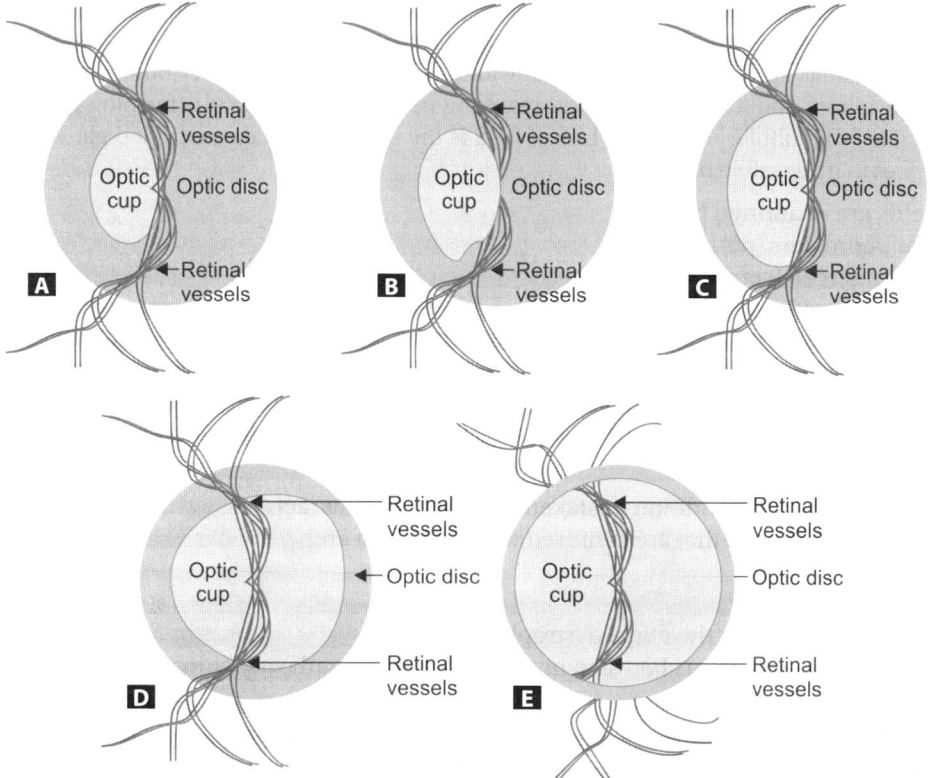

Figs. 16.8A to E: Various types of glaucomatous disc changes in chronic simple glaucoma.

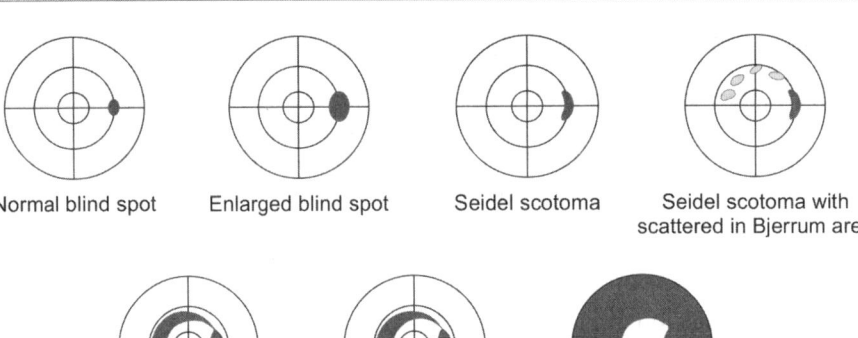
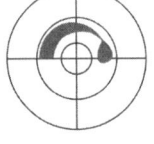
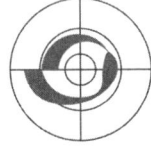
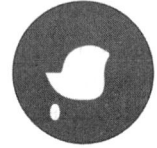

Fig. 16.9: Various stages of field changes in chronic simple glaucoma.

more scotomas and a change in the disc that assumes the shape of a bean with concavity towards the center, called the Seidel scotoma. The next change comprises the Bjerrum scotoma, which fans above the point of fixation with a narrow area on the Seidel scotoma and a wide area on the horizontal raphe and is called the Bjerrum scotoma. It is seen in the above part of the disc. A similar scotoma in the lower half is called a double scotoma. The end of the scotomas forms a step at the horizontal raphe, called Roenne's step. The progress of the scotoma is directly proportionate to the loss of nerve fibers, which in turn depends on raised intraocular pressure. The higher and longer the intraocular pressure, the more the field changes. The circular field caused by double arcuate scotomas spreads both peripherally and centrally, with the outer border reaching the retinal periphery and the central border reaching up to 5° of the macula, forming an island of vision called the tubular field. Total loss of field is the end result of uncontrolled glaucoma that terminates in irreversible blindness.

The fields are examined by:
- Lister perimeters (peripheral)
- Bjerrum screen (central 30°)
- Automated perimeter for both

Note: The Amsler grid is not used in charting glaucomatous field loss. They are used to chart the details of the central field and the presence of metamorphopsia in macular and optic nerve disorders.

Differential Diagnosis

- The most common condition mistaken for immature cataracts
- The other conditions that are confused with glaucoma are:
  - High myopia
  - Pale disc
  - Field changes in early retinal dystrophy

The differentiating points between immature cataracts and early chronic simple glaucoma are as follows:

The points in favor of immature cataracts are:
- Both brisk direct and indirect pupillary reactions.
- Normal intraocular pressure

- Negative diurnal variation
- Normal disc
- Normal cup-disc ratio
- No field changes

There is no treatment to cure chronic simple glaucoma. The treatments used are only to alleviate the condition and stop its progression. Vision loss due to glaucoma is irreversible, in spite of the best treatment, which may be medical or surgical. There is no prophylaxis against chronic simple glaucoma. The best method to avoid it is to raise awareness about the disease.

Awareness

- All persons above 40 years of age should get a complete ocular checkup, including recording of tension and examination of the disc, every year.
- Enquire about the possibility of glaucoma in parents and siblings.
- Enquire about the use of steroids for a long time.
- Getting far and near correction tested every year with suitable changes
- Checking intraocular tension every six months with an applanation tonometer is more important with a positive family history.
- Persons with high myopia and diabetes are more prone to develop chronic simple glaucoma.
- Complete an ocular checkup, including a fundus examination, every six months.

Note: If any of the above points are positive, the patient should undergo a detailed fundus examination in an automated perimeter and get an OCT of the disc done.

Predisposing Factors in Chronic Simple Glaucoma

- Positive family history
- High myopia
- Diabetes
- Patients on prolonged steroid, local or systemic
- Forgotten blunt injury to the eye.

Treatment

- Can either be medical or surgical.
- Most of the time, the tension can be kept under control with drugs. They are put into three broad groups:

1. That decrease the secretion of aqueous under these groups come oral drugs belonging to carbonic anhydrase inhibitors, such as acetazolamide (oral or local), beta-blockers, and alpha-2-agonists.
2. The drugs that increase the outflow of aqueous are miotics and beta-blockers. The only miotic presently used is pilocarpine 2% drop, two to three drops daily. The disadvantage of this drug is that it causes drug-induced miosis. The beta-blockers do not change the size of the pupil. Many times, both drugs are used in combination as they enhance each other's effects.
3. **Prostaglandin analogues:** They increase uveoscleral outflow. The usual dose is 0.005%, once every 24 hours.

In advanced cases, multi-drug therapy may be required. Oral anti-glaucoma drugs are generally kept reserved for tension more than 40.00 mm Hg, and that too for not more than 10 days at a stretch. The drugs require good compliance. Patients in underdeveloped countries may not be able to afford life-long, costly treatment. They would opt for a one-time surgical procedure.

The main principle of surgery is to create a permanent drainage passage by passing the trabecular meshwork. Modern surgery is a microsurgical procedure done under a binocular operating microscope. The most common surgery performed is a trabeculotomy. Lasers used for the same purpose have a limited role.

GLAUCOMA SUSPECT

The following persons are likely to develop chronic simple glaucoma:
- Above 40 years of age in both sexes
- Positive family history
- Myopic
- Diabetic
- Prolonged steroid use in any form
- Ocular hypertension (the conversion rate is 1% every year)
- Blunt trauma

Narrow-angle Glaucoma (Acute Congested Glaucoma)

Narrow-angle glaucoma is less common than wide-angle glaucoma. Previously, it was thought to be 25% of all glaucoma cases; with the advent of better instruments, more causes are being attributed to narrow-angle glaucoma than in the past. It is a worldwide disorder, more common in females, starting earlier than chronic simple glaucoma. It is more common in hypermetropic eyes, eyes with a corneal diameter >10.00 mm and an inherent shallow anterior chamber. Hypermetropic eyes are more prone to develop narrow-angle glaucoma.

The condition is always symptomatic, starting with the prodrome of colored halos around lights. It has been divided into the following stages—prodromal stage, stage of constant instability, acute attack, chronic stage, and absolute glaucoma. The other classification depends on the gonioscopic appearance of the angle of the anterior chamber. If the trabecular meshwork is not visible, it is called narrow-angle glaucoma.

The next classification is based on the degree of closure of the angle; if it is completely closed, it presents as an acute attack; partial closure is called subacute narrow angle glaucoma. which passes off without any treatment. The patients may experience milder symptoms of acute attack, such as colored halo, circumciliary congestion, and headache. The other division of narrow-angle glaucoma is obstructable angle and non-obstructable angle. The most clinically significant classification is gonioscopic grading of angle. The grades are given in **Table 16.2**.

Grade	Clinical feature
Grade 0	(0°) is a closed angle due to iridocorneal contact
Grade 1	(10°) is a very narrow angle in which only Schwalbe's line is visible. The condition is at risk or going into acute attack
Grade 2	(20°) is a moderately narrow angle in which only the trabeculum is visible without possibility of complete closure
Grade 3	(25–35°) is an open angle in which the scleral spur is visible, not capable of closure
Grade 4	(35–45°) is the widest angle where ciliary body is visible common in high myopia and aphakia. The condition is incapable of closure with dilatation of pupil

Table 16.2: Various grades of gonioscopic appearance in narrow-angle glaucoma.

Clinical Features of Narrow-angle Glaucoma

Prodromal Stage

In this stage, the most striking feature is seeing colored halos round artificial light and the moon. The patients may have a mild headache, circumciliary congestion, and watering. The phenomenon happens mostly in the evening, while doing near work for hours or staying in a semi-dark area, such as a cinema hall. The halos disappear as the patient stops near work or steps out of a semi-dark area. The episodes are repeated with irregular intervals. The patient remains symptomless in between attacks. As days pass, the incidence increases with a shorter interval until an acute attack sets in.

Stage of the Acute Attack

This is a sudden episode that may/may not follow the prodromal stage. In this stage, there is a rapid loss of vision, copious watering, redness, headache, and pain in the eye. Examination at this stage shows patients in pain with swollen lids, congested conjunctiva, hazy cornea, shallow anterior chamber, sluggish vertically oval pupil, and high tension. The fundus is not visible; the pain is so intense that the patient seeks medical help. The condition should be differentiated from (**Table 16.3**) all cases of acute congested eyes with/without diminished vision.

Management of the acute stage consists of:
1. Oral analgesics are taken three times a day to relieve pain.
2. **Acetazolamide tablet**: Two tablets twice a day. Acetazolamide reduces intraocular pressure by decreasing the formation of aqueous solutions. This prevents further damage. The drug

Table 16.3: Conditions that should be differentiated.

	Acute congestive glaucoma	Acute iritis	Acute conjunctivitis
Age	Generally over 40 years	Any age	Any age, from neonate to old age
Sex	More common in females	Equal in males and females	Equal in males and females
Onset	Sudden, within one to two hours	Gradual, within eight to ten hours	Gradual, within eight to ten hours
Laterality	Generally unilateral	Generally unilateral	Bilateral mostly
Pain	Severe	Dull	Foreign body sensation
Vision	Very low	Normal or slightly low	Normal
Tenderness	+	++	–
Circumciliary congestion	+++	++	–
Cornea	Hazy	Keratic precipitate ++	Bright
AC	Very shallow	Normal	Normal
Pupil	Semi-dilated, sluggish	Constricted, irregular, sluggish	Normal
Tension	High	Normal or low	Normal

acts by blocking the carbonic anhydrase enzyme, which is essential for the production of aqueous solutions. It is also available as a local drop. However, there are reports that acetazolamide taken orally worsens the condition because it is presumed that the edematous ciliary body rotates forward, which reduces the angle width.
3. If tension does not lower with oral acetazolamide, the next step is to start intravenous mannitol.
4. Frequent installation of 2% pilocarpine eye drops to constrict the pupil
5. There is a tendency to use beta blockers, alpha-2 agonists, prostaglandin analogues, and local carbonic anhydrase inhibitors along with pilocarpine.
6. Local corticosteroid drops; this does not have any effect on intraocular pressure or the size of the pupil. The main function of steroids is to control associated inflammation of the iris secondary to raised intraocular pressure.
7. If the condition does not improve within 3 days with medical treatment, the eye should be subjected to a laser iridotomy.
8. The signs of improvement are a reduction in pain, lacrimation, and redness; a bright central cornea; improved vision; and lowered intraocular pressure.
9. The patients should be followed every three months and evaluated for pressure and angle width.

Chronic Congestive Stage

This happens if the tension has not been brought to a lower level or has failed to be lowered. This also happens following the discontinuation of anti-glaucoma treatment following an acute attack. All eyes following an acute attack should be put on any of the following drugs for months until a definitive laser iridotomy has been performed. The drugs are beta blockers, alpha-2 agonists, prostaglandin analogues, and local carbonic anhydrase inhibitors.

On examination, the eye in the chronic congestive stage has lowered vision, which is better than during an acute attack but not normal. The eye has circumciliary congestion; the anterior chamber remains shallow with a semi-dilated, sluggish pupil. The tension remains moderately high. The funds, when visible, show glaucomatous changes with corresponding field losses. The definitive treatment is a trabeculectomy.

Stage of Absolute Glaucoma

Absolute glaucoma is the end result of all glaucomas, primary or secondary, which may be congenital or acquired. The eye is not only blind but also painful, with very high tension. The eye has circumciliary congestion round the cornea and prominent episcleral vessels. The cornea may show bullous keratitis, superficial vascularization, and band keratopathy, which is more frequent in congenital glaucoma. The corneal sensation is reduced, and the eye may develop an indolent ulcer. In the long run, the eye may develop ciliary and intercalary staphylomas, which are more frequent in buphthalmos. The condition does not respond to medical or surgical treatment. Retrobulbar injections of absolute alcohol may give a short-term respite. Enucleation of the eye is the ultimate relief.

Secondary Glaucoma

Secondary glaucoma constitutes a large group of eyes with raised intraocular tension, the common factors being changes in the angle. The angle is generally absent or very narrow in most of the cases except steroid-induced, post-traumatic, and aphakia. They are seen in all ages, right from infancy to old age. Glaucoma generally presents as a chronic rise in tension or is rarely

acute. They may not only have trabecular block but also pupillary block. The condition may be overshadowed by primary causes, such as anterior uveitis and lens-induced glaucoma. The following are common causes of secondary glaucoma:
- Lens
- Injury
- Steroid
- Uveitis
- Neovascularization
- Malignant glaucoma

Lenses can cause glaucoma in the following ways:
- **Congenital:**
  - Microphakia
  - Spherophakia. The lens is, such as a small ball that closes the pupil, pushing the iris forward, and closing the angle.
  - Dislocation of the lens and subluxation of the lens.
- **Cataract:**
  - Change in the size of the lens. Intumescent cataract (swollen). This can happen in senile cataracts and traumatic cataracts.
  - Leak of cortex. The cortical matter blocking the angle.
  - Allergy to cortical matter resulting in severe iridocyclitis and rise of tension.
- Aphakia and pseudophakia

Traumatic Glaucoma

This occurs more commonly with blunt injuries. Tension may rise within a few days due to the following causes:
- Swollen lens
- Dislocated lens, blocking the pupil, or obstructing the angle
- Cortical matter blocking the angle
- A large hyphema in the anterior chamber blocks the angle of the anterior chamber.

The management of lens-induced glaucoma is surgical. The aim should be to remove as much cortical material as possible, managing the vitreous when it prolapses in the anterior chamber.

In the second type, the tension rises weeks to months after a blunt injury. The anterior chamber is deeper on the side of the injury. The angle is damaged. The condition is called a recession of the angle. This is best seen on gonioscopy. The management is generally medical.

Steroid-induced Glaucoma

This type of glaucoma has been very common in persons on local steroids for a long time. It is more severe in children. The children who developed steroid-induced glaucoma are those being treated for vernal catarrh and following the removal of congenital cataracts. Glaucoma is wide-angle glaucoma. Wide-angle glaucoma may be associated with the steroid-induced cataract. The tension generally comes down to normal after stopping the steroid, leaving an already damaged disc and a loss of field. Otherwise, the patients may have to be put on anti-glaucoma drops and monitored for rises in intraocular tension, disc, and field changes. These children are prone to going into the stage of primary open-angle glaucoma in later life. Hence, all children under prolonged steroid use should be monitored for the chance of developing glaucoma.

Uveitis-induced Glaucoma

About 10% of all eyes suffering from acute or chronic anterior uveitis are likely to develop secondary glaucoma. There are three modes of developing glaucoma following or during anterior uveitis. They could be both open-angle or narrow-angle glaucoma. The third type is steroid-induced. The wide-angle glaucoma in iridocyclitis may be present as an acute episode or a chronic sequel. The rise in tension is due to acute inflammation of the trabecular meshwork, the deposit of inflammatory cells in the trabecular meshwork, or scarring of the angle. The cause of close-angle glaucoma may either be pupillary block or angle closure.

The treatment is surgical after the eye has been free of inflammation for at least three months.

Neovascular Glaucoma

With an increase in the incidence of diabetic retinopathy, the glaucoma produced due to neovascularization is showing an upward swing. In contrast to uveitis-induced glaucoma, where the pathology lies in the iris, the cause of neovascularization in the retina is from where the new vessels grow on the surface of the iris, reaching the angle. The two common causes of neovascular glaucoma are proliferative diabetic retinopathy and central retinal vein obstruction.

The treatment of neovascular glaucoma is difficult; it generally gets worsened by the use of miotics. The present trend of treatment is the use of cycloplegic along with steroids; beta-blockers and other anti-glaucoma drugs are not very effective. Administration of oral acetazolamide gives temporary relief. The treatment of choice is pan-retinal photocoagulation. The results of which too is unsatisfactory.

Malignant Glaucoma

The term malignant glaucoma is a misnomer because malignancy does not cause this type of glaucoma. It is better to call it aqueous misdirected syndrome. The disorder develops following many intraocular surgeries, which may include simple lens extraction, pseudophakia, or fishtulizing surgery. There is a history of intraocular surgery in the recent past, with the patient complaining of unexplained pain, watering, and diminished vision. The mechanism consists of a blockage of normal aqueous flow due to a blockage in the ciliary body, lens, and vitreous complex. The aqueous, instead of finding its way into the angle, seeped backward in the vitreous, expending the vitreous all round. Resulting in extreme shallowing of the anterior chamber with a fast rise in intraocular pressure. The treatment is difficult and consists of dilatation of the pupil by a strong cycloplegic instillation of a strong steroid and the administration of a systemic ocular hypotensive. If all these fail, the treatment is extensive vitrectomy.

17 CHAPTER

Squint

INTRODUCTION

Squint is one of the most common disorders of the eyes seen in all races the world over. In both sexes, it may be present from birth (rare congenital) to ripe old age. It is mostly seen in children; adults may continue to have squint if it has not been corrected in childhood. The other mode of presentation in adults is paralysis of the extraocular muscle. The non-paralytic squint is either unilateral or alternate; the bilateral squint is rare and generally seen as a congenital malformation. The squint is defined as the malalignment of one of the visual axes in relation to the other. The non-squinting eye is called the fixing eye, and the other is the squinting eye. The visual axes of the two eyes are parallel to each other in all directions of movement of the eye, except in convergence and divergence. A slight divergence between the two eyes is physiological and called the position of rest, without any clinical significance.

To understand squint, it is better to understand the following commonly used terms:

Orthophoria

This is a physiological, ideal position of the eyes in relation to each other; such as all physiological states, it is a rarity. The eyes are parallel without fixation when looking at a distant object; in convergence, the two eyes move nasally to the same degree; this is also physiological. The orthophoric eyes do not move under cover.

Heterophoria

Heterophoria is a pathological condition where the two visual axes of the eyes are not directed towards the point of fixation when the fusion is broken. It is divided into the following groups—esophoria is the inward turning of the eye under cover, and exophoria is the outward turning of the eye under the same conditions. Hyperphoria is the upward shift of one eye. The term hypophoria is no more in vogue. Cyclophoria, which is turning in or out of the eyeball in the anteroposterior axis, is rarest and most difficult to test.

Heterotropia

In simple terms, heterotropia is a visible squint; it is also known as lazy eye or crossed eye. As per the direction of the deviating eye, the squint may be called esotropic when one eye turns in and the other eye fixes. Similarly, exotropia means outward deviation, while hypertropia means upward deviation **(Fig. 17.1)**.

The terms used in the movement of the eyes.

Duction

This denotes uniocular movement and consists of adduction, abduction, supraduction, infraduction, and cycloduction.

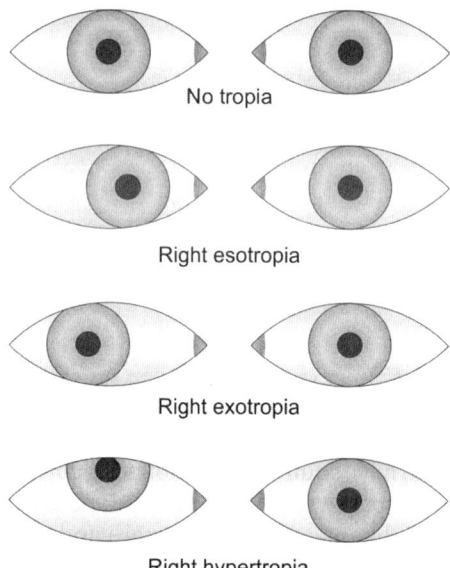

Fig. 17.1: Various types of tropias.

Version

Version is binocular movement when the two eyes move simultaneously, synchronously, and symmetrically in the same direction **(Fig. 17.2)**. They are:
- Dextroversion (right-gaze)
- Levoversion (left-gaze)
- Supraversion (up-gaze)
- Infraversion (down-gaze)

The above are secondary position of gazes
- Dextrodepression (gaze-up and right)
- Dextrodepression (gaze-down and right)
- Levoelevation (gaze-up and left)
- Levodepression (gaze-down and left)

The above are oblique movements called tertiary gazes.

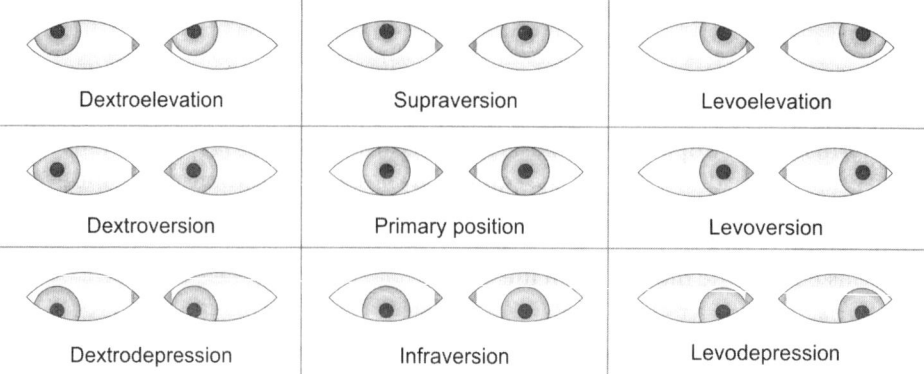

Fig. 17.2: Various position of version in cardinal gazes.

Chapter 17: Squint

Vergences

These are binocular movements that shift the eye in the opposite direction at the same time and are symmetrical. They are convergence and divergence.

Agonist, Antagonist and Synergist Muscles

Agonists are the main muscles that move the eye in any direction.

Antagonists are the muscles that act in the opposite direction of the agonist. When a person looks right, the right lateral rectus acts as the agonist, and the right medial rectus and left lateral rectus are the antagonists.

Synergist muscles are those muscles that act along with agonists.

Binocular Single Vision

This is one of the most important faculties of vision to produce a single image of the object seen by each eye separately. The following features must be present to have binocular single vision:
- Sharp image on the macula.
- Coordinated movement of both eyes in all directions.
- The brain should be able to superimpose two identical pictures into one.
- The result of the absence of binocular single vision is diplopia. The brain tries to overcome this by: suppression, amblyopia, and deviation.
- The binocular single vision is not present at birth. It develops between 12 to 16 weeks after birth.

The advantages of binocular single vision are:
- Increase in field of vision.
- It compensates for the two blind spots.
- Binocular single vision is more than uniocular vision.
- It creates depth with stereopsis.

Grades of binocular vision **(Figs. 17.3A to C)** show different grades of binocular vision.

Grade 1: Simultaneous macular perception: This is the ability to see two different images at the same time and superimpose them.

Grade 2: Binocular fusion: This is the ability to see two dissimilar images formed by two eyes and mix them into one.

Grade 3: Stereopsis: This is the ability to appreciate depth.

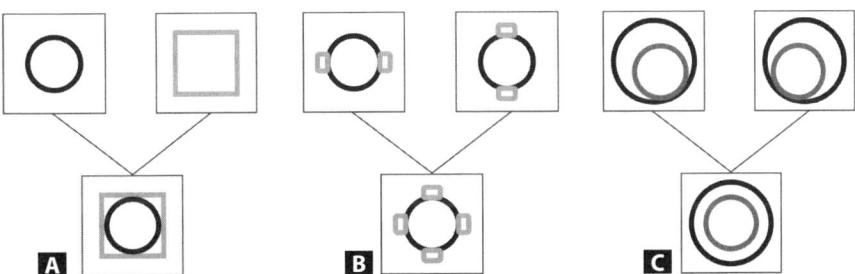

Figs. 17.3A to C: Three grades of binocular vision; (A) Simultaneous macular perception; (B) Binocular fusion; (C) Stereopsis. *(For color version, see Plate 7)*

DIPLOPIA

Diplopia in the common language means seeing two. It is defined as seeing two images of a single object when both eyes are open with equal vision in two eyes. It can be binocular or uniocular; the latter is far less common than the former and has less clinical significance. A diplopia is called binocular when it is present with both eyes open, only to disappear by closing any of the two eyes. The most common cause of binocular diplopia is paralytic squint. The other less common causes are displacement of the globe by any mass in the orbit or restriction of action muscle by injury, entrapment, or involvement in dysthyroid orbitopathy and myasthenia. A person with diplopia tries to overcome it by many methods. The most common of them is closing any eye. The others are turing the head towards the action of the paralyzed muscle or tilting the head in an appropriate position, i.e., tilting the head on one side and depressing/elevating the chin. The naturally occurring aftermath of the phenomenon is amblyopia, which creates a difference in vision between two eyes. Therapeutically, diplopia can be managed by prescribing suitable prisms with an appropriate position at their base.

The causes of uniocular diplopia are—subluxated lenses, iridodialysis, large iridectomy, and recent corneal opacity.

The term polyopia is used to denote a condition where a shining object looks more than two at any given time. The most common cause is incipient immature cataract.

The term haplopia is less commonly used in clinical practice. It means a state of binocular, single vision. The least commonly used term is oxyopia, which means vision better than 6/5 with sharpness of vision and the ability to resolve fine details.

AMBLYOPIA

Amblyopia is a common cause of unilaterally diminished vision in children, developing before 8 years. The condition is often missed; it is treatable before 8 years of age. It is a chronic or subacute condition seen equally in boys and girls; it is a more neglected condition in children in developing countries. The cause of the condition is often not apparent on examination, but the predisposing factors are too obvious. Rarely, it can be bilateral. The most common predisposing factor is squint. The most important age to develop amblyopia is before 6 months of age, when the macula is still developing. The causes of amblyopia can be either congenital or acquired; the congenital causes are congenital cataracts and ptosis. The acquired causes are central corneal opacity, unequal error of refraction in two eyes with a difference of more than 2D to 3D, unilateral error of refraction, uncorrected aphakia following surgery for congenital cataract, and acquired squint. Squint is the most common cause of amblyopia. The amblyopia persists even after a successful cosmetic correction of the squint. If amblyopia has not been treated before surgery, this is true for congenital ptosis as well.

The symptoms of amblyopia—most of the time, the child is not aware of the disorder, though he is aware of his squint. The other clinical features are:

Diminished distant vision—not more than 2 to 3 lines in Snellen's chart. The diminished vision is not correctable with glasses. The visual acuity is better when examined on a single optotype rather than a complete line on the Snellen chart. The near vision and colour visions are unaffected.

Neutral density filter test—this is a specific test for amblyopia if a child with normal vision looks through a neutral density filter. The vision diminishes by 1–2 lines. A child with amblyopia looking through a neutral density does not show any difference.

Eccentric fixation—this is tested on a specialized direct ophthalmoscope called a visuoscope that evaluates the position of light on the ophthalmoscope in relation to the fovea by projecting a sharp light on the macula of the unoccluded eye.

Management of Amblyopia

Management of amblyopia is simple, long-drawn, and often taken half-heartedly without immediate results. The principle of management consists of the removal of amblyogenic factors, such as opacities in the media, obstruction on the visual axis, and correction of refractive error, specially if the error is uniocular or there is a difference of >2D to 3D, with special attention to cylindrical error. The gold standard of treatment is occlusion. which should be started as early as possible because the results are directly proportionate to the age of the child. Younger the child faster is the improvement.

The treatment consists of occlusion of the better eye (non-squinting). The child initially resents this. The parents also generally initially do not approve of the procedure. wondering why the non-squinting eye has been closed. This hesitancy can be removed by counseling the parents prior to occlusion.

The principle of the treatment is to force the squinting eye to be used. The treatment should be started before 6 years of age for the best results. Results with 6/18 or less are less likely to improve. There are two methods of occlusion, i.e., conventional and non-conventional. The latter is also called inverse occlusion. The conventional method can be total or partial. The total occlusion blocks both form and light sensation, while the non-conventional blocks only form sense. If the vision in the amblyopic eye is less than 6/18, the eye should be totally occluded. Otherwise, partial occlusion may suffice. The occlusion should be continued till the vision has developed fully or to a level beyond which it has no chance to improve after three months of occlusion. The correction of amblyopia will not correct squint, which has to be managed either optically or surgically.

SQUINT

Squint is a very common disorder of the position of one eye in relation to the other. It is a loss of parallelism between two eyes in all directions. In this case, only one of the visual axes is directed towards the object of interest, allowing the other eye to drift from its normal position. Except in convergence and divergence. The main symptoms that bring the child for consultation are an obvious deviation of one eye or a deviation alternating between two eyes; the squint may be constant or intermittent. The obvious squint is called heterotropia. The other deviation seen following the breakdown of fusion is called heterophoria. The child and the parents are not aware of heterophoria (latent squint). The squinting eye often has diminished vision and is amblyopic. The vision in alternate squints is generally normal, or when the loss is equal in two eyes, the heterotropia can be pseudo-squint or true-squint **(Flowchart 17.1)**.

Pseudosquint

Pseudosquint is a state of misalignment between two eyes when they are actually straight. The most common cause of this is the epicanthic fold, which causes pseudoesotropia. The squint disappears if the epicanthic fold is pushed towards the nose. As the epicanthic fold gradually disappears by 7–8 years, the eye seems to be normal without any treatment. If it persists after 8 years, it requires surgical correction. The epicanthic fold is generally associated with congenital ptosis. If the eyes are set apart, it produces pseudoexotropia. The other features of a pseudosquint are that none of the eyes deviates under cover, the movement of the eyes is normal, and the corneal reflex is central. The distance between the limbus and the canthus are equal in two eyes **(Fig. 17.4)**.

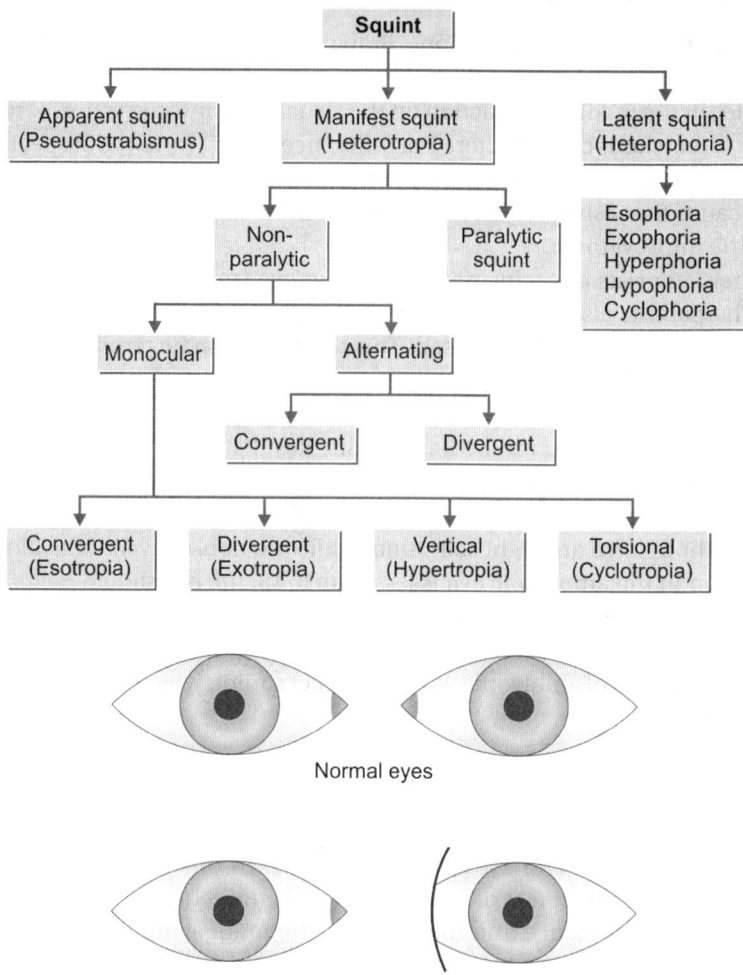

Flowchart 17.1: Broad classification of squints.

Fig.17.4: Pseudoesotropia.

Manifest Squint (Heterotropia)

This type of squint is visible to the onlooker. The child becomes aware of it as he grows and may be embarrassed about it. The vision in the squinting eye is variable; it may range from normal to gross loss. The tropias are visible in photographs. The tropias may be unilateral or alternate. The tropias can be non-paralytic, called concomitant, or paralytic, called incomitant. The deviation remains the same in all directions of gaze in the concomitant squint. The ocular movements are almost normal in all gazes. About 80% of concomitant squints are horizontal. They can rarely be congenital, develop in early childhood, and remain the same for the rest of life if not corrected in childhood. The other type of manifest squint is seen as a paralytic or restrictive squint.

The prevalence of concomitant squint ranges between 2.5% to 6% in children, equally in boys and girls. The squint may be present in one eye and be called a monocular squint, or it may alternate between the two eyes and be called an alternate squint. The straight eye is called a fixing eye, while the other is called a squinting or non-fixing eye. The tropia may be constant or intermittent, i.e., the squint is present only during a particular period. Intermittent squints are known to be converted into constant squints. The squint is called alternate when the two eyes with fixation alternate between the two eyes to the same degree when one eye deviates and the other eye fixes.

Causes of Heterotropia

- All heterophorias have a fair chance of being converted into heterotropia.
- There is an abnormal relationship between accommodation and convergence.
- Absence of binocular single vision:
  - Uncorrected error of refraction
  - Anisometropia
  - Opacities in the media
  - Diseases of macula and optic nerve
  - Congenital anomalies of orbit and extraocular muscles

Clinical Features of Heterotropia

The squint, when fairly large, is detected by parents, or the child becomes aware of the defect at a young age.

The adults are always aware of squints. It is obvious in old photographs and visible when looking in the mirror. There may be diminished vision in the squinting eye; there may be a difference in vision between the squinting and non-squinting eyes. The vision in a squinting eye may/may not be correctable by glasses. There is no diplopia, which differentiates between paralytic and non-paralytic heterotropia. There is no binocular single vision or abnormal head posture; the movements are normal in all directions.

Signs

A deviation of one eye that is most often horizontal may be esotropia or exotropia; less common is a vertical deviation called hypertropia or hypotropia as per the position of the eye (**Fig. 17.1**).

Once it has been confirmed that the child has tropia, the next step is to find out if it is true or a pseudosquint. The next step in true squinting is to find out if the squint is uniocular or alternates between two eyes. This is confirmed by a simple office procedure called a cover test and a cover-uncover test. The cover-uncover test differentiates between phoria and tropia. The alternating cover test measures the amount and direction of a deviation, irrespective of its nature, i.e., phoria or tropia. The cover test measures the deviation; it is done in two steps. In the first, the child is asked to fix a distant object, and the examiner covers one eye and looks for movement of the other eye. The occluder is removed, and movement of the previously covered eye is noted (**Fig. 17.5**). In alternate squints, the eye under the cover remains deviated even after the cover has been removed (**Fig. 17.6**).

Measurement of Squint

It is of utmost importance to have knowledge of the direction and amount of deviation of the eye to decide on the mode of treatment.

The amount of deviation can be measured by the corneal reflex test, the prism test, and the synoptophore. The corneal reflex test depends on the position of the corneal light reflex in relation to the pupil/limbus. In orthophoric eye, the corneal reflex is formed in the center

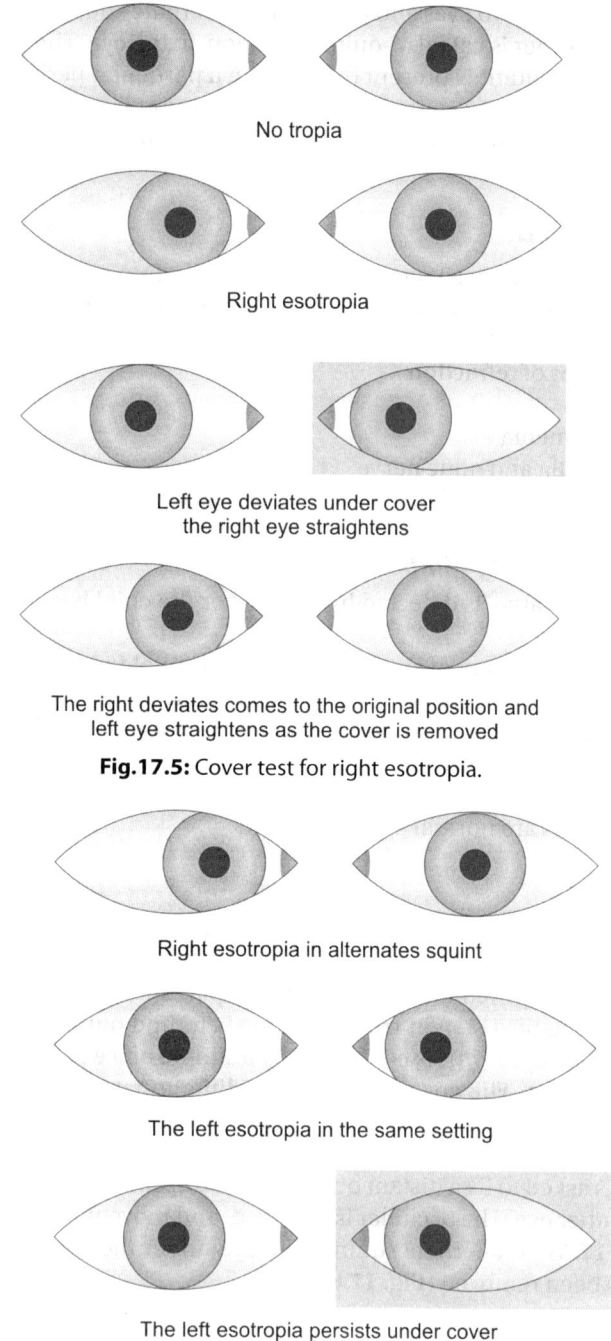

Fig.17.5: Cover test for right esotropia.

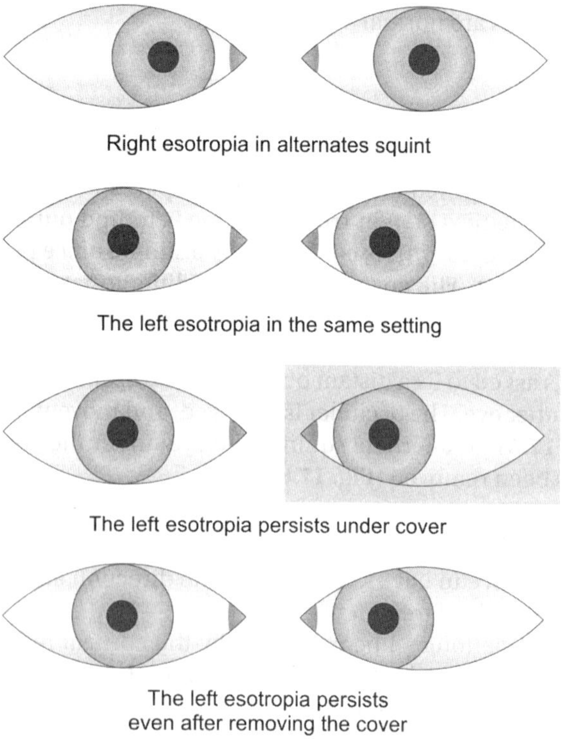

Fig. 17.6: Cover test for alternates isotropia.

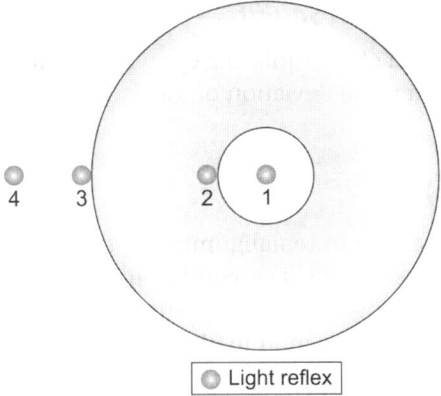

1. Light reflex in the center = no deviation
2. Light reflex at pupillary margin = 20° deviation
3. Light reflex at limbus = 45° deviation
4. Light reflex away from the limbus = deviation >45°

Fig. 17.7: Various positions of corneal reflex in Hirschberg test.

of the pupil. In the case of a squint, the corneal reflex is directed to the opposite side of the deviation. This is called the Hirschberg test (**Fig. 17.7**).

Clinical Features of Alternate Squints

- The deviations are large.
- The deviation is equal in both eyes.
- The eyes have good and equal vision.
- Error of refraction when presents are small
- The eyes do not have binocular vision.
- The alternate's squints are not corrected optically or by occlusion. They are corrected by surgery.

Management of Concomitant Squint

- The aim of treatment for concomitant squint is to give binocular single vision in the straight eye.
- **The treatment consists of four O's:**
  1. Optic (spectacle)
  2. Occlusion (Closing one eye)
  3. Orthoptic exercises
  4. Operation
- Binocular single vision is achieved by correction of the error of refraction and management of amblyopia. Many a time, a proper correction of the error of refraction may suffice to give a straight eye.
- If correction of the error of refraction and occlusion fails to give a straight eye, the treatment of choice is surgery.
- If the child has an error of refraction, it will not be corrected by straightening the eye with surgery. The child will also need to use glasses following surgery.
- Squints do not get corrected except for some pseudosquints caused by the epicanthic fold.
- There is no medical treatment.

Primary and Secondary Deviations in Squint

The primary deviation is the deviation of the squinting eye when the fixing eye fixes the object of interest. The secondary deviation is the deviation of the fixing eye when the squinting eye fixes the object of interest.

Latent Squint (Heterophoria)

Heterophoria, or latent squint, is a type of malalignment of the eyes where the eyes move out of alignment when they are dissociated. The condition is very common but not given much attention because it is not pathological, does not cause amblyopia, and the patients and onlookers are not aware of it. The most common method to break the fusion is to cover any of the eyes for a short period of time and observe the movement behind the cover. If there is a latent squint, the eye behind the cover will move and will be back in its original position when the cover is moved.

The fusion can be broken either by covering one eye or when the two eyes are looking at different targets produced by a prism, red-green glass, or Maddox rod.

The phoria are named as per the direction of deviation, i.e., esophoria when the eye moves in, exophoria when the eye moves out, and hyperphoria when the eye moves up in relation to the other eye when covered. The phorias develop commonly following fever, fatigue, anxiety, or when the child is daydreaming. The binocular fixation has not developed fully in childhood, hence the higher chances of exophoria. In contrast to this excess convergence in nearsighted, school-going children, esophoria is more common.

Symptoms of Heterophoria

The person with heterophoria may be able to overcome the breakdown of fusion and be symptomless. The other symptoms are diminished vision due to stress on the accommodation convergence relation, which decompensates heterophoria. The symptoms of decompasation are:

The primary deviation is the deviation of the squinting eye when the fixing eye fixes the object of interest. The secondary deviation is the deviation of the fixing eye when the squinting eye fixes the object of interest.
* Diminished vision
* Asthenopia*
* Frequent short lived diplopia
* Difficulty changing focus
* Headache
* Recurrent redness and watering of the eyes.

*Asthenopia

Asthenopia is a common, multifactorial ocular discomfort. The condition is presented as tiredness of the eyes, which is absent in the morning but worsens by evening or following prolonged near work. Presenting as running of the letter, headache, after long hours of near-work diplopia in the evening. The asthenopic eyes may pass a period of phorias, which may ultimately be converted into tropia. Asthenopia is treated by changing the reading and near work habits, reducing screening time, correcting errors of refraction, especially astigmatism, and correcting the imbalance between accommodation and convergence. In adults, this is best obtained by prescribing near correction, either in bifocal or progressive glasses; reliving prisms may also help. No surgery is required.

Paralytic Squint

Paralytic squints are less common than non-paralytic squints, and adults more frequently suffer from paralytic squints than children. The paralytic squint is due to the underaction or no action of extraocular muscles. It can be caused by the involvement of either single or multiple extraocular muscles. An example of the first is paralysis of the superior oblique and lateral rectus, which are supplied by the fourth and sixth nerves, respectively. These nerves exclusively supply single muscles. Multiple muscle palsy is seen with involvement of the third nerve. Involvement of multiple cranial nerves at a given time involves muscle supplied by two or three nerves. Involvement of the extraocular muscle is called external ophthalmoplegia. The involvement of the iris and ciliary body is called internal ophthalmoplegia, which may/may not be associated with other extraocular muscle involvement in various combinations. Involvement of both extraocular and intraocular muscles is called total ophthalmoplegia. Bilateral involvement of extraocular muscle is generally seen in a midline intracranial lesion or systemic diseases, such as myasthenia and dysthyroid oculopathy. The paralysis of each extraocular muscle has separate clinical features.

The paralytic squint can be acute or subacute. The lids are involved in paralytic squinting due to the third and seventh nerves. The involvement of the third nerve causes ptosis, while the involvement of the seventh nerve causes lagophthalmos.

The most common symptom of paralytic squint is diplopia, which is reduced by turning and tilting the head in the field of action of the paralytic muscle. The next symptom is the inability to move the affected eye in the desired direction. The result is tropism. In some cases of paralytic squint, there may be associated diminished distant vision if the image is formed away from the macula. Internal ophthalmoplegia causes diminished near vision and iridoplegia. Less common symptoms are vertigo, giddiness, and, rarely, headaches.

Table 17.1 shows difference between paralytic and non-paralytic squint.

Management of Paralytic Squint

Occlusion of the paralyzed eye alleviates the main complaint of diplopia, making the lives of the patients more comfortable. The same can be achieved by prescribing an appropriate prism with an appropriate position for the base.

Table 17.1: Difference between paralytic and non-paralytic squint.	
Non-paralytic squint	**Paralytic squint**
No diplopia	Diplopia is constant feature
No nausea, vomiting or vertigo	Generally present
May have diminished vision in the squinting eye and the diminished vision is the cause of squint	Diminished vision when present is not the cause of squint
No abnormal head posture	Abnormal head posture is always present
Angle of squint is same in all direction	Angle of squint changes with direction of eye
Ocular movements are normal	Ocular movement is less in the direction of action of paralyzed muscle
Primary and secondary deviation are equal	Secondary deviation is greater than primary deviation
No neurological defect is present	Some neurological and myological disorders can be present
All the muscles are fully active	The effected muscle has poor or no action
They generally develop over months	Have sudden onset

All cases of paralytic squint should undergo a complete medical and neurological examination.

The treatment of paralytic squint lies in the management of the systemic cause.

The management of the primary disease may cure the squint, especially in diabetic paralytic squint.

No surgical intervention is recommended until the squint has settled down.

Nystagmus

Nystagmus is a pathological condition that involves both eyes equally and simultaneously. It is a repetitive, uncontrolled movement in any direction. The most common direction is horizontal, followed by vertical, and least cyclic (where the eye turns in or out repetitively). The nystagmus has two components, i.e., a rapid and a slow component. In the case of nystagmus, the extraoculars are normal and fully functioning. The nystagmus can be latent or manifest. In the former, the movements are not present when both eyes are open, but when any of the eyes is closed. In such cases, one eye has less vision.

Clinically, nystagmus has been divided into three groups, i.e., pendular nystagmus, jerk nystagmus, and mixed nystagmus, based on the rhythm of the nystagmus. The ocular causes of nystagmus are mostly congenital, which involves the optic nerve, retina, and macula. The nystagmus is called amblyopic when both eyes have poor vision due to the non-development of the macula within six months of birth. Such cases are very common in albinism and coloboma of the macula. The non-ocular causes are lesions of the eighth cranial nerve, brain stem, cerebellum, and spinal cord. A genetic condition with normal eyes and normal vision without an abnormality of the central nervous system is called ediopathtic nystagmus. The cause of which is not known.

Treatment

There is no treatment for nystagmus due to ocular causes except to give the best corrected vision. Though people with grossly uncorrectable vision should be rehabilitated in a suitable institute, a lesion of the brain may improve with systemic treatment.

The nystagmus may be caused by ocular or non-ocular causes.

Index

Page numbers followed by *f* refer to figure, *fc* refer to flowchart, and *t* refer to table

A

Abscess
  lacrimal 126*f*
  orbital 131
Absolute glaucoma 249
  stages of 258
Accommodation 1, 16, 18, 27, 44
  path of 18*f*
Acetazolamide 257
Acute iridocyclitis 58
  treatment of 203
Acute iritis 201*f*, 257
  differential diagnosis of 203
Adnexa, ocular 12
Air, refractive index of 30
Albinism 198, 198*f*
Allergic conjunctivitis 142, 153
  types of 153*fc*
Allergy 58, 137, 140, 157
Amblyopia 45, 53, 264
  management of 265
Amsler grid 74*f*
Anemia 238
Aniridia 194
Anisometropia 50, 267
Ankyloblepharon 105, 108
  congenital 108*f*
Antagonists 263
Anterior chamber 160*f*, 161*f*, 200*f*
  abnormal contents of 200
  examination of 93
Anti-glaucoma drugs 249
Apert syndromes 129
Aphakia 45, 55, 98, 189, 189*f*
  optics of 47*f*
  signs of 46
Applanation tonometer 82*f*, 103*f*, 248, 248*f*
  principle of 248*f*
Aqueous 1
  chamber 245
  circulation of 15*f*
  humor 14, 24
    circulation of 246*f*
    formation of 247

Arcus senilis 169
Artificial eye 136*f*, 173, 173*f*
Asthenopia 44, 57, 270
Astigmatism 46, 47
  bi-oblique 47
  compound 48
  irregular 47, 49
  mixed 48
  oblique 47
  regular 47
  simple 48
  symptoms of 49
  types of 48*fc*
Autorefractometry 49

B

Band keratopathy 167
Basal cell carcinoma 117, 155
Basal iridectomy 196*f*
Bell's palsy 63
Bell's phenomenon 166
Berlin's edema 231
Binocular corneal loupe 37, 38*f*
Binocular fusion 263*f*
Binocular vision 26, 263
  grades of 263*f*
Biomicroscope 81*f*
Biopsy 135
  excisional 135
Bitot's spots 88, 143
Bjerrum screen 75*f*, 254
Blepharitis 112
  squamous 112, 112*t*
  ulcerative 112, 112*t*
Blepharophimosis 105, 108
  syndrome 107
Blepharospasm 53, 57, 82, 83
Blinding trachoma, management of 152
Blindness 51
  cortical 54
Blood
  dyscrasia 141
  vessels 214
Blunt injury 119, 186, 207, 207*f*, 208, 231

Bones forming orbit 2f
Bowman's membrane 8
Braille letter 52, 52f
Branch retinal vein occlusion 219
Bruch's membrane 15
Bullous keratitis 167
Buphthalmos 156
Burst chalazion 155

C

Canaliculus 121
Carcinoma, epidermoid 118, 155
Caruncle 12
Cataract 97f, 179, 179fc, 180, 185, 186, 259
   advance 55
   blue-dot 185
   central nuclear 56
   complicated 249
   concussion 187, 187f, 188f
   congenital 183, 183f, 196f, 234
   cortical 181, 182f
   immature 97, 97t, 98, 98t, 181f
   lamellar 184f
   mature 97, 97t, 181f, 182f, 200
   posterior subcapsular 182, 183f
   sutural 185, 185f
   symptoms of 180
   traumatic 185, 186f, 234
   treatment of 188
   zonular 184
Catarrh, spring 154
Cavernous sinus thrombosis 131
C-charts 64, 66f
Cellulitis 110
   acute orbital 131
Central field defects 73f
   types of 73f
Central retinal artery 21f
   branches of 21f
   occlusion 232, 238
      clinical features of 228
Central retinal vein
   branches of 21f
   obstruction 238
   occlusion 219
   thrombosis 223
Centrocecal scotomas 241f
Chalazion 114
Chalcosis 92
Chemosis 138, 142
Chemotherapy 134
Chickenpox 111
Chin, position of 79
Chorociliary coloboma 197

Chorioretinal scar 230f
Choroid 15, 208
   disorders of 194
   malignant melanoma of 209
   periphery of 197
Choroidal coloboma 196
   types of 197f
Choroiditis 199, 204
   types of 204f
Chromatopsia 53, 58
Cicatricial ectropion 116
Cicatricial entropion 116
Ciliary body 15, 194, 208
   disorders of 194
Ciliary ganglion 3, 4
Cobalt blue light 162f
Coloboma 93, 105, 108, 183f, 195f, 197, 216
   acquired 196
   congenital 108f
   iris, types of 94f
   peripheral 195f
   typical 195f, 196f
   uveal 195
Color sensation 27
Color vision
   diminished 55
   examination of 70
Computed tomography 211, 238
Concave
   lens 34
   mirror 28, 29t
Concomitant squint 99
   management of 269
Congenital cataract 183, 183f, 196f, 234
   management of 187
Congenital glaucoma 249
   treatment of 250
Congestion 87
   circumciliary 59, 88, 139, 139f, 140, 249
   conjunctival 59f, 139, 139f, 205
   early conjunctival 139f
   episcleral 88, 140
Conjunctiva 10, 24, 120, 140
   benign tumors of 155
   bulbar 10, 11
   congestion, localized 140
   disorders of 137
   examination of 86
   growth of 140, 155
   infective growths of 155
   malignant tumors of 155
   palpebral 10
   parts of 11f, 137f
   swelling of 205
   xerosis of 89, 89f

Conjunctival congestion 59*f*, 139, 139*f*, 205
   characteristics of 88
   types of 138*f*, 140*f*
Conjunctival disorders, clinical features of 138
Conjunctival phlyctens, types of 164*f*
Conjunctivitis 146, 149, 150, 153
   acute 59, 257
      hemorrhagic 149, 150
   allergic 142, 153
   angular 59, 140
   bacterial 146
   chlamydial 150
   chronic 153, 170
   congestion, bilateral 139*f*
   diphtheritic 148
   gonococcal 142, 147, 148
   severe bacterial 142
   simple 142
      allergic 153
   types of 147
   vernal 154
   viral 142, 149
Contact lens 169
   contraindications of 170
   corneal 170*f*
   hygiene of 170
   indications of 170
Convergence 1, 16, 18, 27
Convex lens 34, 36, 45, 45*f*
Cornea 1, 6, 25*f*, 120, 252*f*
   color of 61
   congenital diseases of 156
   conical 168
   deep vascularization of 158*f*
   disorders of 156
   ectasia of 176
   edematous 249
   examination of 90
   fatty degeneration of 168
   haziness of 205
   inflammation of 158
   loss of sensation of 158
   metabolism of 26
   nodular degeneration of 168
   section of 8*f*
   superficial vascularization of 158*f*, 165*f*
   vascularization of 158, 164, 170
Corneal degeneration 167
Corneal disease 171*f*
   common features of 157
Corneal dystrophies 168
Corneal opacity, topographic recording of 91
Corneal phlyctens 164*f*
   types of 164*f*

Corneal reflex test 101, 101*f*, 269*f*
Corneal sensation, diminished 170
Corneal surgery 170
Corneal ulcers 159
   management of 161
   marginal 163
   natural history of 160*fc*
   neurotrophic 166
   phlyctenular 163
Corneoscleral injury, penetrating 206*f*
Cortical cataract 181, 182*f*
   symptoms of 182
Corynebacterium xerosis 88
Cover test 268*f*
Cranial facial injury 142*f*
Cranial nerve 3, 4*t*
Crouzon syndromes 129
Curvature 90, 96
   hypermetropia 43
Cyclitis 199, 203
Cycloplegia 234
Cylindrical lenses 38
   principle of 39*f*
Cystoid macular edema 221*f*, 223
Cysts
   congenital 122*f*, 208
   parasitic 208
   tarsal 114
Cytomegalovirus 217

D

Dacryocystectomy 126
Dacryocystitis 85
   acute 122
   chronic 85, 122, 124, 124*f*, 125, 126*f*, 170
   congenital 123*f*
   neonatal 123
Dacryocystorhinostomy 126
   failure of 122
Deep corneal vascularization 158, 158*t*
Degeneration 157, 220
Dermoids 133
Dermolipoma 155
Descemet's membrane 8
Descemetocele 160*f*
Deviation, angle of 101*f*
Dextrodepression 262
Dextroversion 262
Diabetic retinopathy 219, 223-225, 238
   management of 225
Diopter 36
Diplopia 56, 101, 107, 135, 264
   chart 102, 102*f*
   glasses 102*f*

Disc
- congenital anomalies of 239
- drusen of 239
- inflammation of 238
- redness of 238
- swelling of 238

Disciform keratitis 165, 166
Discoloration 87
Distant vision 50, 64
- diminished 44, 240
- sudden blurring of 44

Distichiasis 105, 108, 109f
Dry eye 170
- syndrome 9

Dull foveal reflexes, cause of 215
Duochrome test 49
Dystrophy 157, 220

E

Eales' disease 219
Early Treatment Diabetic Retinopathy Study 67
E-chart 65, 66f
Ectopia lentis 179, 192
Ectropion 115, 116
- paralytic 116

Edema, retinal 214
Edridge green lantern 72f
Elevators, paralysis of 79
Endophthalmitis 199, 200f, 204, 205f
- acute 190
- endogenous 205
- postoperative 190

Endothelium 8
Enophthalmos 136, 175
- bilateral 136f

Entropion 115
Epicanthus 105, 108, 108f
Epiphora 85
- cause of 59, 121t, 122

Episcleral vessels, prominent 249
Episcleritis 58, 138, 140, 144, 144f, 175, 175f
- cause of 175

Epithelium 8
- development of 24

Esotropia 100f
Exenteration 209
Exophthalmos 79, 86, 128, 128f, 135, 170
Exotropia 100f
Extraocular muscle 3, 9
- action of 10t
- fascia of 4
- insertion of 10t
- nerve supply of 10t

Exudate 214, 215

Eye 39f, 196f
- abnormal movement of 79
- adnexa of 1
- anatomy of 1
- artificial 136f, 173, 173f
- bank 171
- chambers of 245f
- clinical examination of 79
- development of 23
- discharge 59
- dryness of 121
- examination of 63, 64, 76, 84
- gross anatomy of 1
- horizontal deviation of 61f
- injury 59
- internal examination of 104
- nerve supply of 22
- optics of 26, 27
- oscillation of 79
- pain 60
- physiology of 26
- redness of 58
- specific structure of 82
- squint, deviation of 79
- watering of 59, 270

Eyeball
- bulging of 79, 81
- deviation of 60
- hypermetropic 45
- prominent 61
- sinking of 61, 81
- swinging of 61

Eyebrow
- loss of 79, 80
- position of 79, 80

Eyelid, upper 60

F

Face, symmetry of 80
Field defects
- bilateral 74fc
- types of 57f

Fine needle biopsy 135
Flare 200
Fleischer ring 92
Fluorescein 92f
Follicles 87
Fornices 11
Friend test 49
Fundus
- examination 234
- fluorescein angiography 211, 238

Fungal keratitis 163

Index

G

Giant papillary conjunctivitis 155
Glands, inflammation of 113
Glare 53, 57
Glass
  frequent changes in power of 56
  prism 31, 31*f*
Glaucoma 103, 245, 248, 249, 251, 256
  absolute 249
  acute 58, 59
    congestive 256, 257
  applied
    anatomy of 245
    physiology of 247
  bilateral advanced congenital 250*f*
  chronic simple 98, 251, 253, 253*f*, 254, 254*f*
  congenital 249
  examination of 103
  malignant 259, 260
  neovascular 260
  secondary 258
  steroid-induced 259
  traumatic 259
  types of 249*fc*
  uveitis-induced 260
  wide-angle 251
Glaucomatous disc, types of 253*f*
Globe 1, 3, 5
  abnormal length of 40
  examination of 89
  intraocular structures of 1
  parts of 5*f*
Glycolysis, anaerobic 26
Goldmann perimeter 75, 76*f*
Gonioscope
  direct 252*f*, 252*t*
  indirect 252*t*
Gonioscopic appearance, grades of 256*t*
Granuloma, foreign body 155, 208
Growth 58, 82, 83, 116, 138, 146

H

Head
  injury 141, 142*f*
  posture 79
  turning of 80
Headache 270
Hemangioma 117, 133, 155, 208
Hemorrhage 214, 215, 232
  generalized subconjunctival 141
  intraretinal 215
  localized subconjunctival 141
  macular 232
  petechial 141*f*

preretinal 215
subconjunctival 58, 87, 138, 139*f*, 140, 141*f*, 142*f*
subretinal 215
traumatic retinal 232
Herpes simplex 111, 149, 165
  conjunctivitis 150
  keratitis 161
    primary 162
    recurrent 162
Herpes zoster 149, 165
  ophthalmicus 60, 64, 110, 110*f*
  varicella conjunctivitis 150
Hess chart 102
Heterochromia iridium 93
Heterophoria 261, 270
  symptoms of 270
Heterotropia 266
  causes of 267
  clinical features of 267
  symptoms of 101
Hirschberg test 60, 101, 101*f*, 269*f*
HIV retinitis 218
Hordeolum interna 114
Horner's syndrome 107, 136
Hudson-Stahli line 92
Hyperemia 138
Hyperglycemia 56
Hypermetropia 43, 44, 45*f*, 56
  axial 43
  clinical classification of 44
  high 44
  low 44
  moderate 44
  pathological 45
  symptoms of 44
  types of 44*fc*
Hypertension, ocular 249
Hypertropia 101*f*
Hyphema 93, 208
Hypoglycemia 57
Hypopyon 93, 160*f*, 200, 200*f*
  corneal ulcer 159
  treatment of 201

I

Impairment, types of 51, 51*t*
Indirect ophthalmoscope 211, 212*f*, 213*f*, 213*t*, 214*f*, 234
  disadvantages of 213
Infection 84, 122, 137, 140, 157
  acute
    bacterial 58
    viral 58
  severe microbial 141

Inferior rectus 10
Infraversion 262
Injury 58, 59, 141, 259
   penetrating 185, 205*f*
Interpalpebral aperture 79, 80
Intraocular parasitic cyst 234
Intraocular pressure 26, 247
Intraocular structure 1, 14, 22, 177*f*
Intraocular tension 248
Iridectomy
   broad-based 196*f*
   peripheral 196*f*
   surgical 196*f*
Iridocyclitis 199, 201
   acute 58
   chronic 234
   complications of 203
Iridodialysis 186*f*, 207*f*
   traumatic 196*f*
Iris 16, 93, 195*f*, 208
   bombe 201, 202*f*
   coloboma of 93, 183*f*
   disorders of 194
   nodules, types of 202*f*
   prolapse 206*f*
   shadow 97, 181, 181*f*
   surface of 93
Iritis 199
   acute 201*f*, 257
Ishihara plates 72*f*
Isotropia 268*f*
Itching 138, 143

J

Jaeger's near vision chart 70
Jaw winking 107

K

Kaposi sarcoma 119
Kayser-Fleischer ring 92
Keratic precipitates 199, 199*f*
Keratitis 59
   deep 165
   exposure 167
   interstitial 165, 166
   mycotic 163
   neuroparalytic 167
   neurotrophic 166
   viral 161
Keratoconjunctivitis
   epidemic 149
   phlyctenular 59
Keratoconus 168
Keratomalacia 169

Keratometer 6*f*
Keratoplasty 171
   penetrating 171*f*
Krause's glands 13
Krukenberg spindle 92

L

Lacrimal drainage system, diseases of 121
Lacrimal fistula 126*f*
Lacrimal gland
   diseases of 126
   disorders of 126
Lacrimal sac 14, 121
   congenital cyst of 122*f*
Lacrimal sinus 124*f*
Lacrimal system 13, 120
   disorders of 120
   examination of 84
   parts of 14*f*
Lacrimation 85, 138
   causes of 59, 120*t*
Lagophthalmos 135, 170
Landolt chart 65
Lattice degeneration 229, 230*f*
Lens 1, 14, 19, 24, 33, 96, 234, 259
   congenital anomalies of 192
   development of 24
   diseases of 179
   dislocation of 97, 187, 259
   disorders of 179
   displacement of 179
   examination of 96
   extraction 188
   metabolism of 26
   parts of 19*f*
   plate 24*f*
   shapes of 33*f*
   subluxation of 97, 187, 259
   vesicle 25*f*
Lensometer 35, 36*f*, 70*f*
Lenticular curvature, abnormal 41
Levator
   action of 84
   palpebrae superioris 10, 13
Levodepression 262
Levoelevation 262
Levoversion 262
Lid 12, 23, 83, 110, 116, 119-121
   abscess 110
   acquired
      disorders of 109
      structural anomalies of 115, 115*f*
   adenocarcinoma of 118
   coloboma of 108

deformity of 170
disorders of 105
edema of 205
examination of 82
infective conditions of 113*f*
laceration of 119
malignant growth of 117
margin 83, 113
   acquired disorders of 112
   infection of 84
   parasitic infestation of 112
position of 12*f*, 83
skin of 83
tearing of 119
Light 27
  faulty projection of 68
  perception, absence of 68
  reflex 16
    path of 17*f*
  sensation 26
Limbal dermoid 146*f*, 155, 157, 170
Limbal phlycten 144*f*, 164*f*
Limbal spring catarrh 154*f*
Limbus 9
Lipid keratopathy 168
Lister perimeter, early modal of 76*f*
Log-MAR chart 66, 66*f*
Low vision 50, 51
  aids, classification of 51*fc*
  characteristics of 50

M

Macula 215, 232
  coloboma of 197
  detachment of 215
  edema of 215
  examination of 215
  hypoplasia of 215
  swelling of 215
Macular degeneration 55, 215
  age-related 223, 232
Macular disorders 222
Macular hole 232
Madarosis 115, 116
Magnetic resonance imaging 211, 238
Measles 150
Medulloepithelioma 208, 209
Melanoma
  benign 208
  malignant 118, 155, 209
Membrane 88
  formation 215
Meningocele 129*f*, 133
Mesoderm 25

Metabolism 26
Metamorphopsia 53, 57
Methyl alcohol poisoning 54
Microcornea 156
Microphakia 259
Microphthalmos 136*f*, 174
  bilateral 174*f*
  unilateral 174*f*
Miosis, traumatic 207*f*
Mirror retinoscopes 77*f*
Moll glands 113
Molluscum contagiosum 111
Mooren's ulcer 164
Moraxella conjunctivitis 149
Morgagnian cataract 97
Muller's muscle 13
Muscle 10
  agonist 263
  antagonists 263
  extraocular 3, 9
  synergist 263
Myasthenia gravis 107
Mydriasis 201*f*
  traumatic 207*f*
Myopathy, ocular 107, 107*f*
Myopia 41
  clinical types of 41
  congenital 41
  degenerative 42
  high 219, 232
  pathological 42
  progressive 42, 56
  simple 41
Myopic refraction 168

N

Nanophthalmos 45
Narrow-angle glaucoma 256, 256*t*
  clinical features of 257
Nasolacrimal duct 121
  block, neonatal 124*f*
  obstruction 122
    congenital 122
Near reflex 16, 18
Near vision
  chart 70*f*, 71*f*
  examination of 70
Neoplasm 137
Nerve palsy 107
Neuroectoderm, fate of 23
Neurofibroma 155, 208
Neurofibromatosis 117
Neuroretinal defect 57*f*
Nevus 117, 155, 208

Night blindness 55
Nodule 88, 93
    formation 201
Non-uveal tissues 199*t*
Normal center circular pupil 201*f*, 207*f*
Nuclear cataract 180, 182*f*
    natural history of 180
    signs of 181
Nutrition 247
Nystagmus 61, 79, 80
    treatment 272

O

Occlusio pupillae 202*f*
Ocular cicatricial pemphigoid 146
Ocular media, refractive index of 41
Opacity, anterior subcapsular 187
Opaque nerve fibers 214, 239
Ophthalmia neonatorum 147
Ophthalmic artery, branches of 3
Ophthalmic interest, chlamydia of 151
Ophthalmitis, sympathetic 206
Ophthalmoscopes 210
    direct 211*f*, 213, 213*f*, 213*t*, 234
    indirect 211, 212*f*, 213*f*, 213*t*, 214*f*, 234
Ophthalmoscopy 253
Optic atrophy 238, 242
    glaucomatous 243
    primary 243
    secondary 243
Optic disc 197
    coloboma of 239
    drusen of 239, 240
    hypoplasia of 239
Optic foramen 2*f*
Optic nerve 21*f*, 57*f*, 244, 248
    disorders of 236
    glioma of 243
    inflammation of 240
    meningioma of 244
    non-inflammatory disorders of 242
    tumor of 243
Optic neuritis 238, 239
Optic neuropathy
    acute ischemic 243
    hereditary 240
Optic pathway 17*f*, 237*f*
Optic stalk 24*f*, 25*f*
Optic vesicle
    formation of 23*f*
    primary 24*f*
    secondary 24*f*
Optical coherence tomography 211, 238

Orbicularis
    action of 84
    oculi 10, 12
Orbit 1, 2
    apex of 10
    base of 4
    boney rim of 4
    chronic inflammation of 132
    disorders of 128
    examination of 85
    facial part of 4
    hemangioma of 133
    infectious diseases of 131
    position of 2*f*
    pseudotumors of 129
    rim of 10
    superiotemporal 135*f*
    superomedial 135*f*
    surgical spaces of 3*f*
    tumors of 132
Orbital fascia 3
Orbital fat 3, 4
Orbital fissures 2*f*
Orbital injury 141
Orbital lymphoma 134
Orbital septum 4
Orbital tumor
    acquired 133
    classification of 132*fc*
    clinical presentation of 134
    signs of 135
Orthophoria 261

P

Pain 82, 83
Painful symptoms 180
Painless diminished vision, causes of 54
Panophthalmitis 199, 205, 205*f*
Panuveitis 59, 204
Papillae 87, 154*f*
Papilledema 238, 242
Papilloma 155
Paralytic squint 103*f*, 271, 271*t*
    characteristics of 101
    management of 271
Pars planitis 199, 203
Pericystitis 126*f*
Perimeters, automated 75, 254
Peripheral anterior synechiae 202*f*
Peripheral fields 73*f*
    types of 74*f*
Persistent pupillary membrane 197
Pharyngoconjunctival fever 149
Phlyctens 58, 138, 140, 143, 165*f*
    multiple 59

Photophobia 53, 57
Photopsia 53, 58
Phthisis bulbae 175, 175f
Pinguecula 138, 144
Pinhole camera 39f
Placido's disc 7, 7f
Plica semilunaris 12
Polyopia 53, 57
Pregnancy, retinopathy of 224, 226
Prematurity, retinopathy of 224, 226
Presbyopia 50
Prism 30, 33f
    angle of 31
    bar 101
    identification of 31
    uses of 33
Proliferative retinopathy, management of 225
Proptosis 79, 128, 130, 133f, 170
    acquired 129
    acute 130t
    bilateral 129t
    chronic 130t
    congenital 128
    direction of 130
    eccentric 135f
    examination of 86
    inspection of 131f
    unilateral 129t, 130f
Prostaglandin analogues 255
Prosthesis 173
Pseudoesotropia 266f
Pseudohypopyon 161, 200
Pseudomyopia 43
Pseudoneuritis 238, 239
Pseudo-optic neuritis 239
Pseudophakia 47f, 55, 99, 190, 192f
Pseudoproptosis 130
Pseudoptosis 105f
Pseudosquint 265
Pterygium 58, 138, 140, 145, 145f, 170
Ptosis 12f, 79, 105, 106f, 107
    acquired 107
    bilateral mild 106f
    causes of 60
    complicated congenital 106
    congenital 106
    grades of 106f
    myogenic 107
    simple congenital 106
Puncta 121
Punctum dilator 123f
Pupil, color of 61, 97
Pupillary margin, examination of 94
Purkinje images 6, 7f

R

Radiotherapy 134
Rainbow-round artificial light 56
Red spot, causes of 232
Reflection 29f
    law of 27
Reflex lacrimation 59
Refraction 30f, 31f, 234
    abnormal 41
    error of 40f, 78fc
    high errors of 79
    law of 29
    uncorrected errors of 55
Refractive corneal surgeries 171
Retina 14, 20, 210, 211, 214
    development of 210
    disorders of 210, 216
    inflammation of 217
    layers of 20f
    metabolism of 26
    penetrating injuries of 233
    tumors of 233
    vascular disorders of 224, 227
    vessel of 215
Retinal artery
    obstruction 227
    occlusion 224
Retinal degeneration 220
Retinal detachment 214, 228
    symptoms of 230
Retinal disorders, clinical features of 210
Retinal dystrophies 220, 223
Retinal pigmentation, congenital 217
Retinal vein
    obstruction 228
    occlusion 224, 227fc
Retinal vessels
    appearance of 214f
    congenital anomalies of 219
Retinitis pigmentosa 220, 221f
    atypical 222
    treatment of 222
    typical 220
Retinitis
    bacterial 218
    parasitic 218
Retinoblastoma 233, 234f
    bilateral 134f
    differential diagnosis of 234
    signs of 234
    symptoms of 234
    types of 233
    unilateral 134f
Retinochoroidal colobomas 216f

Retinopathy
    central serous 215, 222
    hypertensive 219, 224, 225
Retinoscope 77*f*
Retinoscopy 168, 182*f*, 184*f*, 187*f*
    types of 79*f*
Retraction syndrome 136
Retrobulbar neuritis 241
Retrolental fibroplasia 234
Rhabdomyosarcoma 134
Rhinosporidiosis 122, 155
Ring
    scotomas 221*f*
    synechiae 202*f*
Rubella
    cataract 184
    retinitis 217

S

Sac
    absence of 122
    encysted mucocele of 125*f*
    granuloma of 122
    mucocele of 125*f*
    pyocele of 125*f*
Scar 87, 215
Schiotz tonometer 103*f*, 247*f*
Schirmer's test 9
Sclera 5, 9
    congenital anomalies of 174
    disorders of 174
    ectasia of 176
    examination of 89
    inflammation of 175
Scleral staphyloma 177
    types of 177, 178*f*
Scleritis 58, 59, 176
Sclerocornea 157
Scotomas
    central 241*f*
    paracentral 241*f*
Senile 116
    cataract 180
    ectropion 116
    entropion 115
Sensation 91
Sensory retina 20
Sickle cell anemia 219
Siderosis 92
Skull 2*f*
Slit lamp 81, 81*f*, 103*f*, 199*f*, 211
Snellen's chart 65, 65*f*, 66*f*, 70
    types of 65*f*

Spherical lenses 34
    construction of 34*f*
    parts of 34*f*
Spherophakia 259
Sphincterotomy 196*f*
Squamous cell carcinoma 118
Squint 80, 261, 265, 266, 270
    alternate 269
    broad classification of 266*fc*
    concomitant 99
    convergent 45
    examination of 99
    latent 270
    measurement of 267
    non-paralytic 271, 271*t*
    obvious 101
    paralytic 103*f*, 271, 271*t*
    surgery 136
    types of 100*fc*
Staphyloma 90
    corneal 176
    distribution of 176*fc*
    types of 177*f*
Static methods 75
Stereopsis 263*f*
Steroid 259
Stevens-Johnson syndrome 146
Strabismus 80, 99
Stroma 8
Stycar chart 67, 67*f*
Stye 113
Sunken eyeball 79
Superficial corneal vascularization 158, 158*t*
Superior rectus 10, 79
    origin of 10
Surgery 134
Swelling 82, 83, 205
Swollen disc 238
    causes of 238
Swollen lens 259
Symblepharon 138, 145, 146*f*
Sympathetic chain, branches of 3
Synechiae, posterior 202*f*
Synoptophore 101
Syphilis
    acquired 165
    congenital 165

T

Tarsal spring catarrh 154*f*
Tay-Sachs disease 232
Tear
    drainage of 120
    film 8

functions of 8
layers of 8f
retinal 232
Tenderness 82, 83
Tenon's capsule 4, 6
Tonometers, types of 103f
Total corneal staphyloma 176f
Trachoma 151, 164, 165f
　corneal involvement of 164
　established 152
　management of 151
　WHO classification of 151
Trauma 107, 119, 140, 141, 157, 177, 219, 232, 244
　corneal 172
　retinal 231
　uveal 206
Trichiasis 115
Tropia, types of 262f
Tuberculosis 165
Tumors 132, 208, 233, 239
　primary 129
　retinal 214
　secondary 129
Tylosis 115, 116

U

Ulcer
　corneal 159
　dendritic 162, 162f
　fascicular 164f
Ultrasonography 211, 235, 238
Uniocular corneal loupe 36f
　construction of 37f
　optics of 37f
Upper lid 12f
　vertical section of 13f
Uvea 14, 15, 120
　benign tumors of 208
　blood supply of 18
　blunt injury of 207
　examination of 93
　inflammation of 198
　penetrating injury of 206
　tumors of 208
Uveitis 199, 199t, 259
　acute anterior 59
　anatomical classification of 198f
　anterior 202f
　posterior 204, 223

V

Varicella 111
Vascular retinopathies 224

Vasculitis, retinal 218
Veins, ophthalmic 3
Vergences 263
Verruca 111
Vesicles 110
VIBGYOR 27
Vision 68, 97
　diminished 55, 56, 101, 135, 270
　distant 50, 64
　double 56
　examination of field of 71
　far 55
　field of 58
　loss of upper field of 79
　low 50, 51
　neurology of 27
　painless loss of 230
　physiology of 26
　recording of 64, 234
　subnormal 76
　sudden loss of 54, 230
Visual acuity 51
Visual pathway 27
Visual sensation 26
Visual symptoms 53
　causes of 53
Vitamin, administration of 143
Vitreous 1, 14, 23
　chamber 20
Vossius ring 186, 187, 207, 207f

W

Warts 111
Water, refractive index of 30
Whooping cough 141
Wolfring's glands 10, 13
Wound
　corneal 170
　corneoscleral 172f

X

Xanthelasma 117
Xeroderma pigmentosa 118
Xerophthalmia
　prevention of 143
　treatment of 143
Xerosis 89, 89f, 138, 143

Z

Zeis glands 113
Zinn annulus 10
Zonules 23